*Women Healers and Physicians*

# WOMEN HEALERS AND PHYSICIANS
## Climbing a Long Hill

LILIAN R. FURST, *Editor*

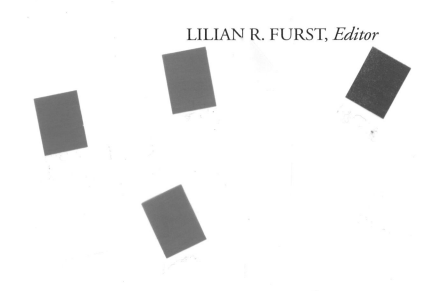

THE UNIVERSITY PRESS OF KENTUCKY

Publication of this volume was made possible in part
by a grant from the National Endowment for the Humanities.

Production of the index was supported in part by the University Research
Council of the University of North Carolina at Chapel Hill.

Scholarly publisher for the Commonwealth, serving Bellarmine College,
Berea College, Centre College of Kentucky, Eastern Kentucky University,
The Filson Club Historical Society, Georgetown College, Kentucky Histori-
cal Society, Kentucky State University, Morehead State University, Murray
State University, Northern Kentucky University, Transylvania University,
University of Kentucky, University of Louisville, and Western Kentucky
University.

*Editorial and Sales Offices:* The University Press of Kentucky
663 South Limestone Street, Lexington, Kentucky 40508-4008

03 02 01 00 99   5 4 3 2 1

**Library of Congress Cataloging-in-Publication Data**

Women physicians and healers : climbing a long hill / Lilian R. Furst, editor.
    p.    cm.
    Includes bibliographical references and index.
    ISBN 0-8131-2011-X (cloth : alk. paper). — ISBN 0-8131-0954-X
(paper : alk. paper)
    1. Women in medicine—History.  I. Furst, Lilian R.
  R692.W676    1997
  610.69'52'082—dc20               96-32389

# CONTENTS

# ACKNOWLEDGMENTS

*First, my thanks* to all the contributors, not only for their sterling work but also for their patience with my requests for cuts and revisions, and with the delays inevitable in a cooperative project such as this. It would be appropriate to include here, too, those who made contributions which could not be accommodated in the final format.

I am grateful to Peter W. Graham for his interest and encouragement, and to the two readers for the University Press of Kentucky who made such valuable, constructive suggestions.

I would like to dedicate this volume to the memory of my mother, Sarah Furst-Neufeld, M.D., who herself, Jewish as well as female, climbed a particularly steep hill at the University of Vienna in the 1920s. Medicine was throughout her life her great passion. Sadly, after the promulgation of the racial laws by the Nazis in 1938 she was never again able to practice her beloved profession. Her continuing commitment to medicine, through reading the journals and discussing the cases presented in them, sparked my earliest interest, which eventually led me to medical history and the possibility of combining it with my own field, literature.

# INTRODUCTION

LILIAN R. FURST

*The subtitle of this volume* comes from Sarah Orne Jewett's novel, *A Country Doctor*, in which the titular figure, Dr. Leslie, warns his young protégée, Nan Prince, that studying medicine, on which she has set her heart, is like "climbing a long hill."[1] *A Country Doctor* was published in 1884, and although no internal date is given for the fictional action, it is evidently contemporaneous, say the early 1880s. At that time the study and practice of medicine was a much steeper and longer climb for women than for men because of the many ideological and practical obstacles that stood in their way.

It is precisely these ideological and practical obstacles that form the focus of this collection of essays as they examine diverse expressions of women's participation in healing activities over the centuries. The specifics of the situation vary from one cultural context to another and from one period to another. Yet an overall pattern does emerge, and it is that of a lengthy uphill struggle as women were subjected to marginalization and, frequently, to attempts to exclude them from independent practice and even from the claim to professional expertise in healing.

However, a paradox immediately becomes apparent because women have traditionally been expected to tend the sick as a normative part of their domestic obligations. While this informal, unpaid, home-based therapeutic care was sanctioned, and indeed approved, any steps taken by women to apply their undeniable skills in the public forum met with an almost ubiquitous opposition which varied only in its intensity, overt pretexts, and underlying motivation. The barriers to women's full acceptance as professional healers were articulated in forthrightly political, feminist terms in 1869 by Sophia Jex-Blake, the British leader in the fight for women's admission to medical schools: "it cannot be commendable to obey instructions as a nurse, when it

1

would be unseemly to learn the reasons for them as a student, or to give them as a doctor."[2] The giving of orders according to their own judgement is the factor common to all the women discussed here. In so doing, either through open acts of self-assertion or through devious strategies, they defy the hierarchically gendered codes that would permit them merely to act in a subservient role under male direction. By affirming their right to autonomous knowledge and its practical implementation, they challenge and transcend the confines that society would impose on them.[3]

This volume is not intended as another history of women's work in the realm of healing, but rather as a complement to existing linear accounts.[4] Its distinctive contribution is to fill in blanks and probe areas hitherto veiled in silence, and to do so by drawing on literary as well as historical sources. Its method is that of a series of cultural frames ranging in time and place from fifth century B.C. Greece to late twentieth century African-American. Each essay examines the situation—or generally, the problematics—at a particular moment and in a particular setting through analysis of a certain healer or group of healers. These individual instances are contextualized in relation to the larger issues and controversies of their respective periods. The interface of prevailing norms, established medicine, and women's healing activities becomes manifest in the intersection not only of historical and literary texts but also in their connections to folklore, the law, and religion in both popular and high culture. The graphic vividness of the discrete episodes gives cumulatively a memorable picture of the continuing struggles of women as healers and physicians in their climb up that long hill. The stories told are at once singular and typical of different but parallel facets of women's history in medicine.

The essays fall into two parts: "Between Magic and Medicine," and "The Emergence of Professionalism." Each of these deals with a certain temporal segment: "Between Magic and Medicine" focuses mainly on the Middle Ages and the Renaissance, while "The Emergence of Professionalism" naturally concentrates on the later nineteenth century, when the battle for acceptance in official medicine was at its height. Within each part the sequence is predominantly chronological, although inevitably, in dovetailing, some of the pieces overlap to a certain extent. More importantly, one essay in each part breaks out of the prevailing temporal parameters to show a continuity prospectively or retrospectively. So the final essay in "Between Magic and Medicine," Gunilla T. Kester's "The Blues, Healing, and Cultural Representation in Contemporary African-American Women's Literature" develops the thesis that

African-American women in our own time have devised for themselves an unorthodox, quasi-magical mode of self-healing through the incantatory effect of music's rhythms. Likewise, the opening piece of "The Emergence of Professionalism" harks back to the ancient world as Holt Parker documents the prevalence of female physicians in ancient Greece, Rome, and the Byzantine Empire, that is, early precedents to women's integration into the medical realm well before the nineteenth century.

The first five essays in "Between Magic and Medicine" all pivot on the controversial status of medicine, and particularly of women healers from the early Middle Ages through the Renaissance. Before the understanding of the mechanisms of disease and treatment resulting from the momentous scientific discoveries that began toward the middle of the nineteenth century and have continued at an accelerating pace into our own time, the causation and course of illnesses were more or less a mystery. As an entity apparently beyond human understanding disease fell into the domain of the Church, which virtually controlled medical study in the early Middle Ages. What is more, as a matter of belief, healing was also strongly imbued with superstition. This constellation is the starting point for Debra L. Stoudt, who outlines the consociation between religion, magic, and medicine, and traces how women modified their healing activities in response to the changing circumstances of the sociocultural environment in which they exercised their powers. Within the same context—Germany—at approximately the same time, Nancy P. Nenno deals with another aspect of the tripartite link between religion, magic, and medicine: the demonization of women healers as witches. She cites two canonical courtly epics, *Êrec* (ca. 1180/1185) and *Tristan* (ca. 1210), as testifying to the cultural tendency to cast women healers in a contradictory, anxiety provoking role on account of their perceived potential to harm, to poison, to enchant as much as to cure, to heal, to release.

By contrast, a much more benign image emerges from Esther Zago's exploration of a number of figures in Boccaccio's *Decameron*. In striking anticipation of Kester's contemporary African-American subjects, these women in mid-fourteenth-century Italy instinctively grasp that they must, through self-understanding, find the form of healing most apposite to themselves, even if it proves to be in opposition to the dominant conventions of the Western text of their time.

But far more common is the branding of the woman healer as a suspect force for evil rather than good, as already suggested by Nenno. In sixteenth-century Spain, Michael Solomon demonstrates, a stringent line was drawn between the legitimate healer and the sinister other who was impugned with what he designates as "the power to disease." In a series of attempts to eliminate all that was dismissed as "charlatanism," the medical faculty, with the full support of the Church, propounded legislation to ban unlicensed healers. Solomon asserts, however, that his campaign stemmed less from the desire to protect the public from incompetent practitioners than from an effort to control the consequential social power of medicine. He cites the writings of an eminent Valencian physician, Jaume Roig, as the prototype of antifeminist literature, which sought to marginalize women healers through the cultivation of distrust and suspicion. It becomes amply apparent at this juncture that the hill that women in the medical field had to climb grew steeper and harder to scale as official (male) medicine reinforced its sway and closed its ranks.

This trend is borne out by the fate of Margaret Kennix in England at the turn of the sixteenth to the seventeenth century. She was indicted as a danger to public health for practicing without legal sanction, primarily, William Kerwin argues, because unauthorized women healers were feared, although they were also much needed, above all by the poor and in rural areas. Like Solomon, Kerwin shows by reference to a number of Renaissance dramas how these women were banished to the margins of medical practice on account of their spiritualism, which was seen as a threat to the conventional medicine of the period. The challenge they were thought to pose to established authority through their unorthodoxy exposed them to the suspicion of malevolence, yet in the plays (all, incidentally, authored by men) they appear as constructive figures, agents for reconciliation and even social reform.

Need and, at least by implication, social reform were the central arguments propounded in the later nineteenth century in favor of the regular medical training of women. Jex-Blake urged vehemently in "Medicine as a Profession for Women" (1869) that women must be enabled "to attend medically to those of their own sex who need them" and to give "sisterly counsel and advice."[5] In order to defuse the menace that Victorian society saw in what was perceived as "unfeminine" and "unladylike" behavior, the pioneer women physicians emphasized their intention of remaining within the female sphere by underscoring their wish to minister only to women and children. This was a telling argument at a time when modesty and shame held many women back from physical examination by male doctors. Invoking the long tradition of women as informal healers, Jex-Blake points out that the "innovation lies in the exclusion of women"[6] as a result of the 1858 British Medical Registration Act, which "was wrested from its original purpose, and made an almost insurmountable barrier to the admission of women to the authorized practice of medicine; and this because the Act made it obligatory on all candidates to comply with certain conditions, and yet left it in the power of the Medical Schools, collectively, arbitrarily to preclude women from such compliance." (65).

Jex-Blake's contentions are confirmed in Holt Parker's insistence that "The history of women as professionals in medicine does not begin in America in 1849 with Dr. Elizabeth Blackwell (1821-1910), the first woman to earn an M.D. in modern times; nor in Naples in 1422, with Costanza Calenda, the first woman we know of to receive a doctorate in medicine from a university; nor in Naples in 1321, with Francesca de Romana, the earliest woman we currently know of to have been licensed to practice medicine generally, nor in Catania in 1276 with Virdimura . . . but extends back to at least the fifth century B.C. in Greece" (131). Parker's model of parity between male and female healers in the ancient world is an important and generally overlooked exception to the convention that encouraged women to act as domestic healers but debarred them from authorized professionalism.

This convention was most vociferously attacked after the mid-nineteenth century with the increasing strenuousness of women's efforts to gain entry into official medicine. On the one hand women's suitability for regular medicine was emphatically denied by the mostly (but not solely) male adversaries of the intrepid young women who were banging on the doors of medical schools. On the other hand, at this same time, women's innate aptitude for informal healing within the circle of family, friends, and community continued not only to be endorsed but even to be systematized in the widely used, influential nineteenth-century manuals of household management. All of them include significant amounts of medical lore, and enjoin women to acquire diagnostic and therapeutic knowledge for the well-being of those under their domestic care. For instance, the third part of Cora-Elisabeth Millet-Robinet's *La Maison rustique des dames* (1844-45) is given to "Médecine domestique,"[7] and covers in its ten chapters the following topics: instruments and medications to be kept in the home; the preparation and administration of medications (including infusions, enemas, pills, baths, leeches, etc.); indications for calling a doctor; infant and child care; children's diseases (convulsions, croup, scarlet fever, chicken pox, worms, etc.); the diagnosis and treatment of medical and surgical conditions ranging from weight loss through chillblains, bleeding, fevers, sciatica, fractures and burns to epilepsy and urinary retention, reviewed in an extensive reference section (48-86); animal and insect bites; poisonings, asphyxiation; and the establishment of death. An even more thorough primer is *Mrs. Beeton's Book of Household Management* (1861) which has separate chapters on "Invalid Cookery," "The Rearing and Management of Children and Diseases of Infancy and Childhood," and "The Doctor." The latter deals with much the same ground as Millet-Robinet's "Médecine domestique," but is more advanced, giving guidance on when and how to bleed,[8] how to distinguish between hemorrhage from the lungs and from the stomach (1066-7), how to handle concussion (1073) and cholera (1073-74), how to differentiate between apoplexy and epilepsy as well as between epilepsy and drunkenness (1077-78) and how to treat each of these conditions, how to set about trying to revive a drowned person (1091-92), and how to cure stammering (1089). "The Sick-Room" is the title of a similar section in Mary Mason's *The Young Housewife's Counsellor* (Philadelphia: Lippincott, 1871). Mrs. Mason offers general advice on hygiene, tact in handling the patient, recipes for the invalid's diet, and directions for preparing and applying various types of plasters, "blisters," and leeches. The woman who mastered the precise instructions in these manuals would clearly be a valuable medical resource. The presence of such detailed medical information in these manuals of household management is strong testimony to the persistence of the tradition of women's healing as located in the domestic, maternal sphere.

It was when women sought to extend beyond these limits that the most violent conflicts arose. "The Emergence of Professionalism," Holt Parker's revealing exposition of the place of female physicians in classical antiquity, is followed by three essays on the nineteenth century examining the various ways in which the gender barrier was confronted in different parts of the world. The German and Russian women, of whom Paulette Meyer writes, attempt to enter the male bastion while simultaneously developing a subculture of their own. Their duality points to one of the foremost and most hotly debated late nineteenth-century issues surrounding women's entry into medicine as a profession: the desirability of integration versus separatism, especially in regard to hospitals.[9] The implications and effects of separatism are shown by Alison Bashford in her comparative study of Australian and British women's hospitals 1870-1920 and the evolution of their feminist culture. On the other hand, assimilation to male models of medical practice and its consequences are the topic of Regina Morantz-Sanchez's analysis of the path chosen by a highly successful woman surgeon, Dr. Mary Dixon Jones, in Brooklyn in the closing decade of the nineteenth century. Jones's career hinges on an unexpected reversal of the traditional gender roles when she is sued by her women patients and defended by her male colleagues.

As a controversial social question of the day, the emergence of professionalism found expression in the literature of the period too. The last two essays are therefore devoted to the portrayal of women doctors in late nineteenth- and early twentieth-century novels respectively. Lilian R. Furst discusses the appearance of the fully qualified "doctress," as she was then called, in a cluster of five American fictions that appeared between 1881 and 1891, following the foundation of women's medical colleges and hospitals in the third quarter of the nineteenth century. Since these works focus on the social more than the professional problems faced by women who were determined to pursue this unconventional way of life, they afford the opportunity to consider the mixed responses they evoked—compounded of curiosity, admiration, and condemnation. The attitude toward the doctress is found to be mostly correlated to the gendered perspectives from which they are presented. Even in the early twentieth century, Elsa Nettels argues in the concluding piece on Virginia Woolf and her doctors, defiance of patriarchal power on both the personal and the societal level still remained at the core of women's quest for professional status. She uses a biographical as well as a literary approach to show how women's individual struggle against their fathers is played out again publicly in the collective challenge to the medical establishment.

But it would be wrong to end on such a negative note, for the situation of women in medicine has changed radically since Woolf's time. In the final decade of the twentieth century the future of women in medicine looks brighter than ever before. Enormous strides have been made toward greater opportunity in the past half century. The figures speak for themselves: in 1944 only 4.6 percent of medical students in the United States were female,[10] and almost none held senior appointments in teaching hospitals. Fifty years later, the enrollment of women in American medical schools has not yet quite attained parity with that of men, but is certainly moving rapidly in that direction. With more women qualifying and moving up the professional ladder, they have also begun to appear, albeit still rather sparsely, on teaching faculties. Nevertheless, complete equality with men has not yet been achieved. The tendency for women physicians to cluster in traditionally "feminine" specialties such as pediatrics, public and preventive health, is still discernible.

However, the areas in which they are concentrated have expanded to include psychiatry,[11] radiology, and anesthesiology, although they remain underrepresented in such "tough" fields as surgery. Yet even there the outlook is hopeful as more young women are given the chance to prove their abilities.

But perhaps precisely because women's rightful place in medicine is taken for granted nowadays, it is well to have the stories documented in this collection as a reminder of the long hill that women had to climb in order to enter the medical profession and also as a testimony to the perseverance, determination, and ingenuity that enabled them eventually to reach their current level of achievement and acceptance.

## NOTES

I would like to express my thanks to Véronique Machelidon, Ian Wilson, and Melissa Moorhead, who gave me such willing assistance with library research.

1. *A Country Doctor,* rpt. (Boston: Houghton Mifflin, 1984), 179.

2. "Medicine as a Profession for Women," in *Women, The Family and Freedom,* ed. Susan Groag Bell, and Karen M. Offen (Stanford: Stanford University Press, 1983), I:476.

3. Both nursing and midwifery, long female territory, remain very much on the periphery of this volume largely for pragmatic reasons. To have tried to include these forms, too, would have excessively expanded the scope of a collection that was already difficult to limit. The history of nursing and midwifery is a separate subject that has been well addressed elsewhere: e.g. Vern L. Bullough, *History, Trends, and Politics of Nursing* (Norwalk, Conn.: Appleton-Century-Crofts, 1984); Josephine A. Dolan, *Nursing in Society: A Historical Perspective* (Philadelphia: Saunders, 14th. ed., 1978); Anne Hudson Jones, *Images of Nurses: Perspectives from History, Art, and Literature* (Philadelphia: Univ. of Pennsylvania Press, 1988); Joan I. Roberts, *Feminism and Nursing: An Historical Perspective on Power, Status, and Political Activism in the Nursing Profession* (Westport, Conn.: Praeger, 1995); Richard Harrison Shryock, *The History of Nursing: An Interpretation of the Social and Medical Factors Involved* (Philadelphia: Saunders, 1959); Isabel Maitland Stewart, *A History of Nursing, from Ancient to Modern Times; A World View* (New York: Putnam, 5th ed., 1962); Jean Donnison, *Midwives and Medical Men: A History of Inter-Professional Rivalries and Women's Rights* (New York: Schocken Books, 1977); Judy Barrett Litoff, *American Midwives, 1860 to the Present* (Westport, Conn.: Greenwood Press, 1978); Jean Towler, *Midwives in History and Society* (London: Croom Helm, 1986); Laurel Ulrich, *A Midwife's Tale: The Life of Martha Ballard, Based on Her Diary, 1785-1812* (New York: Knopf/Random House, 1990).

4. See Regina Morantz-Sanchez, *Sympathy and Science: Women Physicians in American Medicine* (New York: Oxford Univ. Press, 1985), and Mary Roth Walsh, *"Doctors Wanted: No Women Need Apply": Sexual Barriers in the Medical Profession, 1835-1975* (New Haven: Yale Univ. Press, 1977); for England see E. Moberly Bell, *Storming the Citadel: The Rise of the Woman Doctor* (London: Constable, 1953), and Catriona Blake, *The Charge of the Parasols: Women's Entry to the Medical Profession* (London, The Women's Press, 1990).

5. *Medical Women* (Edinburgh: Oliphant, Anderson & Ferrier, and London: Hamilton Adams & Co., 1886; rpt. New York: Source Books, 1970), 44.

6. Ibid., 9

7. 10th ed. (Paris: Librairie agricole de la maison rustique, n.d.), II:1-101.

8. *Mrs. Beeton's Book of Household Management* (rpt. New York: Exeter Books, 1986), 1065-6.

9. See Virginia Drachman, *Hospital with a Heart: Women Doctors and the Paradox of Separatism at the New England Hospital, 1862-1969* (Ithaca: Cornell University Press, 1984).

10. Walsh, *"Doctors Wanted: No Women Need Apply": Sexual Barriers in the Medical Profession, 1835-1974*, 245.

11. See Ilene J. Philipson, *On the Shoulders of Women: The Feminization of Psychotherapy* (New York: Guilford Publications, 1993).

# Part 1

# BETWEEN MAGIC AND MEDICINE

# [ 1 ]

# MEDIEVAL GERMAN WOMEN
# AND THE POWER OF HEALING

DEBRA L. STOUDT

*The role of medieval women* in the healing arts in Western Europe traditionally has been viewed as a modest one, and its characterization has been fraught with myth and assumption.[1] Women healers in works of medieval fiction and noblewomen in the Middle Ages who commissioned medical works often have attracted more attention than the female practitioners themselves.[2] Whereas women in medieval epics appear in the role of healer with some frequency, extant historical documents offer little evidence of a reflex of this situation in medieval reality. The common perception is that women healers of the Middle Ages either were unschooled or their knowledge was limited to folk medicine. Scholars have assumed that medieval women healers served exclusively as midwives, an assumption not borne out by contemporary accounts; although much of the secondary literature on female practitioners of medicine has focused on women as gynecologists or women as gynecological patients, it is apparent that women were involved in all aspects of the healing arts.[3]

This study undertakes a closer examination of the role of women as healers in medieval and Renaissance Germany and focuses on the type of care offered, by whom and to whom it was offered, and the kinds of remedies employed. The first section provides an overview of the medical activity of German laywomen, a phenomenon of the late Middle Ages and Renaissance, with extant records dating only from the thirteenth century. The second section focuses on the role of religious women in the healing arts and examines in detail how such women modified their response to the power of healing in the course of the Middle Ages. The image of female healers that emerges from the study underscores the evolving relationship among religion, magic, and medicine throughout the Middle Ages and the role of women in this evolution.

The traditional role of laywomen as health-care providers is noted by Tacitus in his depiction of Germanic women who treat the wounds of the men and do not shrink from counting and comparing the gashes.[4] Caring for illnesses and injuries among family and friends constitutes a customary domestic duty, a tradition that continues throughout the Middle Ages, as references in works of fiction suggest. By the twelfth century there is evidence to support the thesis that laywomen legally practiced medicine in European cities such as Salerno and Paris, but before the thirteenth century there are only occasional references to laywomen in German-speaking areas renowned for their medical expertise.[5] In the middle of the twelfth century the abbot Rudolf wrote to the provost of a neighboring monastery in Thuringia concerning the "mulier de Sangeherhusen," who was versed in the healing arts and from whom he requested information regarding the preparation and dosage of a certain medication.[6] In the thirteenth century a prescription entry mentions a "Frau von Tesingen."[7] City chronicles and tax registers offer more numerous references to female physicians, particularly Jewish women, beginning in the fourteenth and fifteenth centuries.[8] For example, in 1394 in Frankfurt the daughter of the deceased physician Hans Wolff twice received payment for healing mercenaries who had been wounded in the line of duty, and in Hildesheim two women were compensated for supplying draughts for wounds (*wundentrank*) and otherwise treating wounded soldiers.[9] Bishop John II of Würzburg permitted the Jewish doctor Sara to practice medicine in and around Würzburg in 1419, but at the end of the century, in 1494, an unidentified Jewish woman was forbidden to treat the sick in Frankfurt. Most of the chronicle entries offer few details concerning the nature of the healing the women engaged in, but interestingly many of the women are identified as eye doctors.[10] Because surgery still was considered a skilled trade, women would not have been excluded from practicing it.[11] There is scant reference to the means by which German women received their medical training. Based on evidence in documents from other areas in Europe, many may have been apprenticed to medical masters who instructed them.[12]

That so few female healers can be identified is related to the fact that the practice of medicine developed from a skill into a profession in the High Middle Ages, as John Benton notes.[13] The founding of universities and the licensing of physicians ostensibly barred secular (and religious) women from practicing medicine. Barbara Kroemer claims that the pharmacy guilds excluded women until the seventeenth century, and women knowledgeable about the preparation of medications often were denounced as quacks, herb women, and witches.[14] Although the guilds may have banned women from their membership, by the sixteenth century certain individuals clearly were more tolerant of female herbalists and pharmacologists. In his *Arzneibuch* Anton Trutmann mentions six women whose remedies he has included in his collection; for example, from Klara Friederlerrin he obtained a salve for scabies (*grind*), and an eyewash (*ougen wasser*) was provided by "die Rohrmännin."[15] In the sixteenth and more frequently in the seventeenth centuries women of the aristocracy exhibited considerable interest in pharmacology. Anna Marie, wife of Duke Christoph von Wittenberg, and Duchess Eleonore Marie Rosalie von Jagersdorf und Troppau were two such women who recorded remedies and whose collections achieved renown. Women of commoner social status demonstrated even greater involvement. Two such individuals, Anna Gremsin and Regina Hurlewegin, contributed substantially to the *Zwölfbändiges Buch der Medizin* (*Twelve-Volume Book of Medicine*) of Ludwig V, the elector of the Palatinate from 1502 to 1544. Ludwig's great interest in medicine motivated him to copy three thousand pages of medical tracts and recipes, noting the source of a significant number of the more than twenty-two thousand entries. Anna's name appears in connection with approximately four hundred entries, that of Regina with more than nine hundred. The remedies offered by these women do not differ at all from those attributed to male healers: there are herbal remedies as well as charms such as the following:

> Noch eins fur den wurm[16]
> Schreibe diese wordt an ein zettell: Cardia Caredentia nestia Simponia Caradiaticca Tensatica anos Amos Sanctiuicatio; Oder sprich: Jch beschwer dich, wurm, wo du seiest, Bei dem vatter vnd dem sune vnd dem hailigen gaist Vnd bei dem hailigen man Sant Job, Das du so bald sterbest.
>
> [Another one for the worm
> Write these words on a slip of paper: Cardia Caredentia nestia Simponia Caradiaticca Tensatica anos Amos Sanctiuicatio; or recite: I adjure you, worm, wherever you may be, by the Father and the Son and the Holy Spirit and by the holy man Saint Job, that you die soon.]

15

Ein segen für den augenschweren[17]
Sprich: Sant nicasius het ein flecken in den augen Vnd badt
Godt, wer seinen namen anrüefft, Das der erlöst würde von
dem schmertzen der augen. Sant Nicasie, Gottes merteller, ver-
tilg den schmertzen der augen des N. + Jn dem namen des vat-
ters + vnd des suns + vnd des hailigen gaists, amen. Vnd früm
drej messen Jn Sant Nicasien er.
[A blessing for the pain in the eyes
Say: Saint Nicasius had a sty in his eye and entreated God that
whoever would call his name would be relieved from the pain
of the eyes. Saint Nicasius, God's martyr, destroy the pain in
the eyes of N., + in the name of the Father + and of the Son +
and of the Holy Spirit, amen. And have 3 masses said in honor
of Saint Nicasius.]

Regina's name also is found in Codex palatinus germanicus 1, a collection of
tracts dealing with the salutary effects of bloodletting, baths, and special diet.
Keil maintains that the remedies that appear under her name betray familiarity with collections such as the *Cirurgia* of Peter von Ulm and indicate
medical knowledge beyond that of a dilettante.[18]

The relationship between religion and medicine is a very close one in many
cultures, and the alliance of the two in Western Europe proves no exception.
The intertwining of religion and medicine has led scholars to posit two types
of medicine in the Middle Ages. Loren MacKinney proposes the dichotomy
between supernatural and human medicine; the former relies upon Christian
saints and their relics as well as Christian pagan charms and magical incantations, whereas the latter stresses drugs, surgery, and diet.[19] In her description
of the relationship between Christianity and medicine, Nancy Siraisi characterizes religious and secular healing in terms of the supernatural and natural
means employed; most significant for her argument is the role of miracles as
part of the religious healing process in early Christianity.[20] Throughout the
Middle Ages religious men and women dedicated their efforts to both types of
healing practices. The period from the seventh century to the mid-eleventh
century was the era of monastic medicine; the Council of Aachen of 817
placed the care and healing of the sick squarely in the hands of the religious,[21]
and already in the ninth century the names of male religious healers were

recorded.[22] Despite the meager documentation, most scholars have asserted that religious women also were active in the healing arts at the time. As the best educated members of society, religious men and women functioned as transcribers and disseminators of medical knowledge; their communities were centers of learning, housed scriptoria where medical texts could be copied, and included gardens which served as sources for herbal remedies. The first hospitals were either physically joined to religious institutions or directed by them,[23] and hence the inhabitants served as healers and caregivers, as physicians and as attendants. Although their principal responsibility was to fellow religious, they attended to the laity as well.[24] The hospitals became independent institutions as secular education gained in importance, as Church councils sought to create a dichotomy between the *seelenarzt* and the *leibarzt,* and as urban areas grew. Nonetheless, particularly outside the cities, the religious continued to perform the dual role of spiritual and physical healers throughout the Middle Ages.

The relationship of religious women to the healing arts in medieval Germany reflected prevailing emphases in spiritual life and developed in a parallel fashion to them. In the earlier centuries of the Middle Ages, religious women wielded greater ecclesiastical authority and exercised a greater number of responsibilities within and without their communities.[25] In 657, Hilda, the grand-niece of King Edwin of Northumbria, became abbess of the double monastery at Whitby; recognized for her abilities as a teacher and administrator, she earned the adulation of no less a luminary than Bede himself. Lioba (died 782), a nun from the community of Wimborne, journeyed from her Anglo Saxon homeland to the area around Würzburg at the request of Boniface; she assisted in the conversion of the German people and later directed the abbey at Tauberbischofsheim. At the behest of Queen Hildegard, Lioba visited Charlemagne's court at Aachen on several occasions. In the tenth and eleventh centuries the abbey of Gandersheim was allied closely with the royal family, whose princesses, for example, Gerberg II (died 1001), daughter of the duke of Bavaria, served as the leaders of the community. Because of the special status afforded the institution by Otto I in 947, the abbesses enjoyed greater freedom and additional rights, including the right of ban and representation at the imperial assembly.

However, the Cluniac reforms that began in the eleventh century and the subsequent concerns related to the *cura monialium* relegated religious women to a more subservient role, always under the watchful eye of a male confessor.[26]

Around this same time several council decrees marked the beginning of the decline of monastic medicine. After 1163 monks and canons and in 1219 secular clergy were forbidden to leave the monastery to study medicine. Such bans would not have had an impact on religious women healers since there were no opportunities for religious women to pursue formal medical training in any case. A prohibition of the Fourth Lateran Council in 1215 forbade the religious from practicing surgery that involved "burning or cutting,"[27] yet the clergy continued to minister to the sick. Only with the establishment of universities and the standardization of professional practices through medical licensing did clerical involvement in the healing arts finally begin to wane. Thus, new social strictures in the form of the limitation of the clergy's medical responsibilities by ecclesiastical councils and increased prescription of medical standards by secular sources dramatically diminished the role of religious women in the practice of medicine; nonetheless, as we shall see below, women preserved their role of healer, albeit on a more modest scale than is posited for the earlier Middle Ages.

Despite the barriers that the ecclesiastical hierarchy began to erect in the twelfth century, the members of the leading monastic order of the time, the Benedictines, maintained a tradition of medical study and practice that was fostered by the translation of the works of Avicenna, which began to reach the West around the middle of the century.[28] In his Letters of Direction to Heloise, Abelard describes the role of the infirmarian in the religious community for women:

> Oportet quoque infirmis providam semper assistere custodiam quae cum opus fuerit statim subveniat et domum omnibus instructam esse quae infirmitati illi sunt necessaria. De medicamentis quoque, si necesse est, pro facultate loci providendum erit. Quod facilius fieri poterit si quae infirmis praeest non fuerit expers medicinae. Ad quam etiam de iis quae sanguinem minuunt cura pertinebit. Oportet autem aliquam flebotomiae peritam esse ne virum propter hoc ad mulieres ingredi necesse sit.
>
> [There must also be a watchful nurse always with the sick to answer their call at once when needed, and the infirmary must be equipped with everything necessary for their illness. Medicaments too must be provided, according to the resources of the convent, and this can more easily be done if the sister in

charge of the sick has some knowledge of medicine. Those who have a period of bleeding shall also be in her care. And there should be someone with experience of blood-letting, or it would be necessary for a man to come in amongst the women for this purpose.][29]

Although not extensive, Abelard's advice indicates that women with medical knowledge and even the expertise required for bloodletting would not be rarities in Benedictine communities.

Because members of religious orders customarily fulfilled the role of caregiver, it is not surprising that at least some medical knowledge has been ascribed to almost every renowned religious woman before 1200. The name of Hrotsvith von Gandersheim (935-1000) has appeared in a survey of women in medicine because the Benedictine canoness gathered herbs for medicine and cared for the sick; Mathilda, abbess at Quedlinburg, has been included as well since she ostensibly supplied her cousin Hrotsvith with substantial material for the canoness's medical work.[30]

Although scholars in the past also attributed a knowledge of the healing arts to Herrad von Hohenbourg (died 1195),[31] speculation on the subject today is more circumspect. The name of the Benedictine abbess has been rescued from obscurity because of her role as compiler of the *Hortus deliciarum,* an encyclopedic work presenting a historical and allegorical narrative of selected scenes from the Old and New Testaments in picture and word. Medicine is mentioned in the *Hortus* almost exclusively in connection with the miracles of healing performed by Christ and the Apostles. In her history of women in medicine Hurd-Mead cited Herrad's descriptions of plants and their preparation for medicinal purposes as evidence of the abbess's knowledge of healing, but the 1979 reconstruction of the *Hortus* includes no such texts.[32] Two entries, "De lapsu carnis quo labitur homo de scala caritatis" and "Ritus leprosi,"[33] deal with illnesses, but neither describes the symptoms of any malady nor offers any remedy. Arnald of Villanova is supposed to have alluded to Herrad's medical expertise with his praise for her explication of the relationship between the seven planets, seven maladies, and seven curative plants,[34] but the abbess's text apparently has not survived. Herrad did obtain land for the establishment of a canonical community for men at nearby Truttenhausen, where a hospital for the poor was among the structures erected; in addition, at the neighboring canonical community of Marbach the intellectual activity,

19

including the copying and collecting of manuscripts, likely stimulated comparable activity at Hohenbourg.[35] In such an environment Herrad certainly could have gained medical knowledge and possibly practical experience.

The sole religious woman in the Middle Ages whose medical knowledge remains undisputed and amply documented today is Hildegard von Bingen (1098-1179);[36] however, whether or not she actually practiced medicine is still much debated. In one of the earliest studies devoted to Hildegard as physician, Gertrude Engbring notes that the duties of the prioress of the community at Disibodenberg would have included health care for the servants and workers who lived on the estate of the monastery, as well as that of their dependents; such a responsibility would have afforded Hildegard the opportunity to engage actively in the healing arts.[37] Although known primarily for her mystical works, especially the *Scivias,* Hildegard today is recognized as the author of two scientific works, the *Liber simplicis medicinae* [Book of Simple Medicine], usually called the *Physica,* an encyclopedic work concerned with natural science, and the *Liber compositae medicinae* [Book of Composite Medicine] or *Causae et curae;* originally appearing together under the rubric *Liber subtilitatum diversarum naturarum creaturarum,* the two works later were recorded separately.[38] It is doubtful that Hildegard actually studied medicine, but it is probable that through manuscripts that found their way to Disibodenberg she familiarized herself with the Scholastic medical tradition as well as that of Salerno. Her scientific works focus to a great extent on her cosmological ideas, but as the title suggests, the *Causae et curae* describes specific diseases and offers remedies for them.[39] The basis of Hildegard's characterization of disease is the concept of humors, which had its origins in the Greek tradition.[40] Although Hildegard's ideas concerning the relationship between mankind and the universe are novel, there is nothing unusual or innovative about the medical treatments she proposes; suggested measures include bloodletting, herbal remedies, and cures involving the recitation of incantations and the use of magic stones.[41] Hildegard represents the end of an era in which healers merge their limited and fragmentary knowledge of medical theory with therapeutic practices gleaned from various sources—folk remedies and treatments suggested by authoritative sources—to deal with common ailments and conditions such as fever, broken bones, or childbirth, as well as medical crises; during the period of monastic medicine both medical study and care occur within the walls of the religious community.[42] In subsequent centuries there is a dichotomy between these two aspects of the healing arts: universities become centers of abstract medical study and hospitals serve as institutions where the sick receive care.

Unique to Hildegard among women healers is the attribution of miraculous healing. Twenty-five such incidents are documented in the autobiographical third book of her vita, entitled *de miraculis;* [43] the reports describe how the abbess effects cures by employing gestures, words, and natural objects such as plants and stones. Hildegard is said to have cured a servant in the monastic community of a swelling of the chest and throat by making the sign of the cross over the unhealthy spots. [44] She restored the sight of a blind boy by drawing water from the Rhine with her left hand, blessing the child with her right, and recalling Jesus's words recorded in John 9:7: "Vade ad natatoria Syloe et laua" [Go, wash in the pool of Siloam]. [45] Sibylle, a woman from Lausanne, petitioned Hildegard through a messenger to be healed from a flow of blood; the abbess sent back a letter containing the following: "Hec inquit verba circa pectus et umbilicum tuum pones in nomine illius, qui recte omnia dispensat. In sanguine Ade orta est mors, in sanguine Christi extincta est mors. In eodem sanguine Christi impero tibi, o sanguis, ut fluxum tuum contineas." [46] [Place these words around your chest and navel in the name of Him who ordains all things rightly: In Adam's blood death arose. In Christ's blood death was extinguished. In this blood of Christ I command you, oh Blood, to stop your flowing.] As soon as the words were spoken, the woman was cured. [47] In the *Physica* Hildegard also includes an incantation as part of a headache remedy that employs a topaz. [48]

The incantation cited above, based upon Romans 5:9-12, is a common formula for wounds or the staunching of blood. [49] Healing by the power of the spoken word was common already in pagan societies. By naming the evil force or disease, the healer gained mastery over it and was able to eradicate it. Within the Christian tradition the use of words for healing purposes oftentimes became associated with certain utterances in the liturgy, especially benedictions and prayers; hence, incantations and charms employed by religious and lay healers frequently included the *Ave Maria,* the *Credo,* or a prayer specifically formulated to cure a given malady. For example, in her *Physica* Hildegard recommended that the healer place an emerald in the mouth of an epileptic and that after the attack the afflicted individual pray the following: "'Sicut spiritus domini replevit orbem terrarum, sic domum corporis mei sua gratia repleat ne ea unquam moveri possit;' et sic etiam per novem sequentes dies in mane diei faciat et curabitur"[50] ["Just as the spirit of the Lord filled the circle of the world, thus let His grace fill the dwelling-place of my body, so that it (= the grace) never can be moved;" and let it be done in this way on nine consecutive days in the morning and he will be cured].

As is evident here, religious women like Hildegard demonstrated their curative powers not only through the application of herbs and poultices but through the use of the spoken and written word, which directly linked the healer to the Divine. Thus imbued with God's word and strength, the sisters were empowered to vanquish the physical illnesses that so frequently beset them and their companions and to subdue spiritual adversaries who threatened their relationship with God. The power of the word was a prevalent theme in the works of medieval religious women and one that has served to relate religion, magic, and medicine throughout the ages. Pagan charms and incantations with a palliative purpose had adopted a Christian veneer in German-speaking areas already by the ninth century, for example, "Pro nessia." Healers prefaced the formulations with invocations such as "In the name of the Father and of the Son and of the Holy Spirit," substituted the name of the Christian God for that of the pagan one in the text itself, and appended Christian prayers at the end. The religious women discussed here continued the tradition; although they encroached upon the realm of magic, they did not exceed the confines of Christian orthodoxy because they invoked only the name of God. In his study of nuns and witches, Peter Dinzelbacher notes that whereas both groups engage in the practice of magic, the acts performed by holy women are designated as miracles and are subsumed under the category of "white" magic because of the special relationship between the women and God.[51] The ancient practice of reciting and writing words with sacred power provides religious women of the Middle Ages with a basis for authority, an authority that ultimately is divine and hence cannot be questioned; the appeal to the word is one way in which they redress the curtailing of their ecclesiastical rights and the limiting of their role as healers.

By appealing to the word and thus to God, the women place the ultimate burden to heal on God Himself; as His servants, they seek to cure, but it is only at His pleasure that the remedies are effective. In Matthew 8:8 the centurion whose servant was sick of the palsy said to Jesus: "but speak the word only, and my servant shall be healed." Nonetheless, the word is not only with God, the Word is God (John 1:1). God is the Great Physician (Exod. 15:26,

Mal. 4:2, Matt. 9:35); only if He wills it is a remedy or incantation effective, as Hildegard declares in her description of the beech tree in the *Physica:*

> et si quispiam homo in illo anno *gelsucht* habet, ex eodem ramo parva frusta abscide, et ea in vasculum pone, ac super ea modicum vini ter funde et totiens haec verba dic, et vinum super eadem frusta fundis. "Per sanctam *scincturam* sanctae incarnationis, qua Deus homo factus, abtrahe ab homine isto N. dolorem *gelsucht,*" et tunc vinum illud cum hastulis illis, quas abscidisti in patella vel in crucibulo calefac, et illi jejuno ita calidum ad bibendum per tres dies da, et curabitur, nisi Deus nolit.[52]
>
> [And when a person suffers from jaundice in that year, cut off little pieces from the branch [of a beech tree], place them in a container, pour some wine over them three times, and repeat these words each time as you pour the wine over the branch pieces: "Through the holy girdle of the holy incarnation by which God became man, carry away this disease of jaundice from this person N.," and then warm that wine in a plate or a crucible with those little branches that you cut off, and give it warmed to the fasting person to drink for three days, and the person will be cured, if God does not will otherwise.]

The cure for jaundice is followed immediately by a similar remedy for a fever:

> Sed et si quis *ridden* habet, accipe de fructu fagi, cum primum procedit et eum in pura aqua, scilicet *springbornen,* commisce; et haec verba dic: "Per sanctam *scincturam* sanctae incarnationis qua Deus homo factus est, tu *riddo,* vos febres, defice et deficite in frigore et in calore tuo in homine isto N.;" et tunc aquam illam da illi ad bibendum; per quinque dies eam parabis, et si aut cottidianam aut quartanam habuerit, ab eis cito liberabitur, aut Deus eum liberare non vult.[53]
>
> [But when the person has a fever, take the fruit of the beech when it first ripens and mix it together in pure water, that is in spring water, and say these words: "Through the holy girdle of the holy incarnation by which God became man, grow weak, you fever and you feverish conditions, and weaken your cold-

ness and heat in this person N.;" and then give this water to
the person to drink; you shall provide it for five days, and if the
person has a quotidian or quartan fever, he will be delivered
from them quickly, or God does not wish to free him.]

The spoken and written word can heal the spirit as well as the body.
Although the practice of exorcism reaches beyond the scope of this study, the
unique extant text by Hildegard of such a ceremony provides additional
evidence of the function of the power of the word. As Dronke notes, the text
itself is recorded in the margins of a single manuscript;[54] indeed, it was commonplace for incantations concerning physical and mental disease to be recorded as marginalia or on the endpapers in manuscripts throughout the
Middle Ages.

Given the comparatively scant manuscript tradition of Hildegard's medical works, her influence on the state of the healing arts of her day probably was
limited.[55] Nonetheless, the fact that such works by a medieval woman were
recorded at all attests to the nun's notoriety and diverse talents and the importance of the healing arts within the religious community. The inclusion of
remedies based not only upon a description of the potency of herbs and the efficacy of medical procedures but also upon the articulation of directions for the
application of cures and the direct naming of the condition or cause demonstrate the role of medical-magical matters in the abbess's vocation. From subsequent centuries there are no other such extant writings by women—religious
or lay. This circumstance is due in part to the practice of licensing healers;
the license necessitated a university education, which was denied to women.
Clearly the religious women's opportunities to heal were affected by social and
ecclesiastical innovations and reforms in the later Middle Ages.

In the second half of the twelfth century new spiritual movements gained
momentum. The Beguine movement began in the Low Countries and between the mid-thirteenth and the mid-fourteenth centuries reached its apex in
German-speaking territory in the cities of Cologne and Strasbourg. The Beguines, women who sought to lead a pious and chaste life in the world, were
not cloistered nor were they part of any established order. They commonly
formed their community, the beguinage, close to an established religious institution or hospital. Although some pursued a contemplative life, many supported themselves by engaging in aspects of cloth-making such as spinning,

weaving, dyeing; others comforted the sick. For example, Marie d'Oignies, along with her husband—with whom she lived a celibate life—attended those afflicted with leprosy. Because the provision of care was a common duty among these pious women, it may be inferred that the Beguines in Germany also nursed the infirm, despite the paucity of records from the beguinages of Cologne and Strasbourg alluding to such activity.[56] However, the care offered was most basic, and no argument can be made that the Beguines actually practiced medicine.

The restrictions imposed by the universities and later by the guilds and the more vocal opposition from within the Church certainly effected change in religious women's roles as healers in the later Middle Ages, but they were not the sole influences. From the twelfth to the fifteenth century, the newly emerging female spirituality dramatically altered the response of religious women in medieval Germany to the power of healing. Whereas in the earlier centuries the religious woman functioned as infirmarian, in the later Middle Ages she appeared more frequently in the role of the infirm. This was not simply a transformation from an active to a passive role; it reflected a transformation in the nature of spirituality and in how the women were permitted to or chose to express it.

Throughout the Middle Ages the relationship of religious women to illness and suffering remained ambiguous and resulted in the emergence of two divergent perspectives. According to the more traditional perspective, which was espoused by the majority of healers—both secular and religious—illness and suffering were viewed as conditions to be alleviated or cured. The second perspective was embodied in the lives of the spiritual elite, most especially the medieval mystics, who sought union with God. Although charged with caring for the sick, these religious women (and men) commonly viewed pain and suffering—both physical and mental—as a prerequisite or concomitant condition to the *unio mystica*.[57] Their works seldom referred to their seeking any physical remedy; the most sought-after cure was consolation from God.

The ambivalent attitude of the religious toward sickness and disease is reflected in their writings. Maladies commonly were attributed to evil spirits and to evil deeds that required punishment. Yet clearly for many religious, particularly the mystics, who played a pivotal spiritual role in medieval Germany, sickness was viewed as a trial permitted and even required by God, just as Job's faith was tested by adversity and disease. Thus, the works of the religious German women after Hildegard focused less on the art of healing than on the art of suffering; the emphasis became more the acceptance of sickness rather than the attempt to cure it.

Because of the nature of their religious calling, the Beguines were less likely to chronicle their experiences; hence, in Germany the words and works of the Beguines were eclipsed by those of religious women who recorded or had recorded their divine experiences: the sisters of Helfta and especially the Dominicans of southern Germany. It is their writings that offer the most substantial evidence of the life of religious women during the later Middle Ages.

Helfta was the life-long home of a triumvirate of women mystics: Gertrud (die Grosse) von Helfta, Gertrud von Hackeborn, and Mechthild von Hackeborn; it also became the retreat of the more well-known Mechthild von Magdeburg, a Beguine.[58] The status of the community of Helfta reflected the dynamic state of affairs regarding the *cura monialium:* following the Rule of St. Benedict, it was nonetheless greatly influenced by Cistercian customs, yet under the spiritual direction of Dominicans. In the thirteenth century Helfta was one of the intellectual and spiritual centers in medieval Germany.[59]

In the *Legatus divinae pietatis* [Herald of Divine Love] Gertrud von Helfta focuses almost exclusively on the spiritual life, as opposed to the physical life, within the religious community. Gertrud suffers various illnesses, although she makes less frequent reference to them in her work than her fourteenth-century counterparts do in their visions and revelations. She is familiar with certain types of remedies, for example an aromatic substance which she sucks on to relieve a headache "ad laudem Dei" [to the glory of God].[60] In her description of the spiritual "wound of love," Gertrud again hints at medical knowledge when she writes: "Et statim incidit memoriae meae quod quandoque audieram, vulneribus necessario adhibendum lavacrum, unguentum, et ligamentum" [At once it occurred to me that I had heard it said that wounds have to be bathed, anointed, and bandaged].[61] Beginning with Gertrud religious women attempt to articulate the undeniable bond between spiritual and physical suffering. In her description of the Lord's two rings of the spiritual espousals, Gertrud relates how she has suffered and what she understands the suffering to mean:

> Cum in quadam oratiuncula offerret Domino omnem
> tolerantiam, qua tam in corpore quam in spiritu gravaretur,
> et omnem delectationem qua tam spiritu quam carne frus-

traretur; apparuit Dominus, illa duo quae sibi obtulerat, scili-
cet delectationem et tolerantiam, in specie gemmatorum annu-
lorum quasi pro ornamento utrisque manibus ferens. Quod
cum intellexisset, praetactam orationem saepius iterans, post
aliquantum temporis cum eamdem recitaret, praesensit Domi-
num Jesum annulo sinistrae manus, quem intellexerat cor-
poralem gravaminis tolerantiam esse, sinistrum oculum ejus
linire. Et ex tunc cumdem oculum, quem Dominus visus est in
spiritu tangere, doluit in corpore, in tantum quod postea nun-
quam plene convaluit ad priorem sanitatem. Hinc intellexit
quod, sicut annulus signum est desponsationis, sic adversitas
tam corporalis quam spiritualis verissimum signum est electio-
nis divinae et quasi desponsatio animae cum Deo.

[While she was offering to God in a short prayer all the
pain she had to endure, of body or soul, and all the joys, spiritual or physical, which were denied her, the Lord appeared. He
was wearing this two-fold offering she had made him—namely,
of joys and of sufferings—in the form of two jeweled rings, one
on each hand. When she had understood the meaning of this,
she often repeated the same prayer. After a little while, she was
reciting it when she felt the Lord stroking her left eye with the
ring on his left hand, which she understood to be a symbol of
physical pain. And from that time, that same eye which she
had seen the Lord touching spiritually, suffered so much physically that it never regained its former health. From this she understood that, just as the ring is the symbol of espousals, so any
trial, whether of body or soul, is the truest sign of divine election and is like the espousals of the soul with God.][62]

The concept of tribulation, including physical pain, as evidence of the woman's
status as one of God's chosen suggests why religious women in the later Middle
Ages were less concerned with cures than with the endurance of physical suffering. Through such trials the women not only imitated Christ but achieved a
closer spiritual union with Him.[63]

The contemplative mood and poetic style of the *Fliessendes Licht der Gottheit* [Flowing Light of the Godhead] by Mechthild von Magdeburg precludes
abundant references to the day-to-day life in the community. Like Gertrud,
Mechthild discusses bodily illness and suffering in terms of service to God. In

her advice to priors and prioresses, Mechthild addresses specifically the care of the sick in metaphorical terms: "Du solt alle tage in das siechhus gan und salben si mit den tröstlichen gottes worten und laben si mit irdenischen dingen miltekliche, wand got ist über alle koste rich" [Thou shalt go daily to the sickhouse / And heal the sick with comforting words of God, / And cheer them gently with earthly joys / For God is rich above all price].⁶⁴ The spiritual comforts and small kindnesses the caregiver is to offer are more efficacious than herbal remedies or dietary recommendations, as Mechthild indicates by using the term *koste,* which conveys the meaning "nourishment" as well as "price." The *Fliessendes Licht* contains several other figurative medical allusions, for example, the reference to the little sack containing healing roots, which the Lord shows her in a vision,⁶⁵ and the description of a spiritual convent founded on the virtues, in which compassion is the infirmarian, "die iemer danach hungeret, das si unverdrossen den siechen si bereit, mit helfe und mit reinekeit, mit labunge und mit vrölicheit, mit troste und mit minnesamkeit. So gibet ir got sin widergelt, das si es iemer gerne tůt"⁶⁶ [who is always eager to aid the sick tirelessly with support and with cleanliness, with refreshment and with a cheerful nature, with encouragement and with kindness. So God gives her His reward, that she always does it gladly]. In a prayer toward the end of the seventh and final part of her revelations, Mechthild describes her love-sickness for the Lord and asserts that He has the ability to cure her if He will anoint her wounds; this can only be accomplished if He covers or envelops her soul with Himself:

Helig engel Gabriel, gedenk min. Miner gerunge botschaft bevilhe ich dir. Sage minem lieben herren Jhesu Christo, wie minnensiech ich nach ime si. Sol ich iemer me genesen, so můs er selber min arzat wesen. Du maht ime in trúwen sagen, die wunden, die er mir selber hat gesclagen, die mag ich nit langer ungesalbet und ungebunden tragen. Er hat mich gewundet untz in den tot. Lat er mich nu ungesalbet ligen, so mag ich niemer genesen. Weren alle berge ein wuntsalbe und allú wasser ein arzatin trank und alle böme mit blůmen ein heilsam wundenbant, da mitte möhte ich niemer genesen; er můs sich selber in miner selen wunden legen.
[Holy Angel Gabriel, remember me!
I commend to thee the mission of my longing;

28

Say to Christ my dear Lord
That I am ill for love of Him.
If I am ever to recover,
He Himself must be my Physician.
Tell Him in secret
That I can no longer bear
The wounds He has given me
Unanointed and unbound.
For He has wounded me
Nigh unto death.
If He leaves me unanointed
I can never recover.
—Were all hills healing ointment,
All waters healing draughts,
All flowers and trees healing unguents—
Even with all that,
I could never recover.
He must lay Himself
In the wound of my soul.][67]

With the rise of the mendicant orders contemplation becomes increasingly important to the religious women, and the sought-after union with Christ produces the blossoming of the mystical tradition. The focus on the *imitatio Christi* leads to contemplation of Jesus's suffering and a heightening of the ambivalent attitude toward the healing arts. Although there are examples of religious women (and men) engaging in physically painful ascetic practices,[68] the mystics do not seek out physical illness, but they anticipate it as a concomitant effect of the mystical experience. This circumstance has led some scholars to claim that these are psychosomatic illnesses,[69] an assertion often presupposing that the maladies derive from physical or psychological weakness. However, for the mystic the illness is a trial to endure or a burden to bear; it is not effected by the individual but permitted by Christ. The general description of the physical symptoms—headaches, fever, profuse bleeding—signifies that it is not the exact nature of the illness that is critical in the life of the individual but rather the endurance of the affliction that these physical manifestations connote.

The references in the autobiographical revelations of the fourteenth-century German mystics such as Margaretha Ebner, Christina Ebner, and Adel-

29

heid Langmann, and in the biographies by and about other sisters in the Dominican province of Teutonia offer insights into how the religious women coped with physical pain and suffering. As in the works of their predecessors at Helfta, there are allusions to their own illnesses and praise for those who tend the sick,[70] but relatively little attention is accorded specific remedies or cures and only seldom is a particular malady identified.[71] Although Margaretha Ebner often alludes to her frail health in her *Offenbarungen* [Revelations], it is the letters of her confessor and friend Heinrich von Nördlingen, a secular priest, that cite medical knowledge and practices in cloistered communities. In Letters II and XV he mentions that he is sending mace [*muszkatplut*] and cinnamon [*zimin*], two spices commonly employed for medicinal purposes,[72] and in Letters XXXII, XLIV, and XLVI he refers to medicinal powders he is supplying to the Medingen community.[73] Heinrich informs Margaretha in Letters XV and XLVI that he is sending along a *binden,* a bandage for use in bloodletting.[74] When the nuns were bled or housed in the infirmary, they commonly donned special gowns; in Letter XXXV Heinrich requests such a gown from Margaretha, so that he may touch it and be purified in body and in soul.[75] There are fewer references to healing in Christina Ebner's visions, but Philipp Strauch, the nineteenth-century editor of her work, relates a vision in which God teaches Christina how to make salutary vapor from cloves (*rauch von negellein*) for physical ailments; the Engelthal sister also recognizes that those afflicted with fever who eat the cloves will be cured, which indeed occurs.[76] Adelheid Langmann's revelations make frequent reference to illness but offer little information regarding treatment. There are, however, two accounts of how devils are exorcised. In the first, the sister describes a vision in which devils surround her and she becomes so ill that she cannot speak or raise her hand to make the sign of the cross, so she makes a cross with her tongue in her mouth. As she loses consciousness, angels come and vanquish the devils.[77] In the second account Adelheid intervenes when the devil possesses the prioress Jeut Pfintzingin; her rebuke of the devil echoes the formulas found in exorcisms and other incantations: "du pöser gaist, ich gepeut dir bei dem lebendigen got daz du stille stest. . . . ich gepeut dir bei dem vater und pei dem sun und pei dem heilgen gaist und pei dem jungsten geriht, daz du still stest und si nindert füerest" [you evil spirit, I adjure you by the living God that you stand still. . . . I adjure you by the Father and by the Son and by the Holy Spirit and by the Last Judgment that you stand still and not lead her further away].[78]

The chronicles or *Schwesternbücher* present a compendium of the lives of several generations of religious women in a given community; they offer few details, but all make reference to care of the sick. Anna von Munzingen refers to the *siechmeisterin* three times in her chronicle of the Adelhausen community; however, in other instances it is clear that the nuns no longer rely on the medical knowledge and abilities of those within their community. In the chronicle of the sisters at Töss, Elsbeth Stagel states that a good male physician ministered to sister Beli von Sure in her suffering.[79] Likewise, when Mechthilt von Stans becomes ill, first the *siechmaisterin*, then a wise male physician, and finally the Dominican provincial come to attempt to determine what is wrong with her.[80] At Weiler, when Elizabeth von Esslingen has been ill for four weeks, the attempt is made to diagnose her malady by sending her urine to a wise doctor for inspection.[81] After an ecstatic experience, the fifteenth-century mystic Magdalena von Frieburg is examined by a male physician, who determines that she is indeed yet alive.[82] In all four situations the nuns are *minnesiech,* physically suffering because of their overabundant love of God. In none of the cases does the physician effect a cure and in fact no treatments are mentioned; nonetheless, except for Beli, all recover. Noteworthy is a reference in Heinrich Seuse's *Vita* to the suffering of his mother from the same affliction. The Dominican priest asserts that she had been bedridden for twelve weeks when "es die arzet kuntlich innen wurden und gŭt bild dar ab namen" [the doctors became aware of it and were edified by her good example].[83] Likewise, in the *Schwesternbücher,* the soliciting of medical help from outside the community may not be an appeal to or reliance on men in positions of authority or knowledge,[84] but rather just the opposite: the suffering of the women exceeds the ken of the learned physicians and has no cure—as the doctors themselves often admit—and because it is an experience permitted by God, the women suffer patiently and willingly, serving as a holy example to others. Although there are references in the chronicles and the revelations to *menschlich ertzni,* the female mystics more commonly resort to prayer and meditation, which are invoked not to cure but to console.

Secular sources also attest to the medical knowledge of religious women. In "The Fever and the Flea," the forty-eighth fable in his collection entitled *Edelstein* (1349/50), Ulrich Boner describes in detail how a nun attempts to combat her fever based upon what she herself has read.[85] Lying under the covers with her entire body shaking, she tells her helper about potential remedies such as rubbing the feet with vinegar and salt, bathing the head with rose water to draw out the bad heat, and partaking of a pomegranate to refresh the mouth. It is unclear which if any of the cures is employed; in any case the nun unfortunately does not experience an immediate recovery. Another source, a "Sermo zum Aderlass" from 1455, contains the following advice: "Es ist gut, dass in Frauenklöstern etliche von den Ältesten wissen und es verstehen, wann und wie und warum man zur Ader lassen soll" [It is good that some of the oldest ones in the convents know and understand when and how and why one lets blood].[86]

Medieval women as well as men were concerned with the wellbeing of the body and the spirit, and throughout the Middle Ages both religious and lay women served as healers. When the religious were the principal custodians of medical knowledge, they also were the principal practitioners. Because of their vocation, the sisters of the regular orders as well as the Beguines were empowered to serve as care providers. However, they were not authorized to act in the capacity of physicians, and, except for Hildegard, there is little evidence to suggest that they disregarded this mandate. In Germany many religious women withdrew to a life of contemplation; instead of tending others in physical need, they sought consolation for their own suffering in Christ their Beloved. This led to a shift in the focus of the healing arts from curative efforts to endurance of the affliction, a physical manifestation of the *imitatio Christi*. Corporeal suffering becomes a familiar, almost conventional aspect of the life of holy women (and some men) of the later Middle Ages, and for the most part the works by and for German religious women of the time describe illnesses, treatments, and cures only in general terms. Some ailments can be remedied, but the lovesickness, the suffering resulting from intimate devotion to Christ, cannot. Indeed, the women who are *minnesiech* do not wish to be cured, since the consequence of recovery or even improvement is alienation from the Beloved. They suffer in imitation of Christ's body, by His will, and for His love.

Social custom caused lay women to pursue medicine in a less conspicuous manner. Although a few gained notoriety for their abilities, more often such skilled women suffered the stigma of the malevolent witch or the unethical procuress [*Kupplerin*].[87] Indeed, the perceived dichotomy between religious and lay women healers is reflected as late as the fifteenth century in the satirical work, *Des Teufels Netz* (1414/20).[88]

Despite the licensing restrictions instituted by municipal authorities, the lack of university training, the cloistered existence of the religious women, and the suspicion and mistrust from society as a whole, women ministered to the infirm by relying primarily, though not exclusively, upon innate ability and tradition. Considering the training and experience of most, it is not surprising that medieval women should have continued to derive their healing power from the same sources they had drawn upon in the early Middle Ages. The essence of the story of medieval women healers does not differ substantially from that of their male counterparts. Faced with the challenge of the power to heal, the women adapted themselves to the task: the few employed innovative procedures and remedies, the majority followed the traditions established centuries before—the traditions of healing through diet, herbal remedies, and the sanctified word.

### NOTES

1. Monica Green's essay, "Women's Medical Practice and Care," *Signs* 14 (1989): 434-73, reprinted in *Sisters and Workers in the Middle Ages,* ed. Judith M. Bennett et al. (Chicago and London: Univ. of Chicago Press, 1989), 39-78, serves as a fine introduction to the subject of women as healers in the Middle Ages. Her footnote 5, p. 41, offers additional secondary literature on the topic, as does footnote 61, pp. 221-22, in Bernard Dietrich Haage, *Studien zur Heilkunde im 'Parzival' Wolframs von Eschenbach,* Göppinger Arbeiten zur Germanistik, 565 (Göppingen: Kümmerle, 1992). To the list may be added Gundolf Keil's 1986 review of selected recent literature, "Die Frau in der alten Medizin. Eine kritische Sichtung der neueren Literatur Teil I und II," *Fortschritte der Medizin* 104.33 (1986): 51-53; and 104.34 (1986): 58-59.

2. Peter Meister, *The Healing Female in the German Courtly Romance,* Göppinger Arbeiten zur Germanistik, 523 (Göppingen: Kümmerle, 1990), characterizes the healing women in Hartmann's *Êrec, Iwein,* and *Der arme Heinrich,* Wolfram's *Parzival,* and Gottfried's *Tristan.* Several other references in Middle High German literature are included in Trude Ehlert, "Die Frau als Arznei. Zum Bild der Fau in hochmittelalterlicher deutscher Lehrdichtung," *Zeitschrift für deutsche Philologie* 105 (1986): 52-53. Additional portrayals of female healers can be found in Wolfram's *Willehalm,* 99, 18-29, in which Gyburg attends to the margrave's wounds with a mixture of vinegar and dittany, and *Diu Crône* of Heinrich von dem Türlin, verses 6721-6733, where Anzansnûse makes for Gawein's wounds a plaster by boiling fine herbs, having learned the secret from Isolde of Ireland.

3. Among studies with a gynecological focus are Britta-Juliane Kruse, *Verborgene Heilkünste. Geschichte der Frauenmedizin im Spätmittelalter,* Quellen und Forschungen

zur Literatur- und Kulturgeschichte 5 (239), (Berlin: de Gruyter, 1996), Monica Blöcker, "Frauenzauber—Zauberfrauen," *Zeitschrift für schweizerische Kirchengeschichte* 76 (1982): 1-39, and Paul Diepgen, *Frau und Frauenheilkunde in der Kultur des Mittelalters* (Stuttgart: Georg Thieme, 1963). John F. Benton evaluates the role of medieval women in medicine in "Trotula, Women's Problems, and the Professionalization of Medicine in the Middle Ages," *Bulletin of the History of Medicine* 59 (1985): 30-53. See also Helen Lemay, "Women and the Literature of Obstetrics and Gynecology," *Medieval Women and the Sources of Medieval History,* ed. Joel T. Rosenthal (Athens: Univ. of Georgia Press, 1990), 189-209; and Merry E. Wiesner, *Working Women in Renaissance Germany* (New Brunswick, N.J.: Rutgers Univ. Press, 1986), 55-73. Green's essay and Gundolf Keil, "Die Frau als Ärztin und Patientin in der medizinischen Fachprosa des deutschen Mittelalters," *Frau und spätmittelalterlicher Alltag. Internationaler Kongress Krems an der Donau 2. bis 5. Oktober 1984,* Veröffentlichungen des Instituts für mittelalterliche Realienkunde Öster-reichs, 9 (Vienna: Verlag der Österreichischen Akademie der Wissenschaften, 1986), 157-211, also shed light on this issue.

4. Tacitus, *Germania,* chapter 7: "ad matres, ad coniuges vulnera ferunt; nec illae numerare aut exigere plagas pavent." For additional comments on the role of Germanic women in the healing arts, see Reinhold Bruder, *Die germanische Frau im Lichte der Runeninschriften und der antiken Historiographie,* Quellen und Forschungen zur Sprach- und Kulturgeschichte der germanischen Völker, N.F. 57 (181) (Berlin and New York: de Gruyter, 1974), 143-45.

5. Green, 45-50, reviews the prosopographical studies of women medical practitioners in western Europe and notes that "no comprehensive archival study has yet been done of medical practitioners in the medieval German principalities" (48-49).

6. Keil, "Die Frau als Ärztin und Patientin in der medizinischen Fachprosa des deutschen Mittelalters," 159-60. See also Werner Gerabek, "'Consolida major,' 'Consolida minor' und eine Kräuterfrau. Medizinhistorische Beobachtungen zur Reinhardsbrunner Briefsammlung," *Sudhoffs Archiv* 67 (1983): 80-93.

7. Keil, "Die Frau als Ärztin und Patientin in der medizinischen Fachprosa des deutschen Mittelalters," 205.

8. The same list is repeated in most of the secondary literature on the subject: Muriel Joy Hughes, *Women Healers in Medieval Life and Literature* (1943; Salem, N.H.: Ayer, 1987), 143; Peter Ketsch, *Frauen im Mittelalter. Band 1: Frauenarbeit im Mittelalter. Quellen und Materialien,* ed. Annette Kuhn (Düsseldorf: Schwann, 1983), 260-76; Georg Ludwig Kriegk, *Deutsches Bürgerthum im Mittelalter. Nach urkundlichen Forschungen und mit besonderer Beziehung auf Frankfurt am Main* (1886; Frankfurt: Sauer & Auvermann, 1969), 34-53, includes male and female physicians before 1500; Mélanie Lipinska, *Histoire des femmes médecins depuis l'antiquité jusquà nos jours* (Paris: G. Jacques, 1900), 122-25; Isak Münz, *Die jüdischen Ärzte im Mittelalter. Ein Beitrag*

*zur Kulturgeschichte des Mittelalters* (Frankfurt: J. Kauffmann, 1922), 56-57; Walther Schönfeld, *Frauen in der abendländischen Heilkunde vom klassischen Altertum bis zum Ausgang des 19. Jahrhunderts* (Stuttgart: Ferdinand Enke, 1947), 77-78; Helmut Wachendorf, *Die wirtschaftliche Stellung der Frau in den deutschen Städten des späteren Mittelalters* (diss., Hamburg, 1933; Quakenbrück i. H.: C.Trute, 1934), 23-26 and 63-65. In addition, Wiesner, 37-73, offers a detailed examination of women's involvement in health care in Renaissance Germany.

 9. Kriegk, 38, and Wachendorf, 24.

 10. Women's involvement in the treatment of eye diseases has an extensive history. See, for example, Schönfeld, 53.

 11. Kriegk, 50, and Wachendorf, 24.

 12. Schönfeld, 54, notes one such example from fourteenth-century France.

 13. Benton, 30.

 14. Barbara Kroemer, "Die Ärztinnen," in *Frauen in der Geschichte II. Fachwissenschaftliche und fachdidaktische Beiträge zur Sozialgeschichte der Frauen vom frühen Mittelalter bis zur Gegenwart,* ed. Annette Kuhn and Jörn Rüsen, Geschichtsdidaktik, 8 (Düsseldorf: Schwann, 1982), 85.

 15. Rainer Sutterer, "Anton Trutmanns 'Arzneibuch'" (diss., Bonn, 1976), 78 and 112; see also 41-42, 122, 126, 145-46, 173, and 182.

 16. Cpg. 266, 143r. The *Zwölfbändiges Buch des Medizin,* Cpg. 261-272 of the Heidelberg Universitätsbibliothek, has not been edited; I am presently completing an edition of the incantations contained in the manuscripts. On Job in worm charms see "Wurmsegen," *Handwörterbuch des deutschen Aberglaubens,* ed. Hanns Bächtold-Stäubli (1941; Berlin and New York: de Gruyter, 1989), vol. 9, 858-61.

 17. Cpg. 271, 132r. For comments on St. Nicasius in eye charms, see "Augensegen," *Handwörterbuch des deutschen Aberglaubens,* vol. 1, 717-18.

 18. Gundolf Keil, "Hurleweg, Regina," in *Die deutsche Literatur des Mittelalters. Verfasserlexikon,* ed. Kurt Ruh, 2d ed., (Berlin: de Gruyter, 1983), vol. 4, 316-17.

 19. Loren C. MacKinney, *Early Medieval Medicine with Special Reference to France and Chartres,* Publications of the Institute of the History of Medicine, Johns Hopkins University, third series, III (Baltimore: Johns Hopkins Univ. Press, 1937), 23.

 20. Nancy G. Siraisi, *Medieval and Early Renaissance Medicine: An Introduction to Knowledge and Practice* (Chicago and London: Univ. of Chicago Press, 1990), 7-9. See also Richard Kieckhefer's discussion of healers and diviners in *Magic in the Middle Ages* (Cambridge and New York: Cambridge Univ. Press, 1989), 56-85; and "Caring and Curing in the Medieval Catholic Tradition," chapter 7 of Darrel W. Amundsen's *Medicine, Society, and Faith in the Ancient and Medieval Worlds* (Baltimore: Johns Hopkins Univ. Press, 1996), 175-221, especially 179-96.

 21. Eduard Seidler, "Heilkunst und Lebensordnung. Die Medizin in der Benediktinischen Tradition," *Erbe und Auftrag* 57 (1981): 23.

35

22. Franz Mone lists more than twenty-five such men in his "Armen- und Krankenpflege vom 13. bis 16. Jahrhundert," *Zeitschrift für die Geschichte des Oberrheins* 12 (1861): 15-16.

23. In his study of the Benedictine tradition of medicine, Seidler, 24, identifies four different care facilities that ideally were part of a monastic community. At the *hospitale pauperum,* located at the gate, the poor, the wayfarer, and the sick (laity) were received. The *domus hospitum* housed distinguished guests and was located near the abbot's house. Within the enclosed area stood the *infirmarium,* intended only for the use of the monks; adjacent to it were the bloodletting house, the bath, the physician's house, and an area to store medication. Behind the hospital was the herb garden. In "Les livres de l'infirmerie dans les monastères médiévaux," *Revue Mabillon,* nouvelle série, 5 (t. 66) (1994), 60-63, Donatella Nebbiai-Dalla Guarda includes a description of the location of such buildings in several different religious communities in western Europe.

24. Wolfgang Hirth, "Popularisierungstendenzen in der mittelalterlichen Fachliteratur," *Medizinhistorisches Journal* 15 (1980): 74.

25. Although somewhat dated, Lina Eckenstein's *Woman under Monasticism: Chapters on Saint-Lore and Convent Life between A.D. 500 and A.D. 1500* (Cambridge, 1896; rpt. New York: Russell and Russell,1963) provides the most detailed information on this era. Another useful monograph is Donald Hochstetler, *A Conflict of Traditions: Women in Religion in the Early Middle Ages 500-840* (Lanham, Md.: Univ. Press of America, 1992). An extensive bibliography of additional works is found in *Women in Medieval History and Historiography,* ed. Susan Mosher Stuard (Philadelphia: Univ. of Pennsylvania Press, 1987), 133-84.

26. Carolyn Walker Bynum discusses this phenomenon in conjunction with her examination of the nature of female spirituality at the Helfta convent in *Jesus as Mother: Studies in the Spirituality of the High Middle Ages* (Berkeley, Los Angeles, and London: Univ. of California Press, 1982), 185 and 250-52.

27. Michael McVaugh, "Medicine, History of," *Dictionary of the Middle Ages,* ed. Joseph R. Strayer (New York: Scribner, 1987), vol. 8, 253.

28. Odilo Engels, "Die Zeit der Heiligen Hildegard," *Hildegard von Bingen 1179-1979. Festschrift zum 800. Todestag der Heiligen,* ed. Anton Brück (Mainz: Selbstverlag der Gesellschaft für Mittelrheinische Kirchengeschichte, 1979), 20.

29. T.P. McLaughlin, ed., "Abelard's Rule for Religious Women," *Mediaeval Studies* 18 (1956): 261; translation from Betty Radice, *The Letters of Abelard and Heloise* (New York: Penguin Books, 1974), 215.

30. Kate Campbell Hurd-Mead, *A History of Women in Medicine from the Earliest Times to the Beginning of the Nineteenth Century* (1938; New York: AMS Press, 1977), 111-12.

31. Scholars now identify the abbess previously known as Herrad of Landsberg as Herrad of Hohenbourg; see Rosalie Green et al., *Herrad of Hohenbourg. Hortus deli-*

*ciarum,* 2 vols., Studies of the Warburg Institute, 36 (London: Warburg Institute, 1979); Michael Curschmann, "Herrad von Hohenburg," in *Die deutsche Literatur des Mittelalters. Verfasserlexikon,* ed. Kurt Ruh, 2d ed., (Berlin: de Gruyter, 1982), vol. 3, 1138-44; and Joan Gibson, "Herrad of Hohenbourg," *A History of Women Philosophers.* Volume II: *Medieval, Renaissance and Enlightenment Women Philosophers A.D. 500-1600,* ed. Mary Ellen Waithe (Dordecht: Kluwer, 1989), 85-89.

32. Hurd-Mead, *A History of Women in Medicine,* 181. The miniatures that Hurd-Mead referred to are included in the reconstruction, vol. 2: evil spirits departing from the possessed can be found in the sketches of Christ Healing the Canaanite Woman's Daughter, p. 193 (fol. 116r), and Christ Healing Two Demoniacs, p. 207 (fol. 123r); I believe the "diagram showing the relation of the planets to the brain" is the sketch of the microcosm on p. 30 (fol. 16v). None of the texts that accompany the sketches makes any reference to medicine.

33. Green, vol. 2, 361-63 (fol. 220r) and 403 (fol. 239r).

34. Hurd-Mead, *A History of Women in Medicine,* 125 and 236. Unfortunately, here as frequently elsewhere Hurd-Mead does not cite her sources.

35. Charles Schmidt, *Herrade de Landsberg* (Strasbourg: J.H. Ed. Heitz, 1926), 8; and Green, vol. 1, 11. Hurd-Mead, *A History of Women in Medicine,* 181, asserts that Herrad "built a large hospital in her monastery at which she was physician in chief." I have found no justification for or corroboration of the assertion.

36. There is a wealth of secondary literature on Hildegard von Bingen and medicine; the list here includes some of the most useful studies: Melitta Weiss Adamson, "A Reevaluation of Saint Hildegard's *Physica* in Light of the Latest Manuscript Finds," in *Manuscript Sources of Medieval Medicine: A Book of Essays,* ed. Margaret R. Schleissner, Garland Medieval Casebooks, 8 (New York and London: Garland, 1995), 55-80; Gerhard Baader, "Naturwissenschaft und Medizin im 12. Jahrhundert und Hildegard von Bingen," *Archiv für mittelrheinische Kirchengeschichte* 31 (1979): 33-54; Joan Cadden, "It Takes All Kinds: Sexuality and Gender Differences in Hildegard of Bingen's *Book of Compound Medicine,*" *Traditio* 49 (1984): 149-74; Gertrude M. Engbring, "Saint Hildegard, Twelfth Century Physician," *Bulletin of the History of Medicine* 8,6 (1940): 770-84; Hermann Fischer, *Die heilige Hildegard von Bingen. Die erste deutsche Naturforscherin und Ärztin. Ihr Leben und Werk,* Münchener Beiträge zur Geschichte und Literatur der Naturwissenschaften und Medizin, Heft 7/8 (Munich: Verlag der Münchner Drucke, 1927); Keil, "Die Frau als Ärztin und Patientin in der medizinischen Fachprosa des deutschen Mittelalters," 157-211; Irmgard Müller, "Krankheit und Heilmittel im Werk Hildegards von Bingen," in *Hildegard von Bingen 1179-1979. Festschrift zum 800. Todestag der Heiligen,* 311-49; George W. Radimersky, "Magic in the Works of Hildegard von Bingen (1098-1179)," *Monatshefte* 49 (1957): 353-60; Peter Riethe, "Die medizinische Lithologie der Hildegard von Bingen," in *Hildegard von Bingen 1179-1979. Festschrift zum 800. Todestag der*

*Heiligen,* 351-70; Heinrich Schipperges, "Krankheitsursache, Krankheitswesen und Heilung in der Kloster-medizin, dargestellt am Welt-Bild Hildegards von Bingen" (diss., Bonn, 1951); and Heinrich Schipperges, "Menschenkunde und Heilkunst bei Hildegard von Bingen," in *Hildegard von Bingen 1179-1979. Festschrift zum 800. Todestag der Heiligen,* 295-310.

37. Engbring, 779.

38. There is at present no critical edition of the *Liber subtilitatum diversarum naturarum creaturarum.*

39. The nature of the illnesses is discussed by Müller, 314-33; a study of the cures is contained in pp. 334-48.

40. See Siraisi, 104-6.

41. Hildegard also discusses the magical properties of certain trees in the third book of the *Physica.* See Müller, 341-42, and the examples below.

42. Seidler, 27.

43. Peter Bernards examines the place of the third book of Hildegard's vita within the contemporaneous tradition of miracle literature in "Die rheinische Mirakelliteratur im 12. Jahrhundert," *Annalen des historischen Vereins für den Niederrhein* 138 (1941): 22-24. In a new edition of Hildegard's life, *Vita Sanctae Hildegardis,* Corpus Christianorum, Continuatio Mediaeualis 126 (Turnhout: Brepols, 1993), 109*-25*, Monika Klaes presents pertinent background information on book 3, especially the issue of the editorial role of the monk Theoderich von Echternach.

44. *Vita Sanctae Hildegardis,* Liber III, Cap. III.

45. *Vita Sanctae Hildegardis,* Liber III, Cap. XVIII. These two incidents are cited without their source by Eduard Gronau in *Hildegard von Bingen 1098-1179. Prophetische Lehrerin der Kirche an der Schwelle und am Ende der Neuzeit* (Stein am Rhein: Christiana-Verlag, 1985), 297.

46. *Vita Sanctae Hildegardis,* Liber III, Cap. X; recorded also in epistolary form in *Analecta Sanctae Hildegardis Opera Spicilegio Solesmensi Parata,* ed. Jean Baptiste Pitra, Analecta Sacra, 8 (1882; Farnborough: Gregg, 1966), Letter XXXVI, 521. The incident is cited by Adolph Franz, *Die kirchlichen Benediktionen im Mittelalter* (Freiburg, 1909; Graz: Akademische Druck- und Verlagsanstalt, 1960), vol. II, 511-12; and Gronau, 297-98. For a description of the tradition of the formula dealing with the blood of Adam and of Christ, see "Blutsegen," *Handwörterbuch des deutschen Aberglaubens,* vol. 1, 1455.

47. All translations are my own unless otherwise noted. The entirety of book 3 of Hildegard's vita has been translated into English by Sister Anna Silvas in "Saint Hildegard of Bingen and the *Vita Sanctae Hildegardis,*" *Tjurunga. An Australasian Benedictine Review* 32 (1987): 46-59.

48. Jacques-Paul Migne, *Patrologia latina,* tom. 197, S. Hildegardis abbatissae Opera omnia (1855; Paris: Migne, 1882), 1255D-1256A; cited hereafter as *PL.*

49. See Franz, II, 511-12; and "Blutsegen," *Handwörterbuch des deutschen Aberglaubens,* vol. 1, 1455.

50. Migne, *PL* 197: 1249C-1250B; cited in Franz, II, 499.

51. *Heilige oder Hexen? Schicksale auffälliger Frauen in Mittelalter und Frühneuzeit* (Zurich: Artemis and Winkler, 1995), 212; pages 212-35 deal with various aspects of magic which women of both types pursued.

52. Migne, *PL* 197: 1235B-C; Radimersky, 359, offers a translation of part of the passage, based on Johannes Bühler's 1922 German edition of selections from Hildegard's works, *Schriften der Heiligen Hildegard von Bingen* (Leipzig: Insel, 1922), 148-49. My translation corresponds with the German translation of Marie-Louise Portmann, *Heilmittel. Erste vollständige und wortgetreue Übersetzung, bei der alle Handschriften berücksichtigt sind,* 1. Lieferung, Buch 3: Von den Bäumen (Basel: Basler Hildegard-Gesellschaft, 1982), 75. In his translation into French, *Hildegarde de Bingen. Le Livre des Subtilités des Créatures Divines. Physique,* vol. 11 (Grenoble: Jérôme Millon, 1989), Pierre Monat suggests "Par le ventre saint" for "Per sanctam *scinturam*"; for *scincturam* Migne's edition offers the conjectures *scissuram* and *cincturam* in the notes.

For more on the role of the beech tree in folk medicine, see "Buche," *Handwörterbuch des deutschen Aberglaubens,* vol. 1, 1693-94.

53. Migne, *PL* 197: 1235C.

54. Peter Dronke, "Problemata Hildegardiana," *Mittellateinisches Jahrbuch* 16 (1981): 118-22 and 127-29.

55. Benton, 51-52, alludes to this circumstance.

56. Ernest W. McDonnell, *The Beguines and Beghards in Medieval Culture. With Special Emphasis on the Belgian Scene* (New York: Octagon, 1969), 271-72.

57. The role of suffering in the lives of the German medieval mystics is examined in Martina Wehrli-Johns, "Aktion und Kontemplation in der Mystik. Über Maria und Martha," Otto Langer, "We ist ein gut wort, we ist ein genadenrichez wort. Zur Spiritualität der Dominikanerinnen im Spätmittelalter," and Alois M. Haas, "Trage Leiden geduldiglich. Die Einstellung der deutschen Mystik zum Leiden," in *Lerne leiden. Leidensbewältigung in der Mystik,* ed. Wolfgang Böhme (Karlsruhe: Tron, 1985), 9-55.

58. Bynum devotes pp. 170-262 of *Jesus as Mother* to a discussion of the Helfta community and the writings of these four women.

59. Although Helfta was undoubtedly the spiritual focal point of thirteenth-century Germany, other monastic communities also served as centers of learning. With regard to medicine, the Cistercian convent of Zimmern deserves special mention. In "Zu den deutschen Bearbeitungen der *Secreta Secretorum* des Mittelalters," *Leuvense Bijdragen. Tijdschrift voor Moderne Filologie* 55 (1966): 44, Wolfgang Hirth asserts that the oldest complete translation of the pseudo-Aristotelian work into Middle High German was accomplished by Hiltgart von Hürnheim, who resided in

this community. See also Gundolf Keil, "Hildegard (Hiltgart) von Hürnheim," *Die deutsche Literatur des Mittelalters. Verfasserlexikon,* ed. Kurt Ruh, 2d ed., (Berlin: de Gruyter, 1983), vol. 4, 1-4.

60. *Revelationes Gertrudianae ac Mechtildianae,* vol, I: Sanctae Gertrudis Magnae, Virginis Ordinis Sancti Benedicti, Legatus Divinae Pietatis. Accedunt eiusdem Exercitia Spiritualia, ed. L. Paquelin (Poitiers and Paris: Oudin, 1875), 36; *Gertrude of Helfta: The Herald of Divine Love,* trans. and ed. Margaret Winkworth, Classics of Western Spirituality (Mahwah, N.J.: Paulist Press, 1993), 74.

61. *Revelationes Gertrudianae ac Mechtildianae,* 69; *Herald of Divine Love,* 102.

62. *Revelationes Gertrudianae ac Mechtildianae,* 119-20; *Herald of Divine Love,* 157.

63. In her introduction to Winkworth's translation, *Herald of Divine Love,* 37, Sister Maximilian Marnau draws attention to this aspect of asceticism: "The point is not an unhealthy desire to suffer for the sake of it, but rather a desire for conformity with Christ and a recognition that suffering can be an excellent instrument for bringing one's own will into harmony with God's and one's whole being into union with him." Langer, 29-32, also examines the two-fold meaning of *líden.*

64. *Mechthild von Magdeburg, 'Das fliessende Licht der Gottheit' nach der Einsiedler Handschrift in kritischem Vergleich mit der gesamten Überlieferung,* ed. Hans Neumann, vol. I, Text, besorgt von Gisela Vollmann-Profe (Munich: Artemis Verlag, 1990), 202. The translation is by Lucy Menzies, *The Revelations of Mechthild of Magdeburg (1210-1297) or The Flowing Light of the Godhead* (London, New York, and Toronto: Longmans, Green, and Co., 1953), 165; her verse translation follows the model of Gall Morel's 1868 edition of Mechthild's work, the Middle High German edition commonly cited before the publication of Neumann's two-volume work.

65. Neumann, 283-84; Menzies, 234.

66. Neumann, 285.

67. Neumann, 304; Menzies, 253-54.

68. The most commonly cited examples are Heinrich Seuse, who describes such practices in chapters 15-18 of his *Vita,* and his spiritual daughter, Elsbeth Stagel, who, in an attempt to follow the example of the desert fathers and of Seuse himself, imitates these practices, as the Dominican priest notes in chapter 35 of his life; see *Henry Suso. The Exemplar, with Two German Sermons,* trans. and ed. Frank Tobin, Classics of Western Spirituality (Mahwah, N.J.: Paulist Press, 1989), 87-97 and 139-41.

69. One such psychoanalytical study is that of Oskar Pfister, "Hysterie und Mystik bei Margaretha Ebner (1291-1351)," *Zentralblatt für Psychoanalyse. Medizinische Monatsschrift für Seelenkunde* 1 (1911): 468-85.

70. For example, see *Der Nonne von Engelthal Büchlein von der Genaden Uberlast,* ed. Karl Schröder (Tübingen: H. Laupp, 1871), 24, 28-30, and "Die Chronik der

Anna von Munzingen. Nach der ältesten Abschrift mit Einleitung und Beilagen," ed. Josef König, *Freiburger Diöcesan-Archiv* 13 (1880): 169, 15 and 34.

71. References to specific illnesses include: *wassersucht* "dropsy," Karl Bihlmeyer, "Mystisches Leben in dem Dominikanerinnenkloster Weiler bei Esslingen im 13. und 14. Jahrhundert," *Württembergische Vierteljahrshefte für Landesgeschichte* N.F. 25 (1916): 73, 6; *veltsiech* "leprosy," "Die Nonnen von St. Katarinental bei Dieszenhofen," ed. Anton Birlinger, *Alemannia* 15 (1887): 162, 41, and *Das Leben der Schwestern zu Töß beschrieben von Elsbet Stagel samt der Vorrede von Johannes Meier und dem Leben der Prinzessin Elisabet von Ungarn,* ed. Ferdinand Vetter, Deutsche Texte des Mittelalters, 6 (Berlin: Weidmann, 1906), 50, 25; and *ungewúrm* "worms," *Das Leben der Schwestern zu Töss,* 22,21.

72. In *Deutsche Mystikerbriefe des Mittelalters 1100-1550* (Munich: Georg Müller, 1931), 783, note 74, Wilhelm Oehl claims that Christina von Stommeln also sent spices to Petrus Dacus for the same purpose. The reference is found in Letter 4 by Christina (Oehl, 261): "Durch den Überbringer dieses Briefes schicke ich Euch einige Geschenke: ein Birett zum persönlichen Gebrauch für Euch und eine Glocke, und in dieser sind Gewürze drin für Euch zum Essen."

73. Philipp Strauch, *Margaretha Ebner und Heinrich von Nördlingen. Ein Beitrag zur Geschichte der deutschen Mystik* (1882; Amsterdam: Schippers, 1966), 171, 24-25, 194, 46, 248, 47, and 253, 71. Strauch's notes on pp. 324 and 358 offer additional commentary.

74. *Margaretha Ebner und Heinrich von Nördlingen,* 336.

75. *Margaretha Ebner und Heinrich von Nördlingen,* 228.

76. *Margaretha Ebner und Heinrich von Nördlingen,* 358; there is no critical edition of Ebner manuscript 90, from which Strauch quotes. Appended to his abridged version of her work, *Leben und Gesichte der Christina Ebnerin, Klosterfrau zu Engelthal* (Nürnberg: Recknagel, 1872), 48 and 50, Georg Wolfgang Karl Lochner includes a report from 1487 by the physician Hartmann Schedel, in which Schedel refers to this episode; Lochner also suggests possible sources for Schedel's assertion.

77. *Die Offenbarungen der Adelheid Langmann, Klosterfrau zu Engelthal,* ed. Philipp Strauch, Quellen und Forschungen zur Sprach- und Culturgeschichte der germanischen Völker, 26 (Strassburg: Trübner, 1878), 75, 22-76, 11.

78. *Die Offenbarungen der Adelheid Langmann, Klosterfrau zu Engelthal,* 79, 15-20.

79. *Das Leben der Schwestern zu Töss,* 42, 29.

80. *Das Leben der Schwestern zu Töss,* 66, 15-67, 6.

81. Bihlmeyer, "Mystisches Leben in dem Dominikanerinnenkloster Weiler bei Esslingen," 69, 14-15.

82. W. Schleussner, "Magdalena von Freiburg. Eine pseudomystische Erscheinung des späteren Mittelalters, 1407-1458," *Der Katholik* 35, 87 (1907): 215.

83. *Heinrich Seuse. Deutsche Schriften,* ed. Karl Bihlmeyer (Stuttgart 1907; rpt. Frankfurt: Minerva, 1961), 142, 29-30; *Henry Suso,* 167. Bihlmeyer notes this reference in "Mystisches Leben in dem Dominikanerinnenkloster Weiler bei Esslingen," 69, footnote 29.

84. The scant references in the chronicles to male spiritual guides supports this assertion. I have noted this circumstance in "'ich súndig wip mŭs schriben': Religious women and Literary Traditions," in *Women as Protagonists and Poets in the German Middle Ages. An Anthology of Feminist Approaches to the Study of Middle High German Literature,* ed. Albrecht Classen, Göppinger Arbeiten zur Germanistik 528 (Göppingen: Kümmerle, 1991), 163.

85. Ulrich Boner, *Der Edel Stein,* ed. George Friederich Benecke (Berlin: Realschul-Buchhandlung, 1816), 151-52, lines 87-116.

86. The sermon is recorded in Cgm. 450; the quotation here is from Johannes Bühler, *Klosterleben im Mittelalter,* ed. Georg A. Narciss (1923; Frankfurt/Main: Insel, 1989), 517.

87. References to such instances in German-speaking Europe of the fifteenth and sixteenth centuries are found in Karl Buxtorf-Falkeisen, *Basler Zauber-Prozesse aus dem 14. und 15. Jahrhundert* (Basel: Schweighauserische Verlags-Buchhandlung, 1868), XII; Carl Theodor Gemeiner, *Regensburgische Chronik* (Regensburg, 1821; Munich: C. H. Beck, 1971), vol. III, 208; and Joseph Hansen, *Quellen und Untersuchungen zur Geschichte des Hexenwahns und der Hexenverfolgung im Mittelalter* (Bonn, 1901; Hildesheim: Olms, 1963), 467, 527, and 561.

88. *Des Teufels Netz. Satirsich-didaktisches Gedicht aus der ersten Hälfte des fünfzehnten Jahrhunderts,* ed. Karl August Barack, Bibliothek des litterarischen Vereins in Stuttgart, 70 (Stuttgart, 1863; Amsterdam: Rodopi, 1968). The sections devoted to regular nuns make no reference to their role as caregivers or healers, but verses 5974-89 describe the charitable activities of the *beginan,* the Beguines or lay sisters, toward the sick. Verses 10297-479 portray the old women who engage in matchmaking and healing, often by means of magic.

# [ 2 ]

# BETWEEN MAGIC AND MEDICINE
## *Medieval Images of the Woman Healer*

NANCY P. NENNO

*In February of 1979,* a traveling exhibition opened at the ethno-graphic museum in Hamburg, Germany, bearing the simple title of *Hexen* [Witches].[1] The displays covered a variety of topics related to witchcraft, from historical accounts in Early Modern Europe to a reassessment of the traditional image of the witch. The visitor to the *Hexen* exhibition first encountered historical and linguistic analyses of the development of the name *witch,* from the Old Norse *hagazussa*[2] to the contemporary German word, *Hexe.* Having established an historical framework for considering the problem, the exhibition then branched into more speculative inquiries of witchcraft. One display advanced the theory that witches had belonged to an older cult of maternity and fecundity centered around the figure of Diana. Another used children's drawings of witches from the late twentieth century to reflect upon the popular folklore surrounding witches and their craft. But the entire exhibition was dominated by a massive reproduction of a painting by Michael Herr dating from around 1650. This terrifying image of a witches' sabbath was the visual and thematic center of the entire exhibition. It not only illustrated a particular seventeenth-century construction of the witch as demonic and bloodthirsty, but because this conception remains dominant today, it brought visitors to rethink their assumptions about witches.

The socio-cultural function of witches and their demonization formed a coherent subtext linking the exhibition's various displays. *Hexen* not only traced the traditional representations of the witch from the late Middle Ages through the late twentieth century, but specifically addressed the histories of the groups that had been demonized as practitioners of witchcraft. These

43

groups included the insane, Jews, midwives, and women healers. The last two groups—both composed of women involved in medical practices—proved to be the only ones whose marginalization seemed based at least in part upon their gender.[3]

Such displays illuminated one of the primary subtexts of the *Hexen* exhibition. The relationship between gender and power struggles was a primary motivation for the witch trials, the exhibition suggested. This interpretation was scarcely surprising in 1979, at the height of the German women's movement and the new interest in women's history. In the *Hexen* exhibition, witches were not merely the subjects of historical inquiry, but were icons of an increasingly politicized women's movement. Thus, the witch represented a focal point not only for re-evaluating the history of witches and the marginalization of particular social groups; she also seemed to provide a mirror of contemporary concerns about gender and power and the history of women in general. As an outsider, the witch served as a figure of identification for the German women's movement, which saw itself as presenting a radical alternative to a male-dominated society. And one of the targets within that patriarchal order was the institution of modern medicine.

The desire to read the past through the lens of contemporary concerns is, however, a dangerous one. Medieval scholar R. Howard Bloch has cautioned against this temptation—especially prevalent in medieval studies—to link the medieval period to the late twentieth century, to perceive and insist upon "a certain identity between the medieval period and our own."[4] Certainly our own interests and needs decide what will interest us in a medieval text. However, the danger remains that these same interests will erase all awareness of historical difference. Instead we might ask why particular narratives and characters draw our attention in the first place. Renaissance scholar Stephen Greenblatt has suggested that, in literary and visual texts such as Herr's painting, figures like that of the witch are filled with what he calls "social energy." "[We] are interested in such cultural expressions as witchcraft accusations, medical manuals, or clothing not as raw materials but as 'cooked'—complex symbolic and material articulations of the imaginative and ideological structures of the society that produced them."[5] Such characters seem to have a life beyond the bounds of the text or the image because they mean something within a larger cultural context. The difference between this kind of interpretation and that of the *Hexen* exhibition lies in how the knowledge of historical distance between then and now is incorporated into the interpretation itself.

*Hexen* presented a trans-historical look at witches that suited the political agenda of its authors. It foregrounded the way in which female medical practitioners were marginalized in the sixteenth and seventeenth centuries because they were women. But it neglected to examine the history of medicine in and of itself, and its relationship to magic. The exhibition also neglected to sustain an historical awareness of the term witch and how it has shifted over the past six centuries in different political and institutional contexts. In regard to the figure of the woman healer, such attention to historical minutiae is particularly important. The relegation of the woman who practiced medicine to the position of outsider evolved over time, and was influenced by the development of the European institution of medicine. To understand why she came to be regarded as an outsider by this medical profession requires an examination not only of that institution, but also of the concept of magic in relation to that medicine, and the role gender played in the definition of these terms.

In this essay, I will examine the figure of the woman healer in two medieval German courtly epics from the early thirteenth century: Hartmann von Aue's *Êrec* and Gottfried von Strassburg's *Tristan,* both of which have powerful women healers at their centers. I will suggest that both epics participate in a larger discussion about the status of the woman who practices healing prior to the Inquisitions of the fourteenth and fifteenth centuries. By examining not only her construction in these texts, but also medieval literary traditions and the historical situation of magic vis-à-vis medicine, I will question why the woman healer seemed so problematic both within these texts and within the larger cultural context.

As the *Hexen* exhibition suggested, women healers were merely one of several groups demonized at the time of the Inquisitions. The question is why? What was at stake? What kinds of conflicts existed in the admittedly heterogeneous culture of thirteenth-century Europe that the woman healer, her skills and practices produced anxiety? Traditionally, the woman healer was the primary medical caretaker of the poor and the unimportant who, unlike the emperors, kings, and popes, could not afford to pay the graduates of medical schools like Salerno or Montpellier. The medicine that dominated these medical schools was intellectual, based upon newly-translated texts of Arab and Greek medical theory. In contrast, the medicine practiced by laywomen was empirical, based in a hands-on knowledge of plants and herbs. The herbal preparations concocted and used by these *Kräuterfrauen* (women versed in the

45

use of herbs) often seemed to be both magical and medicinal, since there was no popular understanding of the chemistry that made the drugs effective.[6] Certainly the mystery surrounding the origins and workings of her medicines contributed to the ambivalence with which the woman healer was often seen. While successful treatments brought her adulation, failure could turn this ambivalence into outright distrust, often resulting in her being denounced as a witch.[7]

While the ambivalent attitude towards the woman healer was not new, the politicization of both her existence and her craft expanded during the High Middle Ages (ca. the twelfth and thirteenth centuries). Prior to this period, healing practices had been evaluated according to the intent of the practitioner. However, by the thirteenth century, the source of these powers became of primary importance, and with this shift in emphasis, the nature of the individual woman healer herself was called into question. At a time when nascent medical institutions were attempting to establish an independent realm of authority, when Church authorities sought to eliminate, absorb, or demonize pre-Christian traditions, and states began to regulate medical practices, the woman healer became a target for anxieties about autonomous medical practice, pagan traditions, and demonic magic.

The lack of a strict division between magic and medicine in the medieval period is indicated in the very names given to the woman healer, many of which she shared with the magical fays of Celtic literature: *saga,* wise woman, and *belladonna.*[8] Practitioners of the healing arts, the fays were usually seen as man's helpmates, aiding him in his difficult life. Although generally portrayed as benevolent, they were also believed capable of malicious intent and evil magic.[9] Perhaps the most famous example of this dual personality is the Welsh water deity who appears as both the beautiful and benevolent Morgain and the evil, ugly hag, Morrigan.[10]

It has been suggested that medieval conceptions of magic, medicine, and science were not separate fields of knowledge, so that often the borders among them became blurred and uncertain.[11] The dynamic of this model is especially jarring to late twentieth-century readers, accustomed to viewing medicine as discrete from magic, as "scientific," rather than "magical" practice. And yet precisely this lack of distinction during the High Middle Ages meant that magical and medical practices often appeared to overlap—particularly when healers, both men and women, were not licensed by the state and also employed treatments and remedies based upon superstition.

46

That superstition often accompanied herbal medicine is borne out in compendia of folk medicines from this period. Numerous remedies called for the use of plants and herbs, supplemented by pious (Christian) invocations and superstitious (pre-Christian) practices.[12] One collection of German folk medicine from the late eleventh or early twelfth centuries, the *Mülinen Rotulus,* illustrates the way in which Christian belief, sympathetic medicine, and folk superstitions were combined in medieval medical practice. In one example, the treatment for nosebleed [*ad sanguinem de naribus*] calls for both an incantation and the invocation of Christ's healing powers.[13]

Written records of medieval folk medicine are not the only indication of the interrelation of the fields of science, medicine, faith, superstition[14] and magic in the Middle Ages. An examination of literary texts of the same period in which one of the main characters is a woman who heals leads to similar conclusions. The two literary texts that I have chosen as examples also suggest how conceptions of magic and medicine overlapped in this period. The figures of Queen Îsôt in Gottfried's *Tristan* and Feimurgan in Hartmann's *Êrec* already indicate how, by the early thirteenth century, the field of medicine was beginning to attempt to define itself as a discrete field, one in which women should have no part. The power negotiations which accompanied this self-definition are evident in the descriptions and actions of the woman healer in these literary texts. Both Gottfried von Strassburg and Hartmann von Aue maintain a narrative fidelity to their sources that was common in the tradition of medieval literature. But their adaptations, rewritings, and additions already suggest ways in which the cultural context cast the woman healer as suspect. Similar to the way in which the *Hexen* exhibition used the rhetoric of the women's movement to revamp the centuries-old tradition of the witch, Gottfried's and Hartmann's participation in the rewriting of Celtic lore betrays a cultural and political agenda. As Michael Batts has suggested, such changes in the constructions of the characters from their Celtic source-texts are significant because they reflect the concerns and desires of the contemporary audience.[15]

Canonical texts of Middle High German literature, the courtly epics *Êrec* and *Tristan* were written within twenty-five years of each other, around the turn of the thirteenth century. Both Feimurgan in *Êrec* (ca. 1180/1185) and Queen Îsôt in *Tristan* (ca. 1210) originated in Celtic literature and tradition, although the character of Feimurgan more strongly resembles the mythological figure of the fay than does Queen Îsôt.[16] From the beginning of *Êrec,* Feimurgan appears not quite human, something different, a marginal figure in the world of mortals. Like the Celtic fay, whose name she bears in Hartmann's source text—Chrétien de Troyes' Arthurian epic, *Érec et Énite* (ca. 1165/1170), in which she is called Morgain la Fée—Feimurgan possesses magical abilities. These include not only an extensive knowledge of the healing properties of plants and herbs, but also shape-shifting and the ability to live underwater. Feimurgan does not appear as an active participant in the story of *Érec;* nonetheless, it is her healing bandage that saves the life of the wounded hero, thus ensuring the continuation of the story. The *deus ex machina* appearance of this bandage merely serves to underscore the magical quality of Feimurgan.

Similarly, the character of Queen Îsôt in Gottfried von Strassburg's courtly epic *Tristan* is also drawn from Celtic legend.[17] She, her daughter Îsôt, and the maid, Brangæne, form a triad of women in the story that recalls the *Matronæ* or *matres* in Irish and Welsh legend.[18] Through her knowledge of herbs, the queen possesses the dual ability to heal and to harm, powers strongly linked to magical practices. Like Feimurgan's, her powers also ensure the life of the story, as she first heals the hero's wounds, and then prepares the love potion which initiates the tragic love story of Tristan and her daughter, Îsôt.

Queen Îsôt's powers bear a stronger resemblance to those of the more traditional woman healer in the Middle Ages than do those of Feimurgan.[19] The queen has extensive knowledge of herbs and plants, such as theriac, which can both harm and heal, and in *Tristan* she uses her knowledge to both ends. She creates the poison on the tip of her brother Morôlt's sword, with which he mortally wounds Tristan, and she is said to be the only person capable of healing this wound.

> ich eine enwende ez danne,
> von wîbe noch von manne
> sone wîrdest dû nie mêr gesunt:
> du bist mit einem swerte wunt,
> daz toedec unde gelüppet ist.
> árzât noch arzâtes list
> ernert dich niemer dirre nôt,
> ez entúo mîn swester eine, Îsôt,
> diu künegîn von Îrlande:
> diu erkénnet maneger hande
> wurze und allér krûte kraft

und arzâtlîche meisterschaft;
díu kan eine disen list
und anders niemen, der der ist.
diu ennér dich, dû bist ungenesen.
wil dû mir noch gevolgic wesen
und mir des zinses jehende sîn,
mîn swéstér, diu künegîn,
diu muoz dich selbe heilen [*Tristan,* ll. 6943-6961][20]
[Unless I alone manage it,
Neither woman nor man,
You will never be cured:
you have been wounded by a sword
that is deadly and poisoned.
neither doctor nor a doctor's skill
will save you from this,
only my sister, Îsôt,
the queen of Ireland:
she knows many kinds of
roots and the powers of every herb
and medical knowledge;
only she is capable of this skill
and no one else.
If she does not heal you, you are incurable.
If you will serve me
and give me the tribute [you carry]
then my sister, the queen,
will heal you herself]

At this point in the story, the Queen has appeared only *in absentia,* that is, only in name and deed. The creator of the poison on Morôlt's sword, she appears to practice *maleficia,* magic with evil intent. However, Morôlt's boasting of her skills and her knowledge of plants also suggest her skill as a healer. Skill with herbs can thus be construed as either good or evil, as beneficial or malicious, depending upon the intention of the practitioner. However, Queen Îsôt seems to belong more to the sphere of medicine than magic; her skills, neither otherworldly nor intrinsically evil, are identified in line 6954 as "*arzâtlîche-meisterschaft*" [medical knowledge]. The idea that her powers are also magical nevertheless resurfaces when Morôlt declares that Îsôt alone can cure Tristan, for her abilities and knowledge far exceed even those of the *arzâte,* or doctors.

The *minnetrank* [love potion] that she creates further supports this hint of magic. Originally intended to unite her daughter and Tristan's uncle, King Marc, the Queen's potion is mistakenly drunk by Tristan and Îsôt. Love magic was one of the many forms of magic which underwent demonization during the fourteenth and fifteenth centuries.[21] And Queen Îsôt's skill at preparing such a potion, the effects of which prove irreversible and ultimately binding, suggests an acquaintance with not only the medicinal, but also the magical, qualities of plants. The Queen's powers do however appear to be limited, for, ironically, she is unable to control the specificity of the *minnetrank.* Instead of binding Marc and Îsôt, as intended, it links Tristan and Îsôt in their tragic destiny. Thus it would appear that the Queen's magical abilities lie exclusively in her knowledge of the magical properties of herbs, and not in the wider ability to guide the destiny of her preparations. Her magic is circumscribed, limited, and finite, for she is neither omniscient nor all-powerful. Any magical power she has comes from her knowledge and skill as a healer. Perhaps this limitation prevents her from being cast as negatively as Feimurgan and her powers are in *Êrec.*

The narrator of *Êrec* accords Feimurgan powers beyond those of medical skill and herbal knowledge, powers which ultimately mark her predominantly as a magical figure. The author of *Êrec,* Hartmann von Aue, remains faithful to the story he inherited from Chrétien; however, he does embellish the single passage devoted to Feimurgan. In Chrétien's text, the scene that describes the healing bandage or salve [*antret*] created by Morgain la Fée runs a mere thirteen lines; Harmann devotes almost one hundred to her. This expansion is significant as the additional text shifts the emphasis from the healing bandage (in Chrétien's *Êrec et Énite*) to the character of the elusive Feimurgan.[22]

Many of the changes made by Hartmann reflect the shifting relationship between magic and medicine in the late twelfth century. Although he retains the fact that Feimurgan is King Artus' sister, Hartmann is credited with being the first author to cast her as a mortal woman, rather than an immortal.[23] While the narrator of *Êrec* mourns the knowledge and ability that died with her, he also voices a distinct ambivalence about those abilities. Her powers, which are various and extend beyond the capacities of most mortals, seem to fascinate the author of *Êrec,* which perhaps explains why he feels compelled to name the source of these powers.

si lebete ir vil werde:
in lufte als ûf der erde
mohte si ze ruowe sweben,
ûf dem wâge und drunder leben.
ouch was ir daz untiure,
si wonte in dem viure
als sanfte als ûf dem touwe.
diz kunde diu vrouwe.
und sô si des gern began,
sô machete si den man
ze vogele oder ze tiere.
dar nâch gap si im schiere
wider sîne geschaft:
si kunde eht zoubers die kraft.
si lebete vaste wider gotte,
wan ez warte ir gebote
daz gevügel zuo dem wilde
an walde und an gevilde,
und daz mich daz meiste
dunket, die übelen geiste,
die dâ tiuvel sint genant,
die wâren alle under ir hant.
si mohte wunder machen,
wan ir muosten die trachen
von den lüften bringen
stiure zuo ir dingen,
die vische von dem wâge.
ouch hâte si mâge
tiefe in der helle:
der tiuvel was ir geselle. [*Êrec,* 5177-5205][24]
[She lived in great splendor
in the air as on the earth
she could remain quietly suspended,
could live above and below water.
It was also a simple thing for her
to live in fire
as sweetly as on the dew.
This lady could do all these things.

51

When she desired,
she turned a human
into a bird or an animal.
Afterwards she returned to him
his own form.
She was truly powerful in magic.
She lived against God's command,
for to her
birds and beasts were obedient
in forest and field
and what I think the most powerful:
the evil spirits
that one calls devils
were all under her power.
She could perform miracles,
for the dragons
from the air
had to give her aid in her desires
as well as the fish in the water.
Beyond this she had relatives
deep in hell:
the Devil was her companion.]

Feimurgan clearly intrigues the narrator both as a source of healing and as an entity linked to the devil. This passage has a much faster pace than the rest of the text; like its subject, it pulses with energy and power. The enjambed lines communicate a sense of excitement and curiosity, but the narrator's litany of Feimurgan's powers comes to a dead halt when he names the devil as her accomplice. Feimurgan is inexplicable and mysterious, and the narrator of *Êrec* can explain her powers only in terms of demonic aid. In contrast to Queen Îsôt, the evaluation of whose skill can be reduced to the question of intent, what makes Feimurgan herself questionable is the *source* of her powers. As a result, her status as a healer acquires an additional dimension, namely a moral one. Although she too possesses great medical skill, her relationship with the devil negatively influences how her skills are evaluated. Ironically, the narrator does not shy away from accepting the product of this power, despite his rejection of its source.

The interpretation of these women healers thus rests largely upon questions involving the source of power. Whereas demonically-assisted Feimurgan is cast in a negative light, Queen Îsôt, whose powers stem from medicinal knowledge available to many laypeople, remains a predominantly positive figure. Of course, in a text that is not especially concerned with the transmission of Christian ethics and in which adulterers are the sympathetic protagonists, it is scarcely surprising that mild forms of magic are not fiercely condemned. An investigation of the words used to describe each of these characters and their activities further calls attention to a fundamental distinction between the skills of the queen and those of Feimurgan, a distinction that hinges on the question of the source of these powers. The words associated with Feimurgan include *"kraft"* [power], *"arzât"* [doctor], *"wunder"* [miracle], *"list"* [skill], *"sinn"* [knowledge], and *"gewalt"* [power, violence]. And the word around which all the others rotate is *"zouber"* [magic]: *"zouberlist"* [magical skill], *"zoubers die kraft"* [magical powers], *"zouberlich gewalt"* [violent magical power], *"von zouberlichem sinne/nie bezzer meisterinne"* [no greater master of magical knowledge]. In contrast, the words *"wise"* [wise], *"gelerte"* [knowledgeable], *"list"* [skill], *"witze"* [knowledge], *"meisterschaft"* [consummate mastery], and *"wiste"* [wisdom] describe Queen Îsôt. Comparing only these words illustrates how the description of Feimurgan relies upon concepts of power as force, whereas the Queen's power resides in her knowledge.

The different valence accorded each figure resides not merely in the description of the source of her powers; indeed, the structure of the text itself suggests the degree of danger posed by each. Although Queen Îsôt is accorded both beneficial and malicious powers, she is clearly the more sympathetic of the two figures, perhaps precisely because her power is limited to that of a mortal being. The narrator does not attempt to confine Queen Îsôt to a small passage of *Tristan;* indeed, the queen appears several times throughout the text of *Tristan.* In contrast Feimurgan appears in *Êrec* in name only. The mysterious and uncontrollable aspect of Feimurgan's powers makes her appear to be the greater threat; and perhaps this explains, in part, why Hartmann's epic confines her to a specific passage, wherein she can be controlled and limited.

Taking a step back from these two courtly epics, we need to ask what such intensely detailed analyses of these figures and their semantic fields tell us about the way the woman healer was perceived and constructed within the larger context of medieval German culture. What do the differences and similarities between Feimurgan and Queen Îsôt tell us about the relationship of magic and medicine? And what other larger social and political issues influenced the way in which these figures were constructed?

One of the crucial issues is, of course, the definition of magic, its source and its meaning. Although it may be clichéd to dismiss Hartmann as a strict adherent to the Christian world view, it does help to understand his radical demonization of Feimurgan. The progressive Christianization of the Celtic sources in medieval European texts suggests the presence of a larger undercurrent, namely that which French scholar Laurence Harf-Lancner has termed the "satanization" of the ancient pagan deities.[25]

Starting in the mid-tenth century, the Catholic Church began a concerted effort to eradicate heathen beliefs and practices, first by attempting to discredit them, then by a process of appropriating and altering these traditions. In 1048, the *Canon episcopi* initiated this first attack, that of the elimination of pre-Christian systems of belief, by rejecting the belief in magic as "unChristian." Specifically directed against the cult of Diana, it claimed that such beliefs had been made obsolete by Christianity. In a similar manner, the *Corrector* (1008-12) by Burchard of Worms directed its attack against the worship of the Holda, a north German fertility goddess.[26]

However, by the eleventh and twelfth centuries, the Church's position on magic had shifted perceptibly. Instead of merely branding non-Christian cults as heathen or, as in the case of the Catharists, even heretical, the Church proceeded to demonize the practice of, and belief in, magic by explicitly linking it to the concept of the Christian devil. In other words, magic became incorporated into a Christian set of beliefs and then was interpreted within this framework. The appropriation of pagan figures into a Christian world view and their subsequent re-evaluation as overtly negative is evident in the figure of Feimurgan. The tension between the magical fay of pagan legend and its demonization is almost palpable.

A similar process of demonization was occurring within the field of medical practice at the same time. While not directly addressing this issue, the texts of both *Êrec* and *Tristan* suggest just how problematic the woman healer was becoming in the cultural context of medieval Germany. This is particularly evident when both Feimurgan and Queen Îsôt have attributed to them skills said to exceed those of the doctors. In *Êrec,* it appears at the end of the passage devoted to Feimurgan:

Jâ waene man iender vunde
swie sêre man wolde ersuochen
die kraft ûz arzâtbuochen,
sô krefteclîche liste
di si wider Kriste
uopte sô des gerte ir muot.
Daz selbe phlaster machete si guot
von alem ir sinne
dâ mite diu küneginne
Êreche die wunden bant. *Êrec,* ll. 5232-46]
[For I truly believe, one could not find
as much as one sought
in medical books,
such effective skills
as those she performed against Christ's Word
when she so desired.
That same bandage she herself had
made using all her powers,
with which the Queen
bound up Êrec's wounds.]

Although a relatively short passage in a long text, a mere one or two lines out of thousands, this tiny moment opens a window onto the larger cultural discussion of the position in which the medieval woman healer found herself. As scholars like Greenblatt have illustrated, it is precisely such passages, which seem to be merely asides, that can open upon a whole new way of seeing a character or a text. These few lines about Feimurgan's abilities reveal just such a tension: namely, that between the role and skill of traditional healers and those of the graduates of the new, state-sanctioned medical schools. In both epics, the woman healer is invested with abilities that exceed those of the doctors, and this excess retains a magical, and in Feimurgan's case, a demonic, quality. Thus, a look at the political machinations underlying this process of demonization may help to explain why it is present as a subtext in these literary fictions.

In 1159, about twenty years before Hartmann von Aue wrote *Êrec,* the Church writer John of Salisbury published two of his most important works, the *Polycraticus* and the *Metalogican*. The first three books of the *Polycraticus*, a political and philosophical guide for rulers, discusses the "frivolities of court life"—including magic. Following this discussion, John of Salisbury addresses the Church's position vis-à-vis magic: "Long ago, the Christian Fathers condemned those who practiced the more demoralizing forms of legerdemain, the art of magic, and astrology because they realized that all these arts, or rather artifices, derive from unholy commerce between men and demons."[27] In subsequent chapters, the author continues to identify different forms of magical arts, such as enchantment, wizardry, and fortune-telling. Ultimately, however, his point remains that magic, insofar as it originates in demonic aid, must be seen to be illusory and deceptive. This is an interpretation that endured for centuries and echoes throughout the pages of *the* treatise on witchcraft, the *Malleus maleficarum* [The Witches' Hammer]. In the *Polycraticus*, John of Salisbury distinguishes sharply between magic and reason or logic by using a complex wordplay: *ma'thesis* (mathematics) versus *mathe'sis* (astrology).[28] This play on words suggests, in fact, that despite the contemporary distinction made between scientific and divinatory astrology, the difference between science and magic remained unclear. This intimation is further supported by the way the author employs the figure of Mercury in his text.

The first mention of Mercury, the god of illusion, appears in book I of the *Polycraticus*, regarding the invention of the term "*praestigium*," where he is named its source: "The word *praestigium* is said to have been invented by Mercury for the reason that he blinds the eyes. He was the most adept of magicians and could make invisible whatever he desired, or, as it appears, change it into other forms."[29] The second time Mercury appears is in relation to physicians. John of Salisbury criticizes their attention to natural phenomena and their lack of attention to God: "As I listen to them, it seems to me they have the power to raise the dead. They are considered not inferior to Aesculapius or Mercury."[30]

Granted, John of Salisbury's style and tone maintain an ironic edge throughout the text, which diffuses some of the overall seriousness of his argument. Nevertheless, it seems important that the figure of Mercury as magician is connected to practitioners both of magic and of medicine. In each instance, Mercury functions as a figure of criticism, linking magicians and physicians, and condemning them alike as practitioners of illusion. In this manner, a subtle similarity and distant kinship is established between the two groups, permitting the Church to level criticism at once against the practice of magic and the medical profession.

The Church's position relative to medicine was an important one in the Middle Ages, not only because of Rome's power in all realms of life, but also because of its involvement in the institutionalization of the medical school. The Church's relationship to medicine remains a much-debated topic in scholarly circles. Some historians, like Benjamin Lee Gordon, take the position that the Church actively campaigned against medical practice, favoring instead "spiritual cures." Others respond by citing texts and authors, including St. Augustine, that evaluate the practice of medicine positively.[31] But the Church had long been associated with medical care, from the example of physician-turned-gospel-writer, St. Luke, to Benedict of Nursia, who established the first cloister in 525 at Monte Cassino.[32] One of the most important mystics of the Middle Ages and the abbess of her own monastery, Hildegard von Bingen, wrote extensive medical treatises, including *Causæ et curæ* and her nine-volume work *Physica,* written between 1151 and 1158.[33]

However, this tradition officially ended in 1131, when the Council of Rheims forbade the clergy to practice medicine. Not surprisingly, this interdiction closely followed upon the establishment of the first Christian medical schools. The collaboration of the Church leadership with the new medical institutions suggests not only the attempt to consolidate the power of the new medical establishment and its ability to regulate the practice of medicine. It also indicates a desire to clarify the distinctions between magical and medical practices.

A brief glance at the influence and growth of the medical schools during the High Middle Ages helps us to clarify why the woman healer became a target of attack in medieval texts like *Érec* and *Tristan.* The medical school at Salerno, one of the few to admit women students, including the legendary Mæstra Trotula, is first mentioned in 924 by a monk named Richer. Although numerous texts mention these women, including the *Circa instans* and the *Practica,* which praised their skill and effectiveness, the woman healer remains a marginal and questionable figure. In his *Commentaries on the Tables of Master Salernus,* Bernard the Provincial describes these women's cures as mixing scientific and superstitious practices[34]—a combination that bears a remarkable similarity to the description of many traditional treatments practiced by laywomen. Despite her scientific training, the woman physician continued to occupy an ambivalent position because women were linked to magic and superstition, and thus to skills and practices outside of the scientific practice of medicine.

By the twelfth century—a time when medical works by Avicenna, the Arab schools, and Greek texts by Galen and Hippocrates were entering western Europe through the schools in Spain and Italy—the state had also begun its intervention into the regulation of medical practice. In 1134, Roger II of Sicily, who maintained strong contacts with Arab doctors, promulgated a series of laws to govern the medical sphere which required those who practiced healing arts first to obtain the state's permission. Frederick II extended this control to include the study of medicine. The set of laws drawn up under his dictate required physicians to attend a five-year course of studies, followed by a year-long apprenticeship before being granted a license. In addition, the preparation and sale of drugs was to be regulated, and the role of the apothecary to be more carefully monitored.[35] The Church hierarchy supported and actively participated in this institutionalization of medical practice. On August 17, 1220, Cardinal Conrad d'Hurach, bishop of Porta and Santa Rufina, and legate of Pope Honorious III, promulgated the statutes founding the school at Montpellier. In 1289, the faculties at the school were united and Philip the Fair granted Montpellier the status of university, an action supported by Pope Nicholas III in a papal bull.[36]

The intrusion of the state into the sphere of medical practice may indeed have come at the behest of the medical schools themselves. The nascent institutions sensed that the traditional *Kräuterfrauen* were rivals, and so sought to eliminate this competition by enlisting the aid of the state.[37] In addition, most members of the ruling classes at this time maintained personal physicians from schools like Salerno and Montpellier; this suggests the complicity between the political power of the state and the new medical institutions, which sought to establish their own sphere of influence.

But there was a further component in the demonization of the woman healer that did not affect the male lay healer, namely the question of her gender. What was the relationship between gender identification and the demonization of the woman healer? How decisive is it that the healers in our literary texts are women, that it was primarily women who became cast as witches in Europe during the Early Modern period?

Almost three centuries after Hartmann and Gottfried wrote their epics, two Dominican monks in Germany, Heinrich Institorus and Jakob Sprenger, wrote the *Malleus maleficarum* (1487). In their diatribe against witchcraft— including medical activities that had become associated with magic—the two link women to magical practice because of their gender-specific weaknesses:

58

woman's lack of steadfast faith and her intrinsically superstitious nature, both of which automatically render her susceptible to temptation by the devil. In this view, a predilection for demonic magic became a biological, indeed a genetic, trait.

However, Sigrid Brauner has suggested that the construction of the witch as female should be read as expressing the conflict between pre-Christian culture and the medieval Church. In her dissertation, Brauner deals extensively with the image of the witch in Early New High German literature between 1486 and 1560. She concisely formulates what she sees as the function of the female body in this period: namely, as both a site of anxiety and a screen for the projection of these anxieties. "During this period, since she is identified with the ambiguous powers of nature, woman, as nature's representative, becomes a field of projection for all problematic areas emerging in the process of civilization and capitalization. . . . For the new sciences in particular, woman and the female body represent chaotic nature's resistance to scientific inquiry and technical domination."[38] Brauner's work may go a long way toward explaining why women became a focus of the witch hunts in this period. Like nature itself, woman appears mysterious, opaque, impervious to scientific inquiry, and yet also something to be tamed and domesticated.

This interpretation might then be extended to include the woman healer and clarify how she operated within medieval culture. A solitary figure for the most part, she did not have any institutional affiliations, and thus her practices remained unregulated. It was precisely this autonomy that caused so much anxiety on the part of the Church, the state, and the new medical institutions. The activity of women healers conflicted with medical practitioners' desires to consolidate and exercise their institutional power over this field of knowledge at a time when the Church began to campaign against pagan magical practices. The position of the woman healer appeared to threaten a wide range of political powers and spheres of influence.

The ambivalent position of the woman healer in the literary texts of *Êrec* and *Tristan* thus becomes more than simply a narrative device. Rather, it suggests how the figures of Feimurgan and Queen Îsôt register the reverberations caused by the discussion about the relationship between magic and medicine within the larger cultural context. The ambiguity that characterizes their healing practices suggests how conflicts around magic and medicine, women and autonomous medical practice, were in the process of being negotiated during the early thirteenth century. And further, they indicate in retrospect how this negotiation would lead to the demonization of the woman healer as a witch over the next few centuries.


NOTES

1. Thomas Hausschild, Heidi Staschen, and Regina Trotschke, *Hexen. Katalog zur Wanderausstellung "Hexen" aus dem Hamburgischen Museum für Völkerkunde* (Zierling: Verlag Clemens, 1986).

2. The term *Hexe* derives from the Old High German word *hagazussa,* which designated a night spirit, cannibal, or sorceress. In Nordic legend, the *hagazussa* "rides the fence that separates the world from the space of the gods." See Sigrid Maria Brauner, "Frightened Shrews and Fearless Wives: The Concept of the Witch in Early Modern German Texts (1487-1560)," (Ph.D. diss., Univ. of California at Berkeley, 1989), 393, and Edgar Poleme, "Althochdeutsch *hag<a>zussa 'Hexe',*" in *Althochdeutsch,* ed. Rolf Bergman and Heinrich Tiefenbach, vol. 2 (Heidelberg: C. Winter, 1987) 1107-12.

3. For further reading on the connections between midwifery and witchcraft, see Thomas Forbes, "Midwifery and Witchcraft," *Journal of the History of Medicine and Allied Sciences* 17 (1962): 417-39; Monica Green, "Women's Medical Practice and Health Care in Medieval Europe," *Signs* 2 (1989): 434-73; and Gundolf Kiel, "Die Frau als Ärztin und Patientin in der medizinischen Fachprosa des deutschen Mittelalters," in *Frau und spätmittelalterlicher Alltag,* Internationaler Kongress Krems an der Donau, Sitzungsberichte der Österreichischen Akademie der Wissenschaften, Philosophisch-Historische Klasse, no. 473, Veröffentlichungen des Instituts für Mittelalterliche Realienkunde Österreichs, no. 9 (Vienna: Verlag der Österreichischen Akademie der Wissenschaften, 1986), 157-211.

4. R. Howard Bloch, "The Once and Future Middle Ages," *Modern Language Quarterly* 54.1 (Mar. 1993): 69.

5. Stephen J. Greenblatt, "Resonance and Wonder," in *Learning to Curse: Essays in Early Modern Culture* (New York and London: Routledge, 1990), 169.

6. S. Sabatini, "Women, Medicine and Life in the Middle Ages (500-1500 A.D.)," *American Journal of Nephrology* 14.4-6 (1994): 391-98.

7. Jules Michelet, *Die Hexe* (Leipzig, 1861) cited in Hausschild, Staschen, and Trotschke, *Hexen,* 22.

8. Ibid.

9. *Handwörterbuch des deutschen Aberglaubens,* ed. Hanns Bächtold-Stäubli and E. Hoffmann-Krayer (Berlin 1927-46), s.v. "Fee."

10. Roger S[herman] Loomis, *Wales and the Arthurian Legend* (Cardiff: Univ. of Wales Press, 1956), 123.

11. Jeffrey Burton Russell, *Witchcraft in the Middle Ages* (Ithaca, N.Y.: Cornell Univ. Press, 1972), 4.

12. This distinction between piety and superstition, Christian and pre-Christian pagan practice is in and of itself a nebulous region, since Christian systems of belief might be included in the category of superstition. See Marie-Thérèse D'Alverny, "Survivance de la magie antique," in *Antike und Orient im Mittelalter,* ed. Paul Wilpert (Berlin: de Gruyter, 1962), 150.

13. Cited in Lucille B. Pinto, "Medical Science and Superstition: A Report on a Unique Medical Scroll of the Eleventh-Twelfth Century," *Manuscripta* 17.1 (Mar. 1973): 13.

14. By superstition, I mean those folk beliefs that fall neither entirely within the realm of religious faith, nor the strictly formulaic realm of magic.

15. Michael Batts, "National Perspectives on Originality and Translation," in *Chrétien de Troyes and the German Middle Ages: Papers from an International Symposium,* ed. Martin H. Jones and Roy Wisbey, Arthurian Studies, no. 26, Publications of the Institute of Germanic Studies, no. 53 (Cambridge: D. S. Brewer, 1993), 9.

16. "Here, then, is the explanation of Morgain's multiple personality, her infinite variety. She has acquired not only attributes and activities of Macha, the Morrigan and Matrona, but also the mythic heritage of other Celtic deities. She is a female pantheon in miniature." In Roger S. Loomis, "Morgain la Fée and the Celtic Goddesses," *Speculum* 20 (1945): 183-203. See also Rachel Bromwich, ed. and trans., *Troiedd Ynys Pryden. The Welsh Triads* (Cardiff: Univ. of Wales Press, 1961).

17. Scholarship which has been conducted on the Celtic sources for *Tristan* and *Érec* include: Rachel Bromwich, "Some Remarks about the Celtic Sources of 'Tristan,'" *The Transactions of the Honourable Society of Cymmrodorion 1953,* 32-60, and Jean Frappier, "Chrétien de Troyes," in *Arthurian Literature in the Middle Ages: A Collaborative History,* ed. Roger Sherman Loomis (Oxford: At the Clarendon, 1967), 44-57. In addition, the figure of Brangæne represents a secondary connection between Gottfried's *Tristan* and the Celtic legends. Rachel Bromwich has associated the name of Branweg verch Lyr in the Second Branch of the *Mabinogion* with Brengvein in the *Tristan* of Thomas of Brittany, whom Gottfried followed closely in his writing of the Tristan story. The Brangæne of *Tristan* also possesses a knowledge of herbs, and in Thomas' text, Brengvein creates a magic pillow which causes Caerdin to fall asleep. Helaine Newstead has explored the connections between this magic pillow, the Welsh "Y storia Trystan," and the Welsh and Breton traditions of the fays in her article "Kaherdin and the Enchanted Pillow: An Episode in the Tristan Legend," *Publications of the Modern Language Association* 30 (1950): 290-312.

18. This triadic constellation seems to have functioned as a mnemonic device for the oral recounting of the legend. Cynthia B. Caples, "Brangæne and Isold in Gottfried von Strassburg's *Tristan,*" *Colloquium Germanica* 9 (1975-76): 167-76.

19. Muriel Joy Hughes, *Women Healers in Medieval Life and Literature* (New York: King's Crown, 1943).

20. Gottfried von Strassburg, *Tristan,* ed. Peter Ganz, 2 vols., Deutsche Klassiker des Mittelalters, no. 4 (Wiesbaden: F.S. Brockhaus, 1978). Hereafter, all line references to Gottfried's *Tristan* will be from this edition. All translations are my own.

21. Richard Kieckhefer, *European Witch Trials: Their Foundations in Popular and Learned Culture, 1300-1500* (London: Routledge and Kegan Paul, 1976), 48.

22. Hendricus Sparnaay suggests that many of these additional characteristics originate in descriptions of Morgain la Fée in earlier texts, including Geoffrey of Monmouth's *Vita Merlini,* and that her name changes reflect the variations in her attributes. Hendricus Sparnaay, "Hartmann von Aue and His Successors," in *Arthurian Literature in the Middle Ages: A Collaborative History,* ed. Roger Sherman Loomis (Oxford: At the Clarendon, 1967), 430-32. Other texts that deal with these name changes include: Hendricus Sparnaay, "Fâmûrgân," *Neophilogus* 16 (1930-31): 255-61; C. Minis, "Fâmûrgân. *Êrec* 5156," *Neophilogus* 30 (1946): 65-68; Margaret Jennings, "'Heavens Defend Me from that Welsh Fairy.' The Metamorphosis of Morgain la Fée in the Romances," in *Court and Poet: Selected Proceedings of the Third Congress of the International Courtly Literature Society, Liverpool 1980,* ed. Glyn S. Burgess, Classical and Medieval Texts, Papers, and Monographs, no. 5 (Liverpool: Francis Cairns, 1980), 197-205.

23. Lucy Allen Paton, *Studies in the Fairy Mythology of Arthurian Romance,* Bibliography and Reference Series, no. 18, Essays in Literature and Criticism, no. 88 (1903; reprint, New York: Burt Franklin, 1970), 164.

24. Hartmann von Aue, *Êrec,* 6th ed. Christoph Cormeau and Kurt Gärtner (Tübingen: Max Niemeyer, 1985). All subsequent line references to Hartmann's *Êrec* are from this edition. All translations are my own.

25. Laurence Harf-Lancner, *Les fées au Moyen Age. Morgane et Melusine. La Naissance des Fées,* Nouvelle Bibliothèque du Moyen Age, no. 8 (Paris: Librairie Honoré Champion, 1984), 197.

26. Russell, 80-81.

27. Joseph B. Pike, *Frivolities of Courtiers and Footprints of Philosophers: Being a Translation of the First, Second, and Third Books and Selections from the Seventh and Eighth books of the Policraticus of John of Salisbury* (Minneapolis: Univ. of Minnesota Press, 1938), 39.

28. Ibid., 39, n.l.

29. Ibid., 39.

30. Ibid., 150

31. John M. Riddle, "Theory and Practice in Medieval Medicine," *Viator* 5 (1974): 166-67.

32. Pinto, "Medical Science," 12.

33. See Marianna Schrader and Adelgundis Führkötter, *Die Echtheit des Schrifttums der Heiligen Hildegard von Bingen: Quellenkritische Untersuchungen,* Beihefte Zum Archiv für Kulturgeschichte, no. 6 (Cologne: Böhlau, 1956), and Kent Kraft, "The German Visionary: Hildegard of Bingen," in *Medieval Women Writers,* ed. Katharina M. Wilson (Athens, Ga.: Univ. of Georgia Press, 1984): 109-30.

34. Charles Greene Cumston, *An Introduction to the History of Medicine* (London: Kegan, Paul, Trench, Trubner and Co., 1926), 217-18.

35. Claire Parkinson, *Breakthroughs: A Chronology of Great Achievements in Science and Mathematics, 1200-1930* (London: Mansell, 1985), 5.

36. Cumston, *Introduction,* 230-33.

37. Hausschild, Staschen, and Trotschke, *Hexen,* 41.

38. Brauner, "Frightened Shrews," 34-35.

# [3]

# WOMEN, MEDICINE, AND THE LAW IN BOCCACCIO'S *DECAMERON*

ESTHER ZAGO

*In her recent study, Lovesickness in the Middle Ages,* Mary Frances Wack notes that, whereas women as desiring subjects as well as desired objects can be found at any place and at any time in literary texts, women as clinical subjects were absent from medical academic literature until the late fourteenth century. Wack aptly surmises that "the relative silence of the physicians concerning women follows from, in the first instance, their preoccupation with analyzing *amor hereos* from a masculine perspective. . . . Moreover, men's lovesickness needed explanation and cure because it made them 'other.' Its signs and symptoms feminized them, separated them from normal masculine ways of behaving."[1]

Boccaccio's *Decameron* is a salient example of a literary text in which lovesickness in both men and women is sympathetically described. To define this condition, Boccaccio uses the medical term *malinconia* [melancholy] in the preface and on several other occasions; in certain instances the term is used to identify sexual frustration. However, Boccaccio makes a clear distinction between those women who allow themselves to be overcome by their sexuality, and those who acknowledge it and respect it. My inquiry will focus on this second group.

The purpose of this essay is therefore twofold. First, I hope to show that in analogous situations in which men and women fall victims of the melancholy condition caused by lovesickness, the therapy available privileges men, thus excluding women from taking advantage of it. Second, I will argue that

64

precisely because women are not allowed the freedom, the diversions, and the justifications available to men, they are more likely to "listen" to their bodies as well as to their minds; they can also speak in self-defense, thus challenging male authority both in the private space of the home and in the public space of the court of law.

Before examining the tales in question, it may be appropriate to situate the *Decameron* within its social and scientific context.

The importance of this collection of one hundred stories within the western tradition does not need to be emphasized here; it will suffice to remember that it generated the paradigm for a new genre, the short story. Most of the tales are set on the stage of the merchant's world of fourteenth-century Europe, focusing on Italy, with occasional excursions into the larger Mediterranean area. The case of the *Decameron* is of special interest also because it was composed sometime after 1348 and before 1354,[2] at the time of the Black Death. As Glending Olson[3] has pointed out, several plague tracts circulated in Europe. The critic cites in particular what is considered to be "the most influential treatise of its time, the *Compendium de epidimia* of the Faculty of Medicine at the University of Paris, written in 1348 at the request of the King of France." Olson quotes from this tract: "[S]ince bodily infirmity is sometimes related to the accidents of the soul, one should avoid anger, excessive sadness, and anxiety. Be of good hope and resolute mind; make peace with God, for death will be less fearsome as a result. *Live in joy and gladness as much as possible, for although joy may sometimes moisten the body, it nevertheless comforts both spirit and body.*" (emphasis added).

Boccaccio gives similar advice in his preface to the *Decameron,* and in the introduction to the first day. In addition, he dedicates his work to women who love and who need the comfort of literature. More specifically, Boccaccio has in mind women—paraphrasing Dante's address in the famous *canzone* of his *Vita Nuova,* "Donne ch' avete intelletto d'amore"—who have an "understanding of love"; he dismisses all others for whom the solace of needles, reels and spindles provides sufficient diversion. Note that Boccaccio is not here making a distinction of social class, but rather of intelligence, knowledge and sensitivity. The concept of the aristocracy of the mind is never very far from the mercantile world.

The decades that followed the plague epidemic coincided with the first appearance, especially in northern Italy, of health books. The physical condition of the body, the question of nutrition, and norms of hygiene acquired much greater importance than they had had in the past, a phenomenon which points to a decidedly more secular attitude towards the body. The space for such views may have been cleared in literary texts by the absence of the papacy from Rome throughout most of the fourteenth century.[4]

According to medieval medical treatises, based on Greek texts and Arab commentaries, the body's health depended on the equilibrium of each of the four humors, and of the corresponding four temperaments. Any form of imbalance could have pernicious effects on both the body and the mind. Boccaccio's interest in the interdependency of body and mind is apparent at the very onset of the *Decameron* in two famous passages: the preface, and the introduction to the first day. The latter shows the extent to which, in the macrocosm of an epidemic disease such as the plague, men's mental faculties are impaired to the point of subverting moral and social values. The former addresses the complementary phenomenon in the microcosm of lovesickness, where a mental affliction prevents the body from accomplishing its normal functions.

Recognized as disease in all medical treatises from antiquity to the Middle Ages, lovesickness was classified as a malady caused by the overproduction of black bile, which upset the equilibrium of body and mind.[5] As mentioned earlier, medical treatises of the medieval period indicate a certain interest in the *aegritudo amoris*[6] in men, but do not pay much attention to lovesickness in women. Boccaccio makes up for such neglect by dedicating his one hundred tales precisely to women affected by that condition. The passage in question is from the preface:

> E se . . . alcuna *malinconia,* mossa da focoso desio sopraviene nelle lor menti, in quelle conviene che con grave noia si dimori, se da nuovi ragionamenti non è rimossa: senza che elle sono men forti che gli uomini a sostenere. [emphasis added].[7]
> [And if, in the course of their meditations, their minds should be invaded by *melancholy* arising out of the flames of longing, it will inevitably take root there and make them suffer greatly, unless it be dislodged by new interests. Besides which, their powers of endurance are considerably weaker than those that men possess.][8]

It is clear that Boccaccio is not alluding here only to cases of melancholy brought about by a precise object of desire; he addresses also the larger question of sexuality, and of those erotic impulses which, according to a widespread belief, were stronger in women than in men.[9] Boccaccio neither confirms nor denies this assumption, but he perceptively suggests that there may also be a psychological reason for the high frequency of melancholy and sexual frustration among women. In his often quoted preface, he notes that most men, if they choose to do so, can divert their minds from melancholy thoughts by seeking out public spaces, where they can occupy themselves with conventionally masculine activities, such as sports and business. Women, instead, being confined to the private space of the home, have no alternative but to give in to their amorous dreams, hopes, and frustrations. The "new interests," namely the therapy which Boccaccio has in mind, is the solace of literature: the author "prescribes" his own literary corpus as a medical treatment for the mind, which, in turn, may help heal the body. In fact, it would not be too far-fetched to suggest an association between literary intercourse and sexual intercourse. Furthermore, we shall see that the remedy for the corresponding condition in men as prescribed by the medical profession as well as by health books was in fact sexual intercourse.

The number of cases of lovesickness and/or melancholy in the *Decameron* is relatively small, but nonetheless sufficient to mirror medical and social attitudes about that illness, which are clearly gender-determined. Several stories in the collection allude also to the historical reality of gender discrimination within the legal system in medieval Italy. For example, in cases of flagrant adultery, men were generally acquitted, whereas women had to pay a fine; in ecclesiastical law, women, but not men, could be condemned to separation from the family, and charged with financial losses.[10]

I will discuss some specific examples of practices, both medical and legal, which are gender-determined. I will then focus on the cases of three women who appropriate therapeutic and legal measures which are denied to them by male authority.

As stated earlier, such cases are few in number, and, in the complex world of the *Decameron,* they represent the exception rather than the rule; nonetheless, they underscore women's ability to diagnose the symptoms of lovesickness in themselves and in others, and to actively seek a healing solution, even though it may be socially dangerous, and even fatal. In other words, their behavior appears to counter some of Boccaccio's own statements regarding the character of women. For example, in the preface he says that women's "powers of endurance are considerably weaker than those that men possess" (46). And in the introduction to the first day, he has Filomena, one of the ten story-tellers, declare that women are "fickle, quarrelsome, suspicious, cowardly, and easily frightened" (62). However, such statements can be interpreted as public posturing for the sake of prudence: Boccaccio was keenly aware of the misogynist backlash which his work incited.[11] I will argue that several women in the *Decameron* are far more perceptive and steadfast than men; they also have a clear understanding of erotic impulses as psycho-physiological phenomena which can and must be treated before they degenerate into illness, thus causing irreparable damage to body and mind.

Boccaccio's knowledge of the medical literature on the subject of love-sickness has been the object of much speculation in recent years, and Massimo Ciavolella[12] has convincingly showed that the representation of *aegritudo amoris* in Boccaccio's *Decameron* is firmly grounded not only in literary and medical traditions going back to antiquity, but specifically in two late thirteenth-century texts, the *Lilium medicinae* and the commentary to Cavalcanti's famous *canzone,* "Donna me prega," by Dino del Garbo. The first text is of particular relevance to my assumptions, and my discussion in this section is greatly indebted to Ciavolella's article.

The *Lilium medicinae* was a medical encyclopedia written (circa 1285) by Bernard of Gordon (Bernardus Gordonius), one of the most esteemed physicians of the Montpellier school. Therein he defines *aegritudo amoris* as follows: "morbus qui hereos dicitur est sollicitudo melancholica propter mulieris amorem" [The disease, which is called hereos, is a melancholy fixation on the love for a woman].[13] The author goes on to state that men afflicted by the disease, may, if not adequately treated, fall into a manic state or even die. It appears that one of the most appropriate treatments consists in convincing the subject "ad diligendam multas, ut distrahatur amor unius propter amorem alterius" [to make love to many women so that the love for one woman may be diverted in favor of the love for another] (511).

Dino del Garbo, in his commentary on "Donna me prega" by Guido Cavalcanti,[14] follows exactly Bernard of Gordon's discussion of the *aegritudo amoris,* stating unequivocally that love is considered a sickness by the experts of medical science.[15] Boccaccio knew this text, referred to it in the *Teseida* and even recopied it in his own hand. The *Lilium medicinae* is not the only text in which sexual intercourse is indicated as therapy for men afflicted with love-sickness. As Wack (66-67) points out, the remedy is recommended in several medical treatises all through the Middle Ages.

It is a known fact that medical science in antiquity and throughout the
Middle Ages considered women's sexuality with contempt, but the *Decameron* provides a privileged locus for showing that male and female desires are
equal, and that women are justified in appropriating a therapy which the
medical profession prescribed to women only in cases of hysteria. The cases I
propose to study are precisely those of women who have no access to medical
treatment and who have to invent their own cure: women who heal themselves.[16]

Let us now turn to the *Decameron* and examine first two cases, one involving
a man and the other a woman, both struck by lovesickness, and the way in
which the remedy of sexual intercourse is problematized by gender.

Giachetto's love for Giannetta is a story within the story of the vicissitudes
suffered by the count of Anguersa (Day II, 8). Forced to abandon his two children, the count does not know that one of them, the daughter, is living as a
maid in the household of a wealthy and noble couple. The couple's son, Giachetto, falls in love with the girl, but dares not reveal his feelings to his parents
because he is under the impression that the object of his desire is socially inferior to him. He falls seriously ill, several doctors are called, but no remedy is
found. It so happens that a young doctor is at Giachetto's bedside, feeling his
pulse, when Giannetta comes into the room. The young doctor notices that
the pulse rhythm accelerates; when Giannetta leaves the room the pulse
rhythm becomes normal. Resorting to a pretext, the doctor calls the girl back:
once again the patient's pulse accelerates.[17] The doctor is then sure of his diagnosis, which he communicates to the worried parents:

> La sanità del vostro figliolo non è nell'aiuto de' medici ma nelle
> mani della Giannetta dimora, la quale si come io ho manifesta-
> mente per certi segni conosciuto, il giovane focosamente ama,
> come che ella non se ne accorge per quello che io vegga. Sapete
> omai che a fare v'avete, se la sua vita v'è cara. [270-71]
> [Your son's health cannot be restored by any doctor, for it rests
> in the hands of Giannetta. As I have discovered through certain
> unmistakable symptoms, the young man is ardently in love
> with her, though as far as I can tell, she herself is unaware of the
> fact. But you will know now what measures to apply if you
> want him to recover. (198-199)]

The young doctor is somewhat allusive in prescribing the therapy, but quite clear about the outcome if the "cure" is not administered. The mother—not the father—understands perfectly what the doctor is talking about. She sends for Giannetta and tells her that it is time for her, young and beautiful as she is, to have a lover. But the girl refuses: her only richness is her honor, she will take a husband, never a lover. The parents have to consent to the marriage, even though they consider it a mésalliance.

This story is interesting for several reasons. First, Giachetto manifests all the symptoms of lovesickness described in the medical treatises: his humoral imbalance causes him to suffer from an acute case of melancholy, and his mind is deeply troubled by feelings of shame and fear. It is also interesting to note that Boccaccio uses for Giachetto's condition exactly the same vocabulary which he uses for women in the preface to the *Decameron*.[18] What we have here is classic case of the "feminization" mentioned by Wack, which so intrigued medieval doctors.

Boccaccio's scientific knowledge concerning *aegritudo amoris* is further evidenced by the behavior of Giachetto's mother. The promptness with which she reacts to the doctor's speech clearly indicates that he is suggesting a therapy which is familiar to her. She doesn't stop for a moment to question its morality, and she immediately tries to arrange, more or less tactfully, for her son to "take his pleasure" with Giannetta.

A similar situation, this time with a young girl as protagonist, occurs in the seventh novella of the tenth day. Lisa, an apothecary's daughter, falls in love with Peter of Aragon, king of Sicily. Painfully aware of her impossible love—not only is the object of her desire a king, but he already has a wife—the girl falls seriously ill. When the king hears of Lisa's story, he is deeply moved; he arranges to visit her and comforts her with such kind words that Lisa immediately begins to get better. When she fully recovers her health, the king visits her again and, right there and then, presents her with the gift of a bridegroom. Ciavolella (499) notes the similarity between the stories of Lisa and Giachetto, but sees the *topos* of lovesickness only as it relates to the theme of the king's nobility and magnanimity. Without denying the validity of this interpretation, I believe it is important to call attention to the fact that, when Lisa is struck by *aegritudo amoris,* neither the doctors nor the parents envisage sexual intercourse as therapy for her. It is the king himself who prescribes it, euphemistically, in the form of marriage. Given the fact that Lisa cannot have the king in her bed, she will have to settle for a husband chosen by the king:

some other lover of her own choice would have been totally out of the question. Within the topos of the *aegritudo amoris,* the stories of Giachetto and Lisa show the extent to which sex as therapy is available only in a man's world, regardless of whether he is the beneficiary or the prescriber of the benefice.

In the preface to the *Decameron* Boccaccio argues that women, subject as they are to male tutelage, have to keep their "amorous flames," their "burning desires," their melancholy spells, well hidden. Let us consider now two of the most famous heroines of the *Decameron* from a social and medical perspective. Ghismonda (Day IV, 1) and Lisabetta (Day IV, 5) represent a polarity in the social scale. Ghismonda is the daughter of Tancredi, prince of Salerno; Lisabetta, an orphan, lives with her merchant brothers in Messina. They do, however, share a similar fate. Ghismonda is a childless young widow who, conforming to the customs of her rank, has returned to live at her father's court. Because of his love—so possessive as to border on incest—the prince neglects to find a new husband for his daughter. Lisabetta is still unmarried because her brothers have not taken the time and care to find a suitable match for her, thus denying her sexuality. Both women lead secluded lives, be it in a princely court or a merchant's house. Both women become aware of their sexual impulses; they sense that unfulfilled desires lead to frustration and melancholy. They cannot, as men do, leave their households and seek diversion elsewhere. But they know their minds and respect their bodies. They reject the simple solution of finding an occasional lover with the complicity of a mercenary servant, as happens in many of the *Decameron* stories (which have given such a bad reputation to their author). Both seek out a young man, worthy of their love, although inferior to their station in life. They take the initiative of making their desires manifest to the men. Both women know that transgressing both male authority and social barriers, with all the dangers inherent in that act, is preferable to suppressing one's own nature. Both men are killed; both women end up paying with their own lives for their transgression, Ghismonda by her own hand, Lisabetta, more fragile, by letting herself die of grief.

Most traditional criticism of the parallel stories of Ghismonda and Lisabetta focused on the way in which Boccaccio shows that Lisabetta, who comes from the lower merchant class, is capable of love just as noble and tragic as that of Ghismonda, a prince's daughter.[19] The tendency of modern criticism, on the other hand, would be to make of Ghismonda the fearless advocate of equality between the sexes in terms of sexual desire. But in the context, and for the purpose of this essay, it is important to analyze the structure of Ghismonda's speech to her father when he discovers her double transgression. She has to articulate her defense on two grounds, and in terms that her father could not possibly refute. Addressing first the question of her sexuality, she reminds him of his own nature and youthful impulses:

> Esser ti dové, Tancredi, manifesto essendo tu di *carne,* aver *generato* figliola di *carne* e non di pietra o di ferro. . . . Sono adunque, sí come da te *generata,* di *carne,* e sí poco vivuta, che ancor son giovane, e per l'una cosa e per l'altra piena di concupiscibile desiderio, al quale maravigliosissime forze hanno date l'aver già per essere stato maritata, conosciuto. [479, emphasis added]
>
> [You are made of *flesh and blood,* Tancredi, and it should have been obvious to you that the daughter you *fathered* was also made of *flesh and blood,* and not of stone or iron. . . . Since you were the person who *fathered* me, I am made of *flesh and blood* like yourself. Moreover, I am still a young woman. And for both of these reasons, I am full of amorous longings, intensified beyond belief by my marriage, which enabled me to discover the marvellous joy that comes from their fulfillment. (337, emphasis added)]

The most striking feature of this first part of Ghismonda's speech rests on the emotional charge with which the words *carne* (flesh) and *generato/a* (fathered) are invested. From a rhetorical standpoint the effect is powerful because it unmasks the father's refusal to face the issue of his daughter's sexuality; from a scientific perspective it establishes the truth of an undeniable natural and physiological process. The medical justification for Ghismonda's desire can be found in an eleventh-century work on women's diseases signed by a woman, Trotula. According to the author, who in turns relies on Galen, women produce a secretion similar to that of the male: "Especially does this happen to those who have no husbands, widows in particular and those who previously have been accustomed to make use of carnal intercourse. It also happens in virgins who have come to marriageable years and have not yet husbands."[20] Trotula goes on to explain that, if such secretion accumulates, it produces hysteria; intercourse and pregnancy can be recommended as therapy. It is safe to assume that the remedy could be administered only in a situation legitimized by marriage. Ghismonda makes it clear to her father that she does not consider her sexuality demeaning in any way; on the contrary, she would appear to be exalting her sexuality by appropriating the vocabulary of the medical treatises.

Ghismonda goes on to remind her father of his own sexuality in his youthful years. In the second part of her speech she addresses the question of her having chosen a lover socially inferior to her. Here again she places the emphasis on the word *carne:*

> [R]iguarda alquanto a' principi delle cose: tu verdrai noi d'una massa di *carne* tutti la *carne* avere e da un medesimo Creatore tutte l'anime con uguali forze, con iguali potenze con iguali virtù create. [480; emphasis added]
> [Consider for a moment the principles of things, and you will see that we are all of one *flesh* and that our souls were created by a single Maker, who gave the same capacities and powers and faculties to each. (338, emphasis added)]

Once more, she hinges her argument first on biological factors, and she uses all her oratorical skills to restate the theory of the nobility of the soul as superior to that of an acquired title.[21]

From a medical perspective, Ghismonda's speech is less revolutionary than it appears at first, since it looks at sexual desire as a natural process that implicates both the mind and the body. As mentioned earlier, its most striking characteristic is the high frequency of the word *carne,* which is endowed with positive connotations. Boccaccio astutely presents Ghismonda as a "virile" personality. When her father confronts her with her "guilt," she understands that her lover's fate is signed, and yet she does not cry as most women would have done in similar circumstances. It is actually her father who bursts into tears. Ghismonda, determined to follow her lover in death, announces her intention to take her own life with "un-feminine" resolution and pride. She even tells him to go off and shed his tears among women. The "masculinization" of Ghismonda stands in opposition to the "feminization" of her father. It is Tancredi who suffers from an acute case of lovesickness and an incestuous one at that. By switching their roles in this manner, Boccaccio reveals the hypocrisy of Tancredi's feelings towards his daughter, and of society towards women. Furthermore, it is significant that Boccaccio should have entrusted Ghismonda, a prince's daughter, with the task of defending women's sexuality: it certainly gives more credibility to the cause. Lisabetta, more feminine and less eloquent, would have been incapable of constructing her self-defense with equal rhetorical ability.

In spite of its rigid structure—ten days, ten stories each day, told by ten different people—the *Decameron* has its own asymmetries, and involves a play of mirrors which, across the boundaries of days and themes, calls attention to the possibility of looking at the same problem from different perspectives. The stories of Ghismonda and Lisabetta are told on the fourth day, which focuses on unhappy or tragic love, so their stories too have the prescribed outcome. But Boccaccio does not neglect the possibility that women's initiative to appropriate for themselves what is typically prescribed for men only may also have a happy outcome.

The narratives of the sixth day focus on the cases of men and women who succeed in escaping from danger by virtue of their intelligence and wit. The seventh story presents the case of a woman from Prato by the name of Madonna Filippa. The location is important: in the thirteenth and fourteenth centuries Prato was one of the busiest centers in Tuscany for cloth manufacture and trade. We can therefore assume that Fillippa's social environment is that of the merchant class. The lady is not too happily married, and she has a relationship with a young and handsome man. Her husband discovers her adultery. Had he killed his wife and her lover on the spot, he would have been acquitted; being too cowardly, he turns her over to the courts, knowing full well that she—not her lover—will be sentenced to death. Pennington[22] reminds us that such harsh law was no longer enforced in the fourteenth century. We might say that Boccaccio makes *fabula* out of history, but we might also notice that Filippa's lover is not summoned to trial, nor is he mentioned again in the rest of the story. In court, Filippa states her case with logical and rhetorical skills worthy of Ghismonda, and according to strict argumentative procedure. She acknowledges the truth of her adultery, but she argues that on that matter, laws which concern women are made by men and favor men. Filippa makes her husband admit that he, her husband, took from her what he needed and wanted. But what about her own needs and desires?

> [I]o che doveva fare di quel che gli avanza? debbolo io gittare a' cani? non è egli molto meglio servirne un gentile uomo che più che sè m'ama, che lasciarlo perdere e guastare? [748]

74

> [What am I to do with the surplus? Throw it to the dogs? Is it
> not far better that I should present it to a gentleman who loves
> me more dearly than himself, rather than allow it to turn bad
> and go to waste? (500)]

Filippa astutely transforms the moral issue of adultery into the economic issue of waste, an argument which was bound to convince the mercantile mentality of Prato's judges and citizens. Filippa obtains the predictable result: she is acquitted, amid the laughter and joking of the public, and she even obtains that the law be changed.

The question of women appropriating a measure available to men only is thus transferred from the medical to the legal field, but the essence of the argument is the same.

The import of this extraordinary story is in a sense confirmed by that of another, more conventional, one. It is the second story of the second day. The situation is far less serious than that in the other cases so far examined, but it has its own contribution to offer. It deals with a man and a woman whose paths cross by chance, and who share a few hours of happiness. The woman is a widow, and the mistress of the local lord. Obviously marriage is out of the question, but the relationship is honorable. One evening the woman is expecting her lord to spend the night with her; she prepares a warm bath and delicious food for him, only to learn that he has been detained by a sudden engagement and will not be able to join her for the night. Greatly disappointed, she hears a noise coming from outside and discovers a wounded man by her house. With the help of a servant she brings him in, gives him a bath, her deceased husband's clothes, the dinner she had prepared for her lord, and finally an invitation to share her bed. On one level, this is the delightful story of a charming and elegant "one night stand without strings attached." On a deeper level, it shows a woman's understanding of her sexuality, and the extent to which she values it. In a sense, it relates to Filippa's argument on waste. Why not make a gift of a surplus which otherwise would be lost? She does more than provide the man with food, clothes and sex: she restores his self-confidence and the trust in human nature, which he had lost when he was attacked. More important, she appropriates sex as therapy to cure her own disappointment and loneliness. What the text is implying here is that a fleeting sexual encounter can be as valid a therapy as a long-term relationship, if it is the result of a conscious, rational, and "generous" (read *noble*) choice.

Healthy sexuality and secular morality seem to share some common ground. It is, of course, a secular morality which closely follows the development of an increasingly secular attitude towards the human body.

Unfortunately, these views could only prosper in the greenhouse of literary imagination. Criticism of Boccaccio's sympathy for women developed early on, and the scriptor deemed it necessary to justify and restate his position in the introduction to the fourth day. Ironically enough, only a few years after completing the *Decameron,* Boccaccio yielded to his own religious scruples and anxieties (too modern a term?) over his corpus of short stories. In the *Corbaccio,* he launched an attack against women worthy of any of the countless misogynist texts of the Middle Ages.

Medical literature was not even remotely touched by Boccaccio's "defense of good women" in the *Decameron.* Yet by the end of the fourteenth century, a more urgent reality probably impelled physicians to recommend sexual intercourse to women suffering from erotic frustration, lovesickness and melancholy, since it had the desirable effect of making women pregnant: in the aftermath of the black plague and with the high index of infant mortality, there was everything to be gained by encouraging women to produce children as often as possible. As a result, medical attention focused more on the uterus and less on the brain. Mary Frances Wack makes an interesting observation about lovesickness in men and women:

> In the Middle Ages a number of academic physicians viewed *amor hereos* as a disease located in the brain rather than in the testicles, and primarily as an affliction of noblemen. . . . The disease gradually shifted "downward" to become, in the estimation of some later writers, an illness of the sexual organs of women. . . . Such a gradual "decline" in the localization of *amor hereos* may help to account for its transformation from a "heroic" malady to a "hysteric affliction." (123)

Wack calls her remark "an admittedly metaphorical description of the change" which occurred in the fifteenth and sixteenth centuries, but it has a ring of truth about it. It also echoes the old medieval prejudice that women's sexual appetites were insatiable by placing a negative psychological connotation on female sexuality. Towards the end of the sixteenth century, the word "hystérique" made its entrance in the French vocabulary to describe "un accès d'érotisme morbide féminin" [an attack of morbid feminine eroticism].[23] Even more than in the Middle Ages, Renaissance women could heal neither themselves nor others: in the next three centuries of scientific progress and intellectual revolution, until the birth of modern medicine in the nineteenth century, they remained marginalized at best or entirely excluded.

NOTES

1. Mary Frances Wack, *Lovesickness in the Middle Ages: The "Viaticum" and Its Commentaries* (Philadelphia: Univ. of Pennsylvania Press, 1990), 175.

2. The precise date of composition of the *Decameron* is the subject of scholarly dispute. There is agreement, however, that the work must postdate 1348, because it opens with a graphic description of the plague that struck Florence that year, which provides the frame for the narration.

3. Glending Olson, *Literature as Recreation in the Later Middle Ages,* (Ithaca: Cornell Univ. Press, 1982), 168-69.

4. The seat of the papacy was transferred to Avignon, France, in 1309, where it remained until 1376.

5. The best study on melancholy remains *Saturn and Melancholy,* by Raymond Klibansky, Erwin Panofsky, and Fritz Saxl (London: Nelson & Son, 1967). Other relevant studies with emphasis on medieval literature include: Giorgio Agamben, *Stanze* (Torino: Einaudi, 1979); and Jacques Roubaud, *La fleur inverse* (Paris: Ramsay, 1986). For the use of the term "melancholy" in the *Decameron,* see Esther Zago, "Gender and Melancholy in Boccaccio's *Decameron,*" *Lingua e Stile* 27.2 (1992): 235-49.

6. Lovesickness was called either *aegritudo amoris* or *amor hereos.* Whereas the first term does not present any problem, the genesis of the second is very complex. See J.L. Lowes, "The Loveres Maladye of Hereos," *Modern Philology* 2 (1914): 491-546.

7. Giovanni Boccaccio, *Decameron,* ed. Vittore Branca (Torino: Einaudi, 1987), 6. All subsequent references in Italian are to this edition.

8. Giovanni Boccaccio, *The Decameron,* trans. G.H. McWilliam (Harmondsworth, England: Penguin Books, 1972), 46. All subsequent references in English are to this translation.

9. On Medieval views of women's sexuality, see Vern L. Bullough, "Medieval and Scientific Views of Women," *Viator* 4 (1973): 485-501.

10. See Kenneth Pennington, "A Note to *Decameron* VII, 6. The Case of Madonna Filippa," *Speculum* 52 (1977): 902-5.

11. See, for example, the following passage from the introduction to the fourth day: "Sono adunque, discrete donne, stati alcuni che, queste novellette leggendo,

hanno detto che voi me piacete troppo e che onesta cosa non è che io tanto diletto prenda di piacervi e di consolarvi e, alcuni han detto peggio, di commendarvi, come io fo" (460-61) [Judicious ladies, there are those who have said, after reading these tales, that I am altogether too fond of you, that it is unseemly for me to take so much delight in entertaining and consoling you, and, what is apparently worse, in singing your praises as I do (325)]. The most plausible explanation for this comment on public reaction to the *Decameron* within the text itself is that some of the stories must have circulated separately, prior to the completion of the work.

12. Massimo Ciavolella, "La Tradizione della *Aegritudo Amoris* nel *Decameron*," *Giornale Storico della Letteratura Italiana* 147, 460 (1970): 496-517. For Boccaccio's interest in science, see also Marga Cottino-Jones, "Boccaccio e la Scienza," in *Letteratura e Scienza nella Cultura Italiana* (Palermo: Manfredi, 1979), 356-70.

13. Quoted by Ciavolella, 511. All subsequent references in Latin are to this article, and all translations are mine.

14. Guido Cavalcanti (1260?-1300) was Dante's "first friend." His celebrated poem, "Donna me priega," is a dark song in which love is described in scientific and astrological terms.

15. Ciavolella, 512.

16. The traditional role of woman as healer is represented in the *Decameron* by Gilette de Narbonne (Day III, 9), the source for Shakespeare's play *All's Well That Ends Well.*

17. For the sources of this case of lovesickness, see Ciavolella, 508-9.

18. Compare the preface, p. 7: "Esse dentro a' dilicati petti, *temendo* e *vergognando,* tengono l'*amorose fiamme nascose . . .* " [For the ladies, out of *fear* or *shame,* conceal the *flames* of *passion* within their fragile breasts . . . (46)]; and in the story under discussion, p. 269: "egli . . . *temendo* non fosse ripreso che bassamente si fosse a amar messo, quanto poteva il suo *amore teneva nascoso*" [since he was *afraid* of being reproached with falling in love with a commoner, he did all he could to keep his *love* a *secret* (198)]. Giachetto's mother urges him to get rid of "la *vergogna* e la *paura*" (172) [the *sadness* and *anxiety* (199)]. Emphasis added in the original text and in the translation.

19. It was a widespread belief in medical literature that only noblemen suffered from lovesickness. In literary texts, women were included, but only in the "noble" genres, such as epic poetry and tragedy, not in comedy or farce.

20. Quoted by Bullough, 495.

21. The concept is certainly not new on the European literary scene, and it has well known antecedents in Boethius, Andreas Cappellanus, Jean de Meung, the Stilnovists, to name a few.

22. Pennington, 902.

23. *Dictionnaire Etymologique Larousse.*

# [4]

# WOMEN HEALERS AND THE POWER
# TO DISEASE IN LATE MEDIEVAL SPAIN

MICHAEL SOLOMON

*In the early Middle Ages,* learned practitioners operated in relative harmony, or at least in harmonious indifference, alongside and in conjunction with empirics, quasi-professional practitioners, and folk healers. Many of these subaltern healers were women who were well-known for their abilities to set bones, remove bladder stones, cure eye diseases, relieve the pains of gout, and treat all kinds of gynecological and obstetric disorders.[1] The major European courts often employed these women healers, allowing them to participate in virtually all aspects of medicine.[2]

From the beginning of the twelfth century legal mechanisms were put into place in Europe to evaluate and limit women practitioners. The earliest recorded attempts to regulate medical practice were those of King Roger II (1130-54) of Sicily and his grandson, Frederick II, who required that all those who desired to practice medicine be examined.[3] Under the guise of acting in the public's best interest, the medical faculty at Paris in the twelfth century began a series of attempts to eliminate all "charlatanism" and medical practice by empirics, and to evaluate and license all "legitimate" medical personnel.[4] In the Iberian peninsula King Alfonso II of Leon (1188-1230) prohibited anyone from practicing medicine without first being examined by an established physician and receiving authorization from the mayor of the town.[5] In 1239 the Valencia court promulgated a *fur* requiring all medical practitioners to possess a university degree and to demonstrate their medical competency by way of an annual examination. The same statute proscribed women from practicing medicine "under penalty of being whipped through the town."[6]

The licensing procedures of the late medieval tribunals were not initially powerful enough to curtail the medicinal practices of women. There were simply not enough university-trained physicians to meet the needs of the sick. In the fourteenth century a thriving port city such as Valencia only had nineteen physicians and eight surgeons available for the thirty thousand inhabitants. This ratio of roughly eight physicians for every ten thousand citizens was one of the highest in Europe.[7] Many smaller towns complained bitterly of the lack of physicians and urged the authorities to make exceptions to the law. The onset of plague epidemics from the mid-fourteenth century further diminished the number of licensed physicians, leaving many areas with "no one to cure the ill and take care of their needs."[8] Even in areas where authorized practitioners were available, their services were often simply too expensive for the poor. Women healers were praised because "they attend the sick poor and incapacitated who lack the means to pay."[9] The paucity and high costs of licensed practitioners assured an ongoing demand for women and other subaltern practitioners even in times when their activities were challenged by new legal constraints.

Perhaps the greatest impediment to controlling the activities of women practitioners was that university-trained and licensed physicians had no monopoly on curing disease and easing pain, nor were they able to consistently demonstrate that their skills were more efficacious than those of other healers. Modern medicine has evolved into a highly specialized enterprise that rigorously distinguishes its technology and practitioners from alternative healers and non-medical personnel. Although it draws its initial authority from the privileged epistemological status of science—which pretends to be an accurate reading of the Book of Nature—it also makes powerful claims of therapeutic efficacy. Medieval physicians, regardless of the number of years of university training, could not demonstrably make the same assertions. Complaints of the inefficacy of medical treatment were so common during the late Middle Ages and the Renaissance that they emerged as a literary trope in the sixteenth century.

In defense of non-licensed medical personnel, many pointed to the effectiveness of their cures. In Paris, for example, during the early fourteenth century (1322), Jacqueline Félicie de Almania was cited for the illegal practice of medicine (practicing without a license) and duly excommunicated. John of Padua, surgeon to the king of France, Philip IV, insisted that empirics, such as Jacqueline, practiced in ignorance of the art of medicine and in so doing could easily kill a patient by incorrectly applying clysters and potions. Countering these arguments, Jacqueline's defending council produced witnesses whom she had successfully treated. During the course of her trial, testimony from former patients expressed overwhelming confidence in her ability to cure their ailments. Many of the witnesses emphatically described the way licensed physicians had failed to cure them, listing by name those professionals who had unsuccessfully treated them. The defense council reiterated the ineffectiveness of licensed professionals, adding that, unlike many licensed physicians, Jacqueline, "cared for her patients assiduously until they were cured."[10]

I contend that the ultimate goal of medical legislation and its subsequent marginalization of women healers in the later Middle Ages was less an attempt to protect the public from incompetent practitioners than an effort to control the tremendous social power of medicine. To do this, authorized physicians participated in an ongoing production of an imaginary otherness that was thought to oppose malevolently the objectives and ideology of legitimate medicine. In the later Middle Ages the licensed practitioner began to define himself in contrast to a body of women practitioners whose goals and techniques where shown to resist those of authorized healers. If medical authorities could not clearly and consistently demonstrate that their methods or their learning were effective, they could at least fortify their claims of legitimacy by casting a shadow on the activities of subalterns. If they were unable to stop the sick from seeking the help of unauthorized healers, they could discourage this practice by creating or retelling stories and anecdotes that impugned the character and methods of these healers, forcefully drawing a line between the legitimate healer and the sinister other.

One of the most powerful examples of this technique appears in the writings of the fifteenth-century Valencian physician, Jaume Roig. Trained in the prestigious medical faculty of Paris, Roig repeatedly served as the official Examiner of Physicians in Valencia until his death in 1478.[11] He was head physician for the Valencian hospitals of En Claper, and En Bou, and held the administrative position of "desospitador" in the Hospital d'Inocents, the hospital often celebrated as the first mental institution in the West.[12] In these official capacities, Roig not only fully participated in the institutional mechanism of the medieval clinic, but also was called upon repeatedly to differentiate between clinical healers and "illegitimate" practitioners. This distinction is fully present in Roig's most celebrated work, the *Spill o Llibre de les dones [1460: The Mirror or Book of Women]*.[13]

81

In the tradition of medieval antifeminist literature, such as the works of Walter Map, Andreas Capellanus, Jehan le Fèvre, and Boccaccio, Roig sets out in the *Spill* to denounce the evil nature of women. Using an autobiographical format, Roig creates a protagonist who recounts a series of painful encounters with manipulative women who trick and abuse him. Because he was a physician, it is not surprising that much of Roig's condemnation focuses on women's illicit attempts to practice medicine.

Throughout the *Spill* Roig establishes a firm distinction between the authorized physician and the antithetical subaltern, describing the former as good and competent while denouncing the later as evil and inept. For example, in his account of his second wife's frustrated efforts to conceive a child, he details the way women doctors, midwives, apothecaries, herbalists, and astrologers not only failed to cure her, but caused her to suffer from additional illnesses.[14]

> a tots arreu / recorregue, / tots los cregue: / huns calda deyen, / altres la feyen / ffreda y himida / o adormida; / tots variaven / hi la 'nguanaven; / d'ells ser liguada / enfitillada / li feyen creure; / fferen-li beure / mil beuratjades / prou mal forjades / en banys, huntures / he faxadures, / perfums, e cales; / ulçers males / li concriaren, / he li causaren / salt de ventrell, / en lo çervell / malencolia / he mirarchia; / molt la guastaren, / he la creamaren. / Tota secada, / prop heticada, / per lo parir / cuydà perir.[15]
> [she turned to all of them, believing each one. Some said she needed warmth; others wanted to treat her with cold, humidity, and sleep; they all disagreed, each one denying the treatment of the other. Some made her believe that she was bewitched. They made her drink a thousand poorly-mixed potions. With their baths, ointments, bandages, perfumes, and suppositories, they produced terrible ulcers and spasms in her stomach, and melancholy and *mirarchia*. Their remedies depleted and consumed her, leaving her dehydrated and consumptive. In her attempts to give birth she almost gave away her life.]

In opposition to these inept practitioners and their dangerous therapies, Roig tells how a "valent metge" [a worthy male physician] finally cured her liver problems and stomach spasms, while freeing her from the pains of consumption.

For Roig, women are simply too incompetent to participate in the healing arts. Moreover they are naturally inclined to invert the therapeutic structure by misdiagnosing diseases and misapplying medicines. In a dream vision retold in the third book of the *Spill,* the biblical Solomon appears to the protagonist complaining that when wives are allowed to treat their sick husbands they do more harm than good. Solomon tells us that a woman will force her husband to recuperate in the worst bed in the house or constantly order him to get up and move from bed to bed. She will dispute the doctor's diagnosis, telling him that he has no fever when in truth he is burning up. She will offer him all kinds of false remedies, feeding him unhealthy food or starving him as she sees fit.[16]

Throughout *Spill,* Roig reminds the reader that women are ill disposed and disinclined to act as legitimate healers. If the etiology of disease could be explained in the Middle Ages as the intervention of devils, demons, and wicked spirits, then it stood to reason that women, who according to Roig have been "friends of the Devil" (10438-39) from the beginning, are more likely to make men sick than cure their ailments. Likewise, if ancient and medieval deontologists were correct when they claimed that the efficacy of the physician was contingent on his moral character and great virtue, then women, who according to Roig are greedy, dishonest, envious, unscrupulous, manipulative, disobedient, and deceitful, have no place wielding surgical instruments, compounding medicines, and checking pulses.[17]

Although Roig repeatedly decries the damage caused by incompetent women healers, his greatest condemnation is reserved for women who appropriate medical postures with the hope of deceiving and injuring men. He tells of a woman who kills her sick husband by offering him a poisonous drink that she calls medicine. After her husband's death she creates a perfectly acceptable clinical explanation for her suspicious neighbors: "D'un gras porçell e vi novell [h]a mort traguat es s'ofeguat de poplexia" (1573-77) [After having consumed much pork and new wine, he suffocated during an attack of apoplexy]. According to the medieval medical theorist, Bernard of Gordon, apoplexy (stroke) was thought to be caused by the excessive consumption of food and drink, and by a life of idleness and leisure.[18] A double diseasing takes place in this anecdote. First the wife poisons her husband and then she appropriates a malady to justify his death.

I use the verb "to disease" here in two ways. First, in its most literal sense of to make someone sick, or to infect, inflict or otherwise dispose someone to an illness. The concern of medical professionals, a concern that fully motivates today's rigorous control over drugs and medical technology, consists of the fear that the ignorant and misinformed can do more harm than good by misapplying or misusing pharmaceutical and medical instruments. In effect, by misadministering a drug, or incorrectly prescribing a therapeutic strategy, one can actually harm another human being. The second meaning of "to disease" is to impose a pathologically significant meaning on a person's biological being, granting that person all the privileges and limitations of this socially defined phenomenon. The power to disease can be an instrument of both oppression and liberation. Feminists have argued convincingly that the medical profession, through its power to pathologize, has historically attempted to control women's desires by casting their discontents into pathological molds. But this power, to the degree that it functions in direct correlation to the rights and privileges that society grants the sick, can be a source of liberation, freeing the individual from difficult or unpleasant situations. The exemption from military service, release from work, monetary compensation, and deference of debt are only a few of the privileges granted to those who have been officially diagnosed as suffering from a biological disorder.[19]

Individuals who diagnose their own ailments and prescribe their own therapy are often deemed to be suspect. It is not enough for a worker to tell his employer that he is suffering from muscle pains and thus needs to spend a few weeks recuperating at a health spa. It is not enough for an airline passenger to say that she was too sick to fly and therefore must be reimbursed for her "non-refundable" ticket. These ailments, real or feigned, require the legitimizing confirmation of an authorized physician if the patient is to be fully liberated from his or her normal responsibilities. The same is true of the diagnoses and therapies of subaltern healers. This reliance on the word of the orthodox physician over the impressions of the patient and the claims of the subaltern healer clearly points to the successful struggle of Western medicine during the past five hundred years to limit the practice of medicine to a select group of healers. The origin of this opposition between authorized physicians and unorthodox practitioners emerges from institutional conventions and discursive practices that arose in the later Middle Ages as an attempt to control the power to disease.

It is the liberating aspect of the power to disease that concerns Roig. He complains that women manipulate the signs and symptoms of disease to camouflage their true objectives: "[C]riden que's moren quant son pus sanes, si han terçanes llur mal no colen; e fingir solen tenir dolor, per dar, color a ses empreses" (448-55) [They complain that they are dying when they are completely healthy. If they suffer from the Tertain fever, rather than taking care of themselves, they usually feign pains to disguise their schemes]. Throughout the *Spill* he frequently protests about the way his wives produced the signs of biological disorder to free themselves from work and to enjoy the privileges extended to the ill. His first wife, for example, always feigned sickness on workdays to stay in bed and to avoid completing her daily chores (2503-8). His second wife, similarly motivated, feigned the signs of pregnancy, imitating all the symptoms; she padded her breasts with cotton, colored her nipples with henna, and invented cravings for pastries and meats. Roig tells us that she was even able to imitate the complaints of a pregnant woman: "Sent-me llassa hun mes me passa, ja ma camisa de bona guisa he prou purguí due draps n'[h]agui; com so dolenta trop-me calenta, si no vomite tantost m'enfite" (4733-42) [A month has passed and I am worn out, my shirt is already a good size, I just purged myself and it took ten rags; I ache all over and suffer from heat flashes; if I don't vomit, I suffer indigestion].

Roig's observations are backed by examples in misogynist literature and didactic treatises that appeared during the fifteenth and sixteenth centuries. Alonso Martínez de Toledo in his diatribe against women, *El Arcipreste de Talavera o Corbacho* (1466), tells of an adulterous wife who engineers a biological distraction to help her lover flee unnoticed from the bedroom after the husband returns home unexpectedly.[20] As the husband enters the house, the wife tells him that she does not feel well. When he sits on a bench near the bed and orders her to bring him something to eat, the wife nervously moves towards the lover, who is hiding behind a curtain. She secretly explains to him that when she shows her husband her breast, he should flee from the house. The wife then complains to the husband, "Marido, non sabes cómo se ha fichado mi teta, e ravio con la mucha leche" (188) [Husband, you've no idea how my breast is swollen. I'm in agony with so much milk]. Concerned over his wife's affliction the husband asks to see the afflicted breast. At this moment the wife

> sacó la teta e diole un rayo de leche por los ojos que lo cegó del todo, e en tanto el otro salió. E dixo: "¡O fija de puta, cómo me escuece la leche!" Respondió el otro que se iva: "Qué deve fazer el cuerno?"[21]

[took out her breast and shot a stream of milk into his eyes, completely blinding him, while the other escaped. And the husband said: "You daughter of a whore, how your milk smarts!" And the other who was making his escape said: "What can the poor cuckold do about it?"][22]

Again, a double diseasing takes place in the anecdote. First, the wife feigns the malady of excessive breast milk.[23] A second diseasing occurs in the story when the wife squirts milk into her husband's eyes, at least temporarily blinding him. Thus, both physically, through her bodily fluids, and verbally, through her description of her biomedical disorder, the wife employs the art of diseasing to liberate herself from what would have surely been a tragic situation for herself and her lover.

For Roig these examples do not simply illustrate random acts of diseasing perpetrated by a few deceitful women. These schemes are the result of skills that have been handed down from woman to woman, sister to sister and mother to daughter. The convent serves as just one of the places where this instruction takes place. Roig's third wife, who was raised in a local convent, explains that the abbess carefully taught her the strategies of feigning illness, as well as how to use the powders, dyes, and ointments to simulate the symptoms of disease:

> Mas l'abadessa / me doctriná, / consell doná / que'm fes malalta / he qualque falta / en ma persona / alguna stona, / o pus sovent / seguons lo vent, / fingís tenir: / no prou hoyr, / al cap dolor, / he baticor, / esmortiments, / afollaments, / mal de neulella; / en la mamella, / no hulçerat / mas començat, / cançer tenir. / "Molt post fingir / ab gentil art: / secret, apart, / met en l'orina / cendra, farina, / oli, calç, llet, / algun ququet / chich del forment / ffes cautament / metge sabut, / practich, astut, / vell, no la vega: / si la menega, / conexeria, / divulgaria / ton aritifçi. /
>
> Metge noviçi / llaguotegat / he ben paguat / te planyera; / he complaura / per son jovent, / no prou sabent / s'enguanarà: / publicarà / que ten grans mals; / mil cordials, / confits, aloses, / he quantes coses / disigaras, / atenyeras." (6016-66)
>
> [The abbess also indoctrinated me and counseled me as to how to make myself ill, and how to fake momentarily and ca-

priciously some kind of personal defect such as deafness, headaches, heart tremors, dizziness, miscarriages, back pains, breast
cancer (not yet ulcerated, but only in its initial stages). "With
subtle artistry, you can simulate many things. In secret, mix cin-
ders, flour, oil, lime, milk, or one of those wheat worms with
your urine; be careful not to be examined by an experienced or
wise physician, because he will see through your scheme; rather
pick a young doctor whom you can flatter; he will have compassion and will comply; on account of his youth and lack of
experience, he will fall for the trick, making your great disease
known in public, by which you will be able to get tonics and
confections, or whatever you want.]

Roig's wife confesses that with the help of the abbess she learned how to put
blisters on her skin using garlic; how to discolor the skin with mustard; how to
produce ulcers with ground pepper; how to prick her palate with a needle so
as to cough and spit up blood; how to produce the symptoms of consumption. The abbess explains:

> D'enmallatir o del guarir, quant son mester, la qui u [ho] sab
> fer molt se'n ajuda, lo que's vol muda: hun "no u [ho] hoy, lo
> mal [h]aguí, ja so guarida, ja so ferida," la scusarà del que volrà
> (6097-102)
> [She who learns to disease or to cure, whichever be necessary,
> will greatly further her cause: an "I couldn't hear," an "I was
> sick," an "I am cured," or an "I am wounded," will get you what
> you want!]

In addition to these teachings, Roig's wife received training from other nuns
who taught her how to give the evil eye, create spells and charms, to abort
babies and fake virginity, and to administer sleeping potions.

For Roig, women who act in a medical context are always suspect, not
necessarily because they lack the knowledge to administer therapeutic tech-
nologies, but because they use this knowledge irresponsibly, with little regard
for the well-being of the patient or the stability of the social order. He retells
how his second wife, motivated by her efforts to conceive a child, sought the
services of a "metgessa stranya" [strange woman physician] from Bigorra. According to Roig, this old practitioner, who specialized in fertility therapy, had

used her medical skills to trick the entire Kingdom of Aragon. When women came to her for treatment, she would offer an accepted medical diagnosis, explaining that their cold bodies, combined with the impure semen of their husbands, made it impossible for them to conceive. To cure her female patients she first offered them a mixture of cloves and ginger to warm their bodies. She then would direct the patients to her back room where she kept several well-endowed young men. With three or four good thrusts, she claimed, they could make any woman pregnant (4334-4602).

For Roig, this female practitioner and her unorthodox remedies threaten the patriarchal order of the entire Kingdom of Aragon. Rather than curing disease and mitigating disorder, she literally helps plant the seeds of personal and social chaos. Roig tells us how he denounced her practice to the local authorities, who determined that the nature of her therapy required a double moratorium on her activities. Not only did she have to stop administering drugs and supplying illicit semen, she also had to be kept from revealing the true circumstances of her clients' pregnancy in order to "evitar scandelizar tan[t] trist marit" (4591-2) [avoid scandalizing so many pitiful husbands]. The solution was to simply ignore the normal judicial process and permanently silence her. Roig tells us that she was discretely strangled one night in her own house. He adds "!Quant bort secret resta ledesme!" [How many bastards in this way were made legitimate!].

For physicians such as Jaume Roig, these narratives of feigned diseases and misappropriate medical therapies illustrate more than just the particular travesties of deceiving women. They were designed to show men the dangers involved in allowing women to acquire medical knowledge and employ medicinal materials. Moreover, these anecdotes were intended to convince men that women, operating in what seemed to be a medical context, were in reality in direct opposition to the goals of the authorized healer.

Roig's warnings do not represent the isolated fears of one physician. Similar admonitions reappear in some of the most celebrate fictions of the later Middle Ages and early Renaissance. In Fernando de Rojas's *Celestina* (1498), a work that enjoyed an enormous popularity throughout Europe in the sixteenth century, the principal character is an old woman, Celestina, who is extremely skilled in the medicinal arts.[24] In her house, which doubles as a brothel, she warehouses a collection of pharmaceuticals so large as to be the envy of even the richest apothecary. Presented with the opportunity to cure a young man, Calisto, of lovesickness—a medically recognized disorder in the

Middle Ages—she immediately concocts a plan in which she can use the young man's illness for her own profit. She ignores the true nature of Calisto's ailment, offering her patient a counter diagnosis based on coital therapy.[25] Skilled at appropriating erudite as well as popular speech, she gives her patient a rationale for joining men and women sexually:

> [D]os conlusiones son verdaderas: la primera, que es forçoso el ombre amar a la mujer y la muger al ombre; la segunda, que el que veraderamente ama es necesario que se turbe con la dulçura del soberano deleite, que por el hazedor de las cosas fue puesto, porque el linage de los ombre se perpetuasse, sin lo cual perecería.[26]
>
> [And know, if you don't know it already, that these two proposi-tions are true: first, that of necessity man must love woman, and woman, man; second, that he who truly loves is necessarily troubled by the sweetness of that sovereign delight which was ordained by the Maker of all things in order to perpetuate mankind, and without which mankind would perish from the earth.[27]

Her justification is a close paraphrasing of one of the standard medical argu-ments that had been established, elaborated, and widely disseminated through-out the Middle Ages concerning the beneficial nature of moderate sexual intercourse. Constantine the African, for example, begins his treatise *De coitu* explaining:

> Creator volens animalium genus firmiter ac stabiliter perma-nere et non perire, por coitum illud ac per generacionem dis-posuir renovari, ut renovatum interitum ex toto non haberet. Ideoque complasmavit animalibus naturalia membra que ad hoc opus apta forent et propria, eisque tam irabilem vitutem et amabilem delectacionem inservit ut nullum sit animalium quod no pernimium delectetur coitu.[28]
>
> [Desiring the Creator that the animal kingdom persisted in a stable and sure form, and so that it would not perish, He estab-lished its renovation by means of coitus and reproduction so that through this renovation, the human race would not suffer complete destruction. For this reason He incorporated into the

nature of animals the necessary and appropriate members for this function and He infused in them such a worthwhile disposition and such an agreeable pleasure that there is not an animal alive who does not delight exceedingly in coitus.]

Despite her subaltern status, Celestina manipulates the same discourse as educated practitioners. But as the readers of *Celestina* learn, neither these words from the lips of Celestina, nor the drugs from her laboratory, ever produce a cure for Calisto's ailment. Rather, they lead him to his downfall and to his death. What is clearly suggested in *Celestina* is that unauthorized practitioners, despite their ability to speak like physicians and administer drugs like an apothecary, are so intrinsically flawed that their therapy can only result in pain and destruction.

If the works of educated men such as Jaume Roig and Fernando de Rojas have any relevance for the contemporary reader, it is in the way these works helped to foster deep-seated suspicions about a woman's ability to function as healer. Beneath the outrageous anecdotes and seemingly ridiculous descriptions of women who disease their husbands and clients lies a formidable argument against accepting women into the ranks of orthodox medical practice. Medical historians have noted that from the fifteenth century on there is an increased marginalization of women in authorized systems of health care. This is notably true in the area of obstetrics and gynecology, which for many centuries had been controlled almost exclusively by women.[29] Today the tensions between midwives and licensed obstetricians, and the complaints abut gender difference and sexual harassment within the domain of orthodox medical education, acknowledge the persistence of Roig's belief that it is risky business to allow that the materials of medicine and the authority to diagnose disease fall into the hands of women.

NOTES

1. For an overview of women healers in the Middle Ages see Monica Green's "Women's Medical Practice and Health Care in Medieval Europe," *Signs: Journal of Women in Culture and Society* 14 (1989): 434-72.

2. Luis García Ballester, Michael McVaugh, and Agustín Rubio Vela, *Medical Licensing and Learning in Fourteenth-Century Valencia* (Philadelphia: The American Philosophical Society, 1989), 30.

3. Nancy Siraisi, *Medieval and Early Renaissance Medicine* (Chicago: Univ. of Chicago Press, 1990), 17-21.

4. Pearl Kibre, "The Faculty of Medicine at Paris, Charlatanism, and Unlicensed Medical Practices in the Later Middle Ages," *Bulletin of the History of Medicine* 27 (1953).

5. Miguel Parrilla Hermida, "Apuntes históricos sobre el protomedicato: antecedentes y organismos herederos," *Anales de la real academia nacional de medicina* (1977): 477.

6. García Ballester, *Medical Licensing and Learning in Fourteenth-Century Valencia,* 59-61.

7. In other urban areas the number of trained practitioners was much lower. For example, in Barcelona during the fourteenth and fifteenth centuries there were on average less than two doctors for every ten thousand inhabitants. See Luis García Ballester, "Academicism versus Empiricism in Practical Medicine in Sixteenth-Century Spain with Regard to Morisco Practitioners," in *The Medical Renaissance of the Sixteenth Century* (Cambridge: Cambridge University Press, 1985), 247.

8. García Ballester, *Medical Licensing,* 21.

9. Ibid., 22.

10. Kibre, 8-11. Similar arguments were made in the defense of a German midwife in the early fifteenth century. Her defenders claimed that she had successfully performed seven Caesarean births in which both the child and mother remained alive and healthy. See Jaroslov Nemec, *Highlights in Medicolegal Relations* (Bethesda, Md.: U.S. Department of Health, Education, and Welfare, 1976), 23.

11. See discussion and accompanying documentation in volume 3 of Josep Almiñana Vallés's recent edition of Roig's *Spill* (1460; Valencia: Del Cenia al Segua, 1990), 842-56, 960-20.

12. Ibid., 910-16.

13. Unfortunately there is no English translation of the *Spill,* which Roig wrote in Catalan or Valencian. For readers of Spanish there is Ramón Miquel i Planas's translation, *Espejo* (Madrid: Alianza Editorial, 1987).

14. *Spill,* lines 4523-33, 4607.

15. Ibid., 4614-44.

16. Ibid., 8153-76.

17. Ancient and medieval deontological writings emphasize that the character of the physician is directly related to the effectiveness of his therapy. See Owsei Tempkin, *Hippocrates in a World of Pagans and Christians* (Baltimore: Johns Hopkins Univ. Press, 1991), 20-21.

18. Bernardo Gordonio [Bernard of Gordon], *Lilio de medicina,* eds. John Cull and Brian Dutton (Madison, Wis.: Hispanic Seminary of Medieval Studies, 1991), 119.

19. For a recent study of the social implications of "diseasing," see Doroth Nelkin and Laurence Tancredi, *Dangerous Diagnostics: The Social Power of Biological Information* (New York: Basic Books, 1989) and Troy Duster, *Backdoor to Eugenics* (New York: Routledge, 1990).

20. Alfonso Martínez de Toledo, *Arcipreste de Talavera o Corbacho,* ed. Michael Gerli (1466; Madrid: Cátedra, 1981).

21. Ibid., 188.

22. Trans. Lesley Bird Simpson, *Little Sermons on Sin: The Archpriest of Talavera,* Alfonso Martínez de Toledo (Berkeley: Univ. of California Press, 1959), 146.

23. We should keep in mind that this was a pathological condition that was recognized by medical theorists. Bernard of Gordon, for example, in book five, chapter thirteen of the *Lilio,* "De las passiones de la teta" [Of the Diseases of the Breast], explains that the abundance of breast milk was caused, if a woman had not recently conceived or given birth, by the retention of menses or a growing tumor (207-8).

24. Fernando de Rojas, *Celestina: Tragicomedia de Calisto y Melibea,* ed. Miguel Marciales (1498; Urbana: Univ. of Illinois Press, 1985).

25. See my article, "Calisto's Ailment: Bitextual Diagnostics and Parody in *Celestina,*" *Revista de estudios hispánicos* 23 (1989): 41-64.

26. *Celestina,* 43.

27. Trans. Leslie Byrd Simpson, *The Celestina: A Novel in Dialogue,* Fernando de Rojas (Berkeley: Univ. of California Press, 1955), 23.

28. Constantine the African, *De coitu,* ed. Enrique Montero Cartelle (12th century; Santiago de Compostella: Monografías de la Universidad de Santiago de Compostela, 1983), 77.

29. See Renate Blumenfeld-Kosinski, "The Marginalization of Women in Obstetrics," in her *Not of Woman Born: Representations of Caesarean Birth in Medieval and Renaissance Culture* (Ithaca: Cornell Univ. Press, 1990), 91-119. Also Myriam Greilsammer, "The Midwife, the Priest, and the Physician: The Subjugation of Midwives in the Low Countries at the End of the Middle Ages," *Journal of Medieval and Renaissance Studies* 21.2 (fall 1991): 285-329.

# WHERE HAVE YOU GONE, MARGARET KENNIX?

## Seeking the Tradition of Healing Women in English Renaissance Drama

WILLIAM KERWIN

> *I shall conjure him,*
> *And crucifie his crabbednesse: he's my Master,*
> *But that's all one.*
>
> —*Juletta,* The Pilgrim

**Charles Goodall's** early history of the Royal College of Physicians includes an eery outline of one woman's struggle to practice medicine in sixteenth
century London. A section devoted to recording "the colleges proceedings
against Empiricks and unlicensed Practisers" publishes a 1581 exchange of
opinions about the medical worthiness of one Margaret Kennix. Kennix, described by the college's records as "an outlandish, ignorant, sorry woman," herself never speaks. Presenting her case is Francis Walsingham, secretary of state
to Elizabeth I:

> Whereas heretofore by her Majesties commandment upon the
> pityful complaint of Margaret Kennix I wrote unto Dr. Sy-
> mondes then President of your Cellege and fellowship of Phisi-
> tions within the City, signifying how that it was her Highness
> pleasure that the poore wooman shoold be permitted by you
> quietly to practise and mynister to the curing of diseases and
> woundes, by the means of certain Simples, in the applieing
> whereof it seemeth God hath given her an especiall knowledge,
> to the benefit of the poorer sort, and chiefly for the better
> maintenance of her impotent husband, and charge of Family,

who wholly depend on the exercise of her skill: Forasmuch as
now I am enformed, she is restrained either by you, or some
other of your College, contrary to her Majesties pleasure, to
practise any longer said manner of mynistring of Simples, as
she hath doon, Whereby her undooing is like to ensue, unless
she maie be permitted to continue the use of her knowledge in
that behalfe. I shall therfore desire yo forthwith to take order
amongst yourselves for the readmitting of her into the quiet
exercise of her small Talent, least by the renewing of her complaint to her Majesty thorough your hard dealing toward her,
you procure further inconvenience thereby to your selfe, the[n]
perhaps you should be willing should fall out. Whereas con-
trariwise it will be well taken, that you afford her the like favour she hath found at the hands of your Predecesor.[1]

To this threatening endorsement of Kennix the leaders of the College reply
with polite but unflinching boldness, suggesting to Walsingham that he simply
needs a clearer grasp of the facts in order to change his position. They urge that
Kennix be "pited of all" but not "maintayned by others through medical practice," which would be a dangerous precedent violating the "holsome Lawes"
prohibiting practitioners outside of the College, as well as a threat to public
health. The College requests an audience with Walsingham to present their
case.

The outcome of this story is unknown. Perhaps Kennix was allowed the
"favour" of the College. Perhaps she was forced, like many others recorded in
official records and presumably many more besides, to practice clandestinely.
Or perhaps the College succeeded, and drove her away from healing altogether. Margaret Kennix's historical record, only a trace of one woman's story,
is emblematic of the stories surviving of most individual women healers
in early modern England—brief, filtered through official institutions, and
leaving personal history largely untold. The situation resembles what Monica
Green laments concerning women practitioners in the medieval period: "the
silence of the records for England is positively deafening."[2] Somewhere behind
the elliptical transcripts of Kennix's case, left to us solely in the polite conflict
of a politician and a professional governing body, were the lives of an active
woman, of the family she supported, and of the community she served. For
her, as for a wide array of other women, medical practice depended upon eva-

sion or challenge of authority. The leaders of the dominant medical culture usually saw women healers as foolish tricksters.

Given the paucity of the historical record, it is especially important to read the period's rich drama for signs of how people other than medical authorities imagined women healers. Unfortunately, because there are few plays by women from the Elizabethan or Jacobean eras to shed light on this group, we are left with a record of how male authors represent them, which brings to the forefront the symbolic meanings men made of women healers. Those staged women, though given lines by male playwrights and voices by male actors, also took their meaning from women, in both the theatrical space and the historical scene. The playhouses of the period had a sizable female audience and, as Jean Howard writes, "in the theatre women were licensed to look."[3] Plays offered them a very rare chance to see women challenge their officially sanctioned roles.[4] The plays I will discuss show such a challenge, in the form of women healers who continue to practice despite hostility and who reshape the social forces creating the experience of health and illness. The woman healer, in the eyes of the male author, becomes blurred with the surreptitious social reformer. The drama gives us a number of women combining these two roles, imagined in ways that counter the thrust of Tudor and Stuart antifeminist propaganda: some of the women are openly medical in the conventional sense, some are medical but forced to disguise their practice, and some provide an alternative definition of what the "medical" means. In all cases, their work makes them live perilously on the edges of society, but they maintain a powerful role in organizing the worlds in which they live. These characters create a dramatic type, one that has not been sufficiently noted, perhaps because the historical women healers in Tudor and Stuart England were forced to mask their medical work.

## Women Healers and the Historical Record

In the period traditionally given the celebratory label "the Renaissance"—in England, the sixteenth and seventeenth centuries—women who practiced physic or surgery were gradually driven into the shadows, and eventually lost their crucial role in the health care system.[5] But at the end of the sixteenth century they were still doing significant medical work: recent analyses of municipal records find sixty female practitioners in London in 1600, not counting midwives.[6] Historians have seriously challenged previously dominant assumptions about what these practitioners did, such as the belief that most were midwives or that they practiced almost exclusively on other women. Instead, it appears that their tasks included the treatment of men and children, as well as a wide variety of gynecological issues in addition to childbirth.[7] The Elizabethan poor laws often lead to the employment by parish officials of women healers.[8] These women were especially important in the provinces, where access to formally educated practitioners was restricted, but even in cities the relatively small number of physicians (only thirty for a London population of 200,000 in 1600) left open a market for the "wise" or "cunning" woman.[9] They often used techniques later spurned by modern science, such as the use of amulets and other religious elements, and they emphasized "simples," drugs made from a single source in nature. Women of higher social status also practiced medicine. In many homes health care was the charge of women, who—unlike the poorer "wise women" dependent upon oral transmission of knowledge—collected medical recipes and handed down collections of them from generation to generation. Numerous accounts of "the Good Woman" depict her caring for sick neighbors and sick poor.[10] Her methods ranged from humoral advice consonant with the philosophy of the most elite court physicians to amulets and rings worn prophylactically, and her work was grounded in a concern for diet.

Perhaps the most discussed part of women's medical practice in the period has been midwifery, which was in England dominated by women until the eighteenth century.[11] In the sixteenth and seventeenth centuries the practical knowledge and experience of midwives began to be challenged by the prestige and more theoretically and scientifically advanced knowledge of physicians and "man-midwives." Midwives tried to incorporate several times in an effort to protect their rights and improve anatomical training, but were never granted a charter, probably because the College of Physicians did not want their competition.[12] The gradual loss of power in this sphere was also connected to the rise of witchcraft trials and the fear surrounding them. Quite often elderly and poor, midwives were the group most in peril of being executed as witches.[13] The power of midwives over birth, and the fears that they would allow illegitimacy, abortions, or secret baptisms, contributed to their persecution.[14] Feared as transgressors in the realms of paternity, sexuality, and religion, midwives were magnets for a wide range of anxieties. Any practice deviating from rigorous orthodoxy could be interpreted as a sign of demonism.

This fear and persecution met not only midwives, but other female medical personnel as well. Records from the years of William Harvey's tenure as censor of the College show an increasingly vehement effort to eliminate female competitors.[15] A variety of factors other than witchcraft fears contributed to the decline of women healers. One was the rise of a market economy, because even as women began to take money for medical services, and thus professionalize activities formerly performed for free or as part of a barter exchange, they refrained from advertising or other public displays of their practice, not fully adapting to new market roles that required more explicit commercial behavior. The steady centralization of medicine also pushed women healers to the verge, as they were largely excluded from the growing formal training structures of physicians, surgeons, and apothecaries.[16] During plague time it was women who most often filled the role of "searchers," examining the sick and dead, and again their regulation reveals loss of independence. Like most women medical workers these searchers are ill-documented, but most of the evidence remaining is in the form of documents of control, including parish records stating that women who did not adequately perform their work would lose their pensions. Masked in their work, unnamed in the historical record, and under threat of economic disaster, searchers were central to plague practices but without organizational identity or power.[17]

An historical example provides evidence of the way women practitioners held a dual position in the popular imagination: both feared and needed, they were hunted by political authority, but also sought out by sufferers desiring care absent from more scientific medicine. John Stow's *Annales of England* relates the 1594 death of Ferdinando Stanley, the Earl of Derby. The passage has two oddly distinct sections. Stow first records Derby's final eleven days with detachment, describing physical symptoms (for instance, constant vomiting and the cessation of urination four days before death) and therapy (regular enemas, and catheterizing to provoke the flow of liquids). The tone of this passage is measured, describing and tabulating bodily events in exhaustive detail: "the number of his vomits were fifty-two and of his stools twenty-nine." After recording the April 16 death, Stow lists the doctors in attendance.

Then the annalist tells a second narrative, which returns to a point four days before the initial symptoms. Again, Stow proceeds chronologically, but this time with a different set of characters and a different sense of causality. The tone of this passage is a radical shift as well, from a listing of organic facts to a story-telling, implying that illness has several complicating levels of meaning. On April 1 Derby refused lodging to an old woman who claimed she was a seer. In the following nights he had terrifying dreams, and on April 5 fell sick. On April 10 a wax doll with Derby's hair was found, partly burnt and "twisted from the navel to the secrets." On April 12, at the same time that Derby stopped urinating, "a witch demanded" of one of his secretaries whether the Earl "still made water." Another "witch" was questioned about the illness, and was unable when asked to repeat the Lord's Prayer. A third woman was helping to treat Derby: "A homely woman . . . this wise woman (as they termed her) seemed often to ease his honor." She thought Derby was possessed and was blessing herbs as part of a response when she was "rated out of the chamber" by a physician, who also thought Derby was possessed but evidently wanted no help from this woman in treating his patient. Derby, sensing the end, discontinued medical treatment and prepared for death by praying with his wife and a few others. This second story, like the more scientific one preceding it, concludes with a list of actors: a roll call of the "spiritual physitians" who were in attendance for the final scene.[18]

To call this account "conflicted" would be both a colossal anachronism and a colossal understatement. Science and spiritualism existed side by side for all involved—the doctor believed in possession, and the more spiritual "wise woman" believed in drug therapy—so no one was trying to separate the two spheres completely. In fact, Stow as narrator, by deciding to tell the story twice from start to finish, separates the bodily from the spiritual more so than anyone else; perhaps as much as the persecuting College, this narrative method works against the viability of the healing woman. The earl's use of the phrase "spiritual physitian" for his religious counselors was a conventional description conveying the interrelatedness of medical and religious issues. Where conflict did exist, and to a great extent, was in interpreting causality. The first narrative follows roughly the same logic as a modern case history, trying to adjust the mechanism of the body; the second resembles a morality play, describing a Christian torn between the forces of God and Satan.

In the first narrative the characters are exclusively male, while the second is dominated by the threats and consolations afforded by women. In the latter, the earl's illness is implicitly connected to his refusal of charity to a homeless woman. The figure of a witch is present at every further stage of physical decline, and is connected to sexual threats (the twisted doll) and spiritual betrayal (the unspeakable prayer). But the "homely woman" is the only medical practitioner in either account who provides relief to the patient, as she "seemed often to ease" him. In the metaphor of the morality play, women are both good angels and bad, while the male practitioners seem to be neither, but part of a logic of a discreet body. In stark contrast to the method of the first narrative, the second never connects women practitioners with quantification, but with forces out of sight—things that surface in dreams, or spirits called from hell. The narrative because of either Stow's imagination or the evidence available to him, displaces the physical into the spiritual and psychological, and makes little attempt to see death in organic terms. For example, except for Derby's wife the women are all unnamed, as is the recipe being prepared by the wisewoman. The women are also associated with a different sort of interpretation than that of the physicians: the second account is much more connected to the meaning of Derby's life—of his connection to his community, and of his attempts to prepare for death. It goes beyond technical terms—the inductive method which will soon find theoretical defense in Bacon's new science—and attempts to incorporate other meanings in a broader model of medical narrative. Women healers are made into symbols of the spiritual and social sides of life—partly by their chosen activities, partly by the shaping forces of cultural limits and narrative decisions.

Stow's rigidly divided narratives point toward a general cultural pattern of pushing women healers outside the dominant medical discourse and into the symbolic role of a threatening other.[19] In the drama, we see history transformed into a two-sided tradition: women who on the one hand are feared or banished, but who on the other preserve a socially critical healing power.

## Mother Bombie and Helena: A Tradition of Women Healers

Conversion of women healings into symbols is a recurrent theme in the drama, and is so dependent upon male reshaping that it is unrealistic to expect to recover in the plays an antecedent historical reality. But symbols should not be dismissed as thoroughly unhistorical; rather, they're responses to history, reimaginings of social realities and social stereotypes. The ubiquity of the woman healer in early modern England means that a playgoing audience would recognize her on the stage and interpet her actions in some relation to her historical analogues.

A composite portrait of a woman healer emerges from the drama. First, she is a social outcast, and her medical practice places her in great danger because it threatens the vested interests of the community. Second, she has an oracular nature, serving as a medium to spiritual power, in contrast to a medical model that focuses therapy on the body. Third, she refutes specific parts of the Elizabethan and Stuart attacks on women practitioners, especially the supposed malevolence of medical unorthodoxy; she explicitly denies that traditional folk medicine is morally subversive. Fourth, she is remarkably skillful as an artist figure, stimulating the plots of the plays and often crafting reconciliations. And fifth, and most fundamentally, the woman healer attacks the social status quo. These five elements receive different emphases from different authors, but their recurrence demonstrates how evocative and central the image was. Even where the characters' actions exceed limited definitions of the medical, their acts of artistry, sedition or spiritualism are acts of diagnosis which cumulatively expand the historical heritage of women healers. Asserting a broad definition of health and illness, they help perpetuate an important cultural tradition which creates one version of the powerful woman.

John Lyly's *Mother Bombie* (1594[20]) places a woman healer in the center of a typical Elizabethan comedy. Three young couples in a Kent village protest the marriages planned by their autocratic fathers, and after a series of deceptions and recognitions are happily rearranged. Where in other comedies the couples go to a forest to work through their misalliances (as in *A Mid Summer Night's Dream* or *As You Like It*), Lyly's youths all make trips to Mother Bombie, who "will profess cunning for all comers" (II.iii.126-27). Either an historical figure or a folk character, Mother Bombie is referred to in fiction and nonfiction so repeatedly from the 1580s to the 1650s that she can safely be deemed a common emblem of a wisewoman.[21]

In Lyly's play she displays some of the few known characteristics of her historical village counterparts. She lives alone, she is old and—to young men—ugly. Characters come to her to have her interpet; one goes to seek a medicine to test virginity, a practice often associated with women healers. Another, Serena, repeats a local legend: "They say there is hard by an old cunning woman who can tell fortunes, expound dreams, tell of things that be lost, and divine of accidents to come. She is called the good woman who yet never did hurt" (III.i.31-35). Serena's faith in Mother Bombie, however, fades when the prophecies given seem unlikely: "These doggerel rhymes and obscure words coming out of the mouth of such a weather-beaten witch are thought divinations of some holy spirit, being but dreams of decayed brains" (III.i.57-60). Such a volatile shift shows the fragility of Mother Bombie's position, and other characters also quickly demonize her. In another scene, she defends herself bluntly:

> SILENA: They say you are a witch.
> MOTHER BOMBIE: They lie.

Or again:

> HALFPENNY: Cross yourselves; look how she looks.
> DROMIO: Mark her not; she'll turn us all to apes.
> MOTHER BOMBIE: What would you with me?
> RISIO: They say you are cunning and are called the good woman of Rochester.
> MOTHER BOMBIE: If never to do harm be to do good, I dare say I am not ill. But what's the matter? [III.iv.75-81]

This wisewoman repeatedly elicits and refutes cultural stereotypes. Mother Bombie fulfills few of the expectations of her visitants: she does predict the future, diagnose virginity, and help locate a lost spoon. Instead, she is resolutely moral, she chastizes the unchaste, and in arranging the *return* of changelings she reverses a behavior feared by the regulators of Elizabethan midwives. Her art is constructive, as she helps unravel the confusion of her village. Her final appearance, which perpetuates the revelations of the changelings and permits the happy marriages, involves her hearing a woman's confession and encouraging her to make it public; Mother Bombie goes beyond predicting the future and actually helps to arrange it. More than a mystical shaman, she is a community architect.

Probably the most often noted trait of Lyly's art is his sense of wit,[22] and Mother Bombie's verbal play suggests that women healers, as well as university humanist scholars, help construct that quality. Like the well-known Euphuism of Lyly's prose Mother Bombie's speech is balanced, but in a different way, stressing mystery and the dangers of pursuing a control of nature: "In studying to be overnatural, thou art like to be unnatural, and all about a natural. Thou shalt be eased of a charge, if thou thy conscience discharge, and this I commit to thy charge." (V.ii.19-22). The play on words, the parallelism, and the balanced structure echo Lyly's Euphuism, but her use of this rhetoric to undercut the assigned marriages belies a latent anarchism. Her role involves craftily returning people to more natural relations to each other. She helps foster the "art" of choosing marriage partners, which the irate fathers had branded as unnatural. As subverter of patriarchal designs, she directs the community back toward a balance that is free of their restrictions, which in some ways echo the historical restrictions on women practitioners. Far from being a completely marginal figure, she participates in one of the most central Renaissance debates when she finds her own way to reconcile Art and Nature. This cunning woman's cure centers on righting cultural imbalance, not on art separate from social arrangements.

Similarly, Helena in Shakespeare's *All's Well That Ends Well* (1603 or 1604), rebalances individuals' bodies as well as cultural disequilibrium. The daughter of a recently dead physician, Helena cures the French king of a fistula considered incurable by his court doctors. This specifically medical activity has for critics overshadowed her participation in the broader healing tradition of the wisewoman, which is brought out in the second half of the play, where she transforms her husband, Bertram, from a reluctant to a willing lover.[23] Shakespeare gives distinctive twists to the English tradition of the woman healer, as he does with most available material; most notably, Helena is young and fair, unlike the village wisewomen. But similarities lie below the surface.

Choosing to heal means risking death and enduring exile. If her therapy for the king fails, Helena agrees to endure absolute punishment:

> Tax of impudence,
> A strumpet's boldness, a divulged shame,
> Traduc'd by odious ballads; my maiden's name
> Sear'd otherwise; nay worse of worst, extended
> With vilest torture, let my life be ended. [II.i. 169-73]

This heightened isolation is one of Shakespeare's changes of his source. In the earlier version (a translation of Boccaccio into English in 1575 by William Painter), after her husband abandons her, Giletta (Helena's original) rules his land of Rossillion, and in fact does a better job than he has done: "shee like a sage Ladye, with greate dilligence and care, disposed his things in order againe, whereof the subjectes rejoysed very much."[24] Shakespeare leaves her largely powerless, and has Helena choose to depart France almost immediately on a pilgrimage. Shakespeare's deviation from the source not only adds his trade-mark dramatic compression, it also nudges his female character, in her isolation, closer to her historical English healing counterparts. This is a major change, in both its dramatic impact and its sociological alliances.

Another element in the woman healer's tradition helps give meaning to the structure of *All's Well That Ends Well*. This play has been often classified as a "problem play" because of, among other things, the perceived dissonance between two parts of the play, the healing of the king and the romance of Helena and Bertram.[25] But if seen within a tradition of healers whose cures involve social reform, integrating these two parts is less of a problem: in the structure of the woman healer's imaginative mission, physical healing is only the first of a series of increasingly wide-reaching changes. Like Mother Bombie, Helena works as a reorganizer of culture, and her role as healer blends into her work as priestess, reformer and artist. The play emphasizes that her work is of another order than the logic of scientific medicine. Helena, "Doctor She," relies upon much more than the cure given her by her father: her power lies in her "inspired merit" and her active break with popular faith in "the congregated college of physicians" who, despite being "embowel'd of their doctrine" have given up hope in the King's case. After the cure, onlookers speak wondrously of her success:

> LAFEW: They say miracles are past; and we have our philo-
> sophical persons to make modern and familiar, things super-
> natural and causeless. Hence is it that we make trifles of
> terrors, ensconcing ourselves into seeming knowledge when
> we should submit ourselves to an unknown fear.
> PAROLLES: Why 'tis the rarest argument of wonder that hath
> shot out in our latter times.
> BERTRAM: And so 'tis.
> LAFEW: To be relinquish'd of the artists—
> PAROLLES: So I say—both of Galen and Paracelsus.
> LAFEW: Of all the learned and authentic Fellows—
> PAROLLES: Right; so I say.
> LAFEW: That gave him our incurable. (II.iii. 1-14)

Helena rejects both Galenists and Paracelsians, repudiating the sphere in which the debate between them takes place. The men commenting upon this cure ascribe it to the category of "wonder," but Helena soon shows that she is much more than a magician or saint.

Helena's skepticism of the official medicine represented by the "authentic Fellows" (and one can hear in that phrase the same body that attempted to restrict Margaret Kennix) is a prelude to her undermining other social assumptions. One of them is that she is unworthy of marriage to a nobleman; another is that honor is gained through military and sexual conquests. The most basic social assumption she challenges is the issue of marital obedience and order: the supposed subjection of women to the wishes of men. Curing the king is only a first step toward transforming Bertram, just as a wisewoman's work with herbs provides her the status and connections she needs to influence the lives of her fellow villagers. Helena operates along a continuum of reform, one in which the miraculous cure of a king given up for dead is easier than forcing a man to treat her as an equal. Similarly, the play's so-called folk tale elements, the bed trick and the exchange of rings, are not just part of general folk tradition but also examples of a more specific heritage: the English wisewoman's ability to reveal secrets and rearrange people's affections. Mother Bombie's detection of a lost spoon and Helena's retrieval of Bertram's ring are not feats of equal importance, but they share the cunning of the mysteriously powerful local woman healer, who starts with objects and bodies and moves on to the rules governing social relations. By the end of the play she has helped reform Bertram and Parolles, creating a new ethos at the court of Rossillion.

Shakespeare moves the symbolism of the woman healer outward, to blur the distinctions between a wisewoman and any active woman, and to connect healing and sexual politics. Of course Helena can not be reduced to bearing the meaning only of this tradition—she has been cogently read as a commentary on theology, psychology, and love. Shakespeare has drawn upon an additional context and created in her a particularly ambitious and powerful way of imagining a woman healer.

### Jacobean Wisewomen: Healing a Corrupt World

The movement from powerlessness to authority continues to unite representation of women healers in Jacobean drama. Either as a cheat or as an exile, women in plays by Heywood and Fletcher are first seemingly exposed to suffering, but they later recuperate credibility and show an ability to mold cultural arrangements.

A more indirectly heroic portrait than Shakespeare's Helena appears in Thomas Heywood's comedy *The Wise Woman of Hogsdon* (1604). The un-named wisewoman at first seems to confirm some of the more dismissive evaluations of women healers, but eventually manages to orchestrate a grand scene of comic cleansing, so that despite being medically fraudulent she is a successful healer. The play deals centrally with the danger which reckless men, especially one Young Chartley, pose to the institution of marriage, and the house of the wisewoman becomes the locus for taming that danger.

This wisewoman's trade is dependent upon trickery, as she confesses to Luce, the young woman from the country whom Chartley has abandoned, and who, disguised as a boy, has taken a job as her servant. When visitors seek-ing help arrive, the old woman hides in a closet near her front door while Luce inquires what they seek; she then appears and seems to divine that informa-tion. Though illiterate she pretends to read in Latin books for the best cures for patients' troubles. In addition, she keeps rooms for prostitutes, and secretly delivers the babies of unwed mothers, afterwards dropping them at the doors of the prosperous. She herself tallies some of her tasks:

> Let me see how many trades have I to live by: first, I am a wise-
> woman, and a fortune-teller, and under that I deal in physic and
> fore-speaking, in palmistry, and recovering of things lost; next, I
> undertake to cure mad folks; then I keep gentlewomen lodgers,
> to furnish such chambers as I let out by night; then I am pro-
> vided for bringing young wenches to bed; and, for a need, you
> see that I can play the match-maker.
>   She that is but one, and professeth to many,
>   May well be termed a wise-woman, if there be any. [III.i][26]

This list of practices, many notorious, surely confirms the claims of those who regard wisewomen as corrupting and fraudulent, stagers of lies.[27]

But more happens upon this stage than cheating. The wisewoman's house also entertains and purifies, and the surreptitious presence of Luce allows us to be spectators to cathartic rearrangements. We witness a staple of Renaissance drama, the play within a play, as the wisewoman arranges the exposure of the rakish Chartley, the most outrageous abuser of women's trust. She directs his victims to hide in various side rooms to witness his lies in the main hall, and then one by one each appears to disprove them. Finally Chartley breaks down

105

and says, "This woman hath lent me a glass, in which I see all my imperfections" (IV.iv). Consistently the most virulent abuser of the wisewoman, and the most apt to call her a witch and threaten violence, he now sees her practice as a form of teaching folly. Again, as in *Mother Bombie,* the tradition of Renaissance humanism is conflated with the tradition of the woman healer, because the healer redefines true knowledge and its social utility. Chartley closes the play by addressing the wisewoman in terms reminiscent of *The Praise of Folly* or *Twelfth Night:*

> Nay, Mother Midnight, there's some love for you;
> Out of thy folly, being reputed wise,
> We, self-conceited, have our follies found.

Luce is reunited with Chartley, very much like Helena with Bertram. In the disguise of a servant, Luce has become a healer herself, manipulating her older guide. Together, they have become symbols of how even the most unscientific women healers could be seen as artists and reformers. In the pariah roles of wisewomen, they have reversed male control and created a new social order.

In Helena and Luce we have seen young women in exile, using the freedom of disguise to promote change. A similar journey is undertaken by Juletta, a supporting character in John Fletcher's *The Pilgrim* (1621). The play's two plots involve romance and Spanish politics. First, Alphonso, "an angry old gentleman" of Segovia, seeks to force his daughter Alinda to marry Roderigo; loving another, she flees to the countryside. Second, disputes between the governor and a group of outlaws terrorize the people. The drama displays the series of flights, disguises, and revisions of identity that end both familial and national conflict.

*The Pilgrim* is filled with the rhetoric of madness and healing. As is common in the period, Fletcher treats mental suffering as having both physiological and psychological causes and cures. Juletta, a maid to Alinda, sets the plot in motion by recommending a cure for sadness:

> Madam, I think a lusty handsome fellow
> If he be kind, and loving, and a right one,
> Is even as good a pill, to purge this melancholy,
> As ever *Galen* gave, I am sure more naturall:

106

And merrier for the heart, then Wine and Saffron:
Madam, wantone youth is such a Cataplasme. [I.i. 111-17][28]

Alphonso prefers a different mix of imaginative order and physical therapy:
"Let her observe my humor" (I.i.11), and again later:

Is she growne mad now?
Is her blood set so high? I'le have her madded,
I'le have her worm'd.[IV.i.17-19]

In ways much more complicated than this simple Galenic therapy, the
characters' journeys represent them all working through their illnesses. In the
two major settings of the play—a madhouse and a forest—characters have to
confront and change their identities. The strongest agent of that change is the
mercurial and explosive Juletta, one of the most striking women in Jacobean
drama.

As with other women healers I have presented, Juletta reaches deeper into
society in her reforming efforts as the play proceeds. She travels to the woods to
find her mistress, who had become "distracted" by fear, and helps her to recover. Together the two come upon Roderigo and Pedro, the outlaw leader and
Alinda's lover. Juletta and Alinda disguise themselves as old women, and use
their strangeness to minister to them: "They wonder at us; let's maintaine that
wonder" (V.iv.41). The lowly women who provoke wonder (also famously central to *The Winter's Tale*'s resolution) often employ medical language. Here,
Juletta and Alinda convince the two to repent, go to the city, confess, and reconcile with the civic authorities.

Again, healing depends upon reform, and again that reform involves de-
ception. A greater source of joy to Juletta than her healing of romantic and
political division is her successful tormenting of Alonso in punishment for his
mistreating his daughter. She leads him further and further into the woods:

All this long night
I have led him out o'th way, to try his patience,
And made him sweare, and curse; and pray, and sweare againe,
And cry for anger; I made him leave his horse too,
Where he can never find him more; whistled to him,
And then he would run through thick and thin, to reach me,

107

> And down in this ditch; up again, and shake him,
> And swear some certain blessings; then into that bush
> Pop goes his pate, and all his face is comb'd over,
> And I sit laughing: a hundred tricks, I have serv'd him:
> I'le teach his anger to dispute with women.
> But all this time, I cannot meet my Mistresse,
> I cannot come to comfort her; that grieves me,
> For sure she is much afflicted: till I doe,
>  I'le haunt thy Ghost *Alphonso;* I'le keep thee waking. [III.ii.3-19]

Later her treatment of him accelerates:

> I shall conjure him,
> And crucifie his crabbednesse: he's my Master,
> But that's all one. [IV.i.84-86]

She forges a letter that gets him committed to the madhouse, and instructs the keeper: "Let him want nothing, but his will" (IV.iii.198). By the end of the play this "will" has been broken, and Juletta vaunts over her victim, who "has had discipline," in his own initial Galenic image: "I am . . . just such another / As your old worship worm'd for running mad Sir" (V.vi.40, 106-7). She sounds like her contemporary Jacobean revengers, but it is still as wisewoman that Juletta draws her strength to take complete command, and she herself connects that wit to the healing woman tradition:

> I am anything,
> An old woman that tels fortune . . .
> I am anything, to doe her good. (V.vi.110-11,116)

She is a woman Prospero, remaking her society, but she operates from the wings of the stage, and of society, and her power depends not on magic or science but on her wit. That power is not the isolated privilege of one bold individual: Juletta points to the historical woman healer as a source of her authority.

The characters discussed in this essay can be envisioned in terms of other types of dramatic figures, including clowns, witches, revengers, patient women, and magi. But an important source for a pattern of strong female behavior, the actual healing women of England and their symbolic form on the stage, has been overlooked. To treat Helena as a type of "patient Griselda," or the Hogsdon wisewoman as a fraudulent witch, is to see through the eyes of the Renaissance antifeminist authorities, who imagined women only as either passive sufferers or active destroyers. Shakespeare gives Helena formidable and aggressive authority, and Heywood's wisewoman defies the College of Physicians' categories of quack and certified healer. These plays draw upon an historically powerful but persecuted group of women and give them important dramatic roles which define healing not predominantly as the treatment of discreet physical symptoms but as reform of a broad network of social relations and the identities that they produce. Not allowed to work in socially central institutions, the drama's women practitioners labor by indirection, and it is wrong to say that they primarily either endure or bewitch. The drama claims for them, and from them, an irrepressible reframing power.

NOTES

1. Charles Goodall, *The Royal College of Physicians of London* (London, 1684), 316-17.

2. Monica Green, "Women's Medical Practice and Health Care in Medieval Europe," *Signs: Journal of Women in Culture and Society* 14 (winter 1989): 410.

3. Jean Howard, "Scripts and / versus Playhouses: Ideological Production and the Renaissance Public Stage," in *The Matter of Difference: Materialist Feminist Criticism.* ed. Valerie Wayne (Ithaca: Cornell Univ. Press, 1991), 225.

4. Andrew Gurr, *Playgoing in Shakespeare's London* (Cambridge: Cambridge Univ. Press, 1987), provides descriptions of the audiences at the plays, and Howard discusses the social dynamics of playgoing for women.

5. In England, this restriction was produced by a variety of interconnected developments: the politics of Church reformation, which restructured acceptable women's roles, healing institutions, and ideas of personal salvation; the increased fear of witchcraft, often associated with midwifery; the growth of medical monopolies for physicians, barber-surgeons, and apothecaries; and the rise of a modern scientific body of knowledge surrounding chemistry, anatomy, and physiology, which women had little opportunity of studying. All these historical forces helped recast the roles women were allowed to play in medicine. A good overall survey, with fine bibliographical direction, is Betty Travitsky's introductory essay, "Placing Women in the English Renaissance," in *The Renaissance Englishwoman in Print: Counterbalancing the Canon,* eds. Betty Travitsky and Anne M. Haselkorn (Amherst: Univ. of Massachusetts Press, 1990). Two good histories of women and work in the period are Susan Cahn's *Industry of Devotion: The*

*Transformation of Women's Work in England, 1500-1660* (New York: Columbia Univ. Press, 1987), and Alice Clark's *The Working Life of Women in the Seventeenth Century* (London: Routledge and Paul, 1991), especially 253-85.

The best anthology I have come across of English women's writings in a broad spectrum of activities is Charlotte F. Otten's *English Women's Voices: 1540-1700* (Miami: Florida International Univ. Press, 1992). See especially the Introduction to "Part Five: Women Taking Charge of Health Care." Otten anthologizes seven women: Elizabeth Grey, Countess of Kent; Lady Margaret Hoby; Lady Anne Halkett; Mary Trye (a chemical physician); Jane Sharp; Elizabeth Cellier; and Elizabeth Clinton, Countess of Lincoln. Lucinda Beier's study of seventeenth-century illness experiences discusses Hoby as a case study of the woman healer: *Sufferers and Healers: The Experience of Illness in Seventeenth Century England* (London: Routledge and Kegan Paul, 1987), 218-23. Beier also notes the century's gradual exclusion of women from healing: "The evidence suggests that by the seventeenth century both the scope of activities of female healers and the respect generally accorded them was in decline" (211).

6. Margaret Pelling and Charles Webster, "Medical Practitioners," in *Health Medicine and Mortality in the Sixteenth Century,* ed. Charles Webster (London: Cambridge, 1979), 188. Pelling and Webster, with typical demographic exactitude, list the number of female practitioners found in historical records in London and Norwich (186-87, 222). They emphasize the diversity of the medical work women performed, and for Norwich provide a list of seven women who worked for the city corporation. Pelling also outlines medical workers in "Medical Practice in Early Modern England," in *The Professions in Early Modern England,* ed. Wilfrid Prest (London: Croom Helm, 1987), 90-129. Pelling argues that women healers were numerically the most significant healers in rural England. This is also the conclusion of Brian Nance regarding a particular region of England: "Patients, Healers and Diseases in the Southwest Midlands, 1597-1634," (Ph.D. diss., Univ. North Carolina at Chapel Hill, 1991). Finally, Harold J. Cook discusses the prevalence of women healers and the diversity of their practices (which included physic and anatomy) in *The Decline of the Old Medical Regime in Stuart London* (Ithaca: Cornell Univ. Press, 1986), 32-33.

7. Green's research on medieval healers provides a thorough rationale for expanding the sense of what women did.

8. See Cook, 32.

9. Pelling, 188. Wisewomen who played healing roles are not rare in the imaginative literature. Chaucer's Nun's Priest speaks in the voice of one:

> For Goddess love, taketh som laxatyf;
> . . . That both of colere, and of malencolye
> Ye purge you; and for ye shal not tarye,
> Thou in this toun is no apotecarie,

I shal myself to herbes techen you,
That shall be for your hele, and for your prow. [ll 123, 126-30]

And twice in Ben Johnson's *The Alchemist* mention is made of the traditional healing role of women. Epicure Mammon urges Dol Common not to marry and "learn / Physic and surgery, for the constable's wife / Of some odd hundred in Essex" (IV.i.132-34). The gull Drugger remembers a "good old woman" who "dwells in Sea-coal Lane, did cure me. / With sodden ale, and pellitory o' the wall; / Cost me but twopence" (III.iv.120-22). For Jonson, healing women are outside of the market and its distorting forces.

10. As Clark writes, "Every housewife was expected to understand the treatments of the minor ailments at least of her household, and to prepare her own drugs" (254). One particularly well-documented example is that of Lady Grace Mildmay. She was educated at home in "phisicke and surgerie," and often read in the popular *Herbal* of William Turner. After having married into a Puritan aristocratic Northamptonshire family, Mildmay kept a journal from approximately 1570 to 1617, which tells of a wide variety of medical activities. She regarded healing as part of her religious duty: "It is good sometimes to be alone and meditate, but it is also good to call on one's neighbors to comfort their souls and bodies." In a diary relating a wide-ranging number of activities, the recurrence of Mildmay's medical work attests to its centrality in her identity. For excerpts from her diary, and commentary, see Rachell Weigall, "An Elizabethan Gentlewoman: The Journal of Lady Mildmay, circa 1570-1617," *Quarterly Review* 215 (1911): 119-36. Londa Schiebinger provides a much broader angle on this topic in *The Mind Has No Sex? Women in the Origins of Modern Science* (Cambridge: Harvard Univ. Press, 1989), which discusses the entire history of women's roles in science, from the medieval to the modern.

11. The history of midwifery in England has been subject to considerable revision in recent decades. While J.H. Aveling's *English Midwives* (London: Hugh K. Elliot, 1872) provides valuable records, it never questions the control of midwives by such men as Peter Chamberlain. A shot across the bow of such optimistic history was fired in 1973 by Barbara Ehrenreich and Deirdre English in *Witches, Midwives and Nurses* (Old Westbury, N.Y.: Feminist Press, 1973). An evenhanded and rigorous study is Jean Donnison's *Midwives and Medical Men: A History of Inter-professional Rivalries and Women's Rights* (New York: Schocken Books, 1977), especially the introduction.

12. See Donnison, and Thomas G. Benedek, "The Changing Relationship between Midwives and Physicians during the Renaissance," *Bulletin of the History of Medicine* 51 (1977): 550-64.

13. Joseph Klaits writes, "Such poor old women were the prime targets for witchcraft allegations: evidence for France, England, and Switzerland shows an average age

between fifty-five and sixty-five for accused witches." *Servants of Satan: The Age of the Witch Hunts* (Bloomington: Indiana Univ. Press, 1985), 94.

14. Other social changes contributed: demographic shifts produced an increased number of poor women without a family to support them, and a changed religious climate apparently helped spur a dramatic increase in trials for infanticide. See Klaits; Cahn, chapter 2; and Thomas R. Forbes, "Midwifery and Witchcraft," *Journal of the History of Medicine* 17 (1962): 264-83.

15. Charles Webster has evaluated the record of Harvey's tenure and discussed the increased "suppression of medical practice by women"; one instance is the College's warning to one Susan Fletcher "to desist from her practice," as Webster writes, "that consisted primarily of treating sore breasts with a lotion comprising milk, white bread, and herbs" (8). "William Harvey and the Crisis of Medicine," in *William Harvey and His Age,* ed. Jerome J. Bylebyl (Baltimore: Johns Hopkins, 1978), 1-28.

16. See Cook, 23-33.

17. I am in debt for this information about searchers to Richelle Munkhoff and her unpublished paper, "Searchers of the Dead: Women, Surveillance, and the Plague in Early Modern England." Munkhoff argues that these women were treated as expendable by medical and legal authorities, and used as a necessary administrative link between the state and deadly infections.

18. John Stow, *Annales of England* (London, 1601), 1275-77.

19. The death of King James provides another example. Cecil Wall, a historian of apothecaries, tells the story:

> In his *Advancement of Learning* Bacon had freely criticized physicians and had dedicated his book to the King. James, it was said, held the same views. In his last illness, against the advice of Harvey and other orthodox physicians, he allowed Buckingham's mother to make trial of an "infallible" remedy, a plaster and posset which she had procured from an empiric named Remington who lived in Essex and claimed to have cured many agues. When Buckingham was accused of having poisoned the King, Harvey gave evidence before the House of Commons that the plaster had been applied in his presence, that he did not know what it was made of, but that he saw no ill effects from its use. Neither King James nor Bacon had hesitated to show their preference for the Apothecaries in their struggle with the College of Physicians.

Wall's focus is the apothecary, but his account demonstrates the centrality of women healers, practitioners not just for the poor but for a king. *A History of the Worshipful Society of Apothecaries of London* (London: Oxford Univ. Press, 1963), 39.

20. Exact dating for plays of this period is, of course, largely impossible. For the purposes of this essay, I have accepted the conjectural date established in each edition from which I quote.

21. John Lyly, *Mother Bombie,* ed. A. Harriette Andreadis (Salzburg: Salzburg Studies in English, 1975) 29-31, 243-48. The conjectural date, and all line numbers, are from this edition.

22. The most influential statement of this now conventional position is probably G.K. Hunter's *John Lyly: The Humanist as Courtier* (Cambridge: Harvard Univ. Press, 1962).

23. For dating and quotation lines, I follow *All's Well That Ends Well: The Arden Shakespeare,* ed. G.K. Hunter (London: Routledge and Paul, 1959). Note that the idea of the play as moving from two types of healing—from the physical to the spiritual—was put forward by David Bergeron, "The Structure of Healing in *All's Well That End's Well,*" *South Atlantic Bulletin* 27 (November 1972): 25-34.

24. *The Arden Shakespeare,* 148.

25. See for instance W.W. Lawrence, *Shakespeare's Problem Comedies* (New York: Macmillan, 1931). For a fuller discussion see Hunter's introduction to *All's Well That Ends Well.*

26. *The Best Plays of the Old Dramatists: Thomas Heywood,* ed. A. Wilson Verity (London: Vizetelly and Co., 1888).

27. Reginald Scot, *The Discovery of Witchcraft* (London: 1584), provides an example of Elizabethan suspicion of women healers. Scot denies that they are witches but also ridicules their work as being almost uniformly dishonest.

28. *Beaumont and Fletcher: Dramatic Works,* vol. 6, ed. Fredson Bowers (Cambridge: Cambridge Univ. Press, 1966).

# [6]

## THE BLUES, HEALING, AND CULTURAL REPRESENTATION IN CONTEMPORARY AFRICAN AMERICAN WOMEN'S LITERATURE

GUNILLA T. KESTER

*If the blues* is the most prominent and formidable artistic expression of African American culture it is likely that, wherever it plays a significant role, it highlights the issue of cultural representation. In this context, it is important to notice the striking role the blues or jazz play in many of the healing processes portrayed in contemporary African American women's novels. Images of women healing ill or injured women, or of women healing themselves, have become one of the central tropes in contemporary African American women's novels. Authors such as Gayl Jones, Alice Walker, Toni Cade Bambara, and Toni Morrison utilize the trope of healing to measure past and present oppression of women of color and to discuss what can and what cannot be healed, forgotten, or forgiven. Much focus is put on how healing can be accomplished. Some hurt, they say, is so distant that it cannot be reached; other hurt goes so deep that there may be no possibility of healing. But, based on the assumption that writerly versions of black music indicate a wider discussion of cultural belonging, the occurrence of the blues during the healing processes suggests that some pain can only be healed through a reconnection to the history of the African American community and culture.

The presence of the blues tends to take different writerly shapes. In many novels such as *Corregidora*[1] and *The Color Purple*,[2] it is both thematically and metaphorically inscribed. In these novels, where women learn to sing the blues and to confront paralyzing fear, anger, and pain, the blues, to quote Ursa Corregidora, helps them "to explain what cannot be explained" (56). In other novels, such as *The Salt Eaters,*[3] the inscription of the blues seems to both redeem the textual chaos and question the textual structure. The core status of the blues suggests a critique of western cultural forms in which, often, these novels partake. The struggle for cultural survival is cast in the dichotomous relationship between the black music and the western text. In these cases, healing often comes about at the expense of the text, as if, inextricably, the literary text is a part of the illness which must be overcome. Healing, then, seems surrounded by a certain ambivalence since its prize is silence and the end of the story.

Many contemporary African American authors have testified to the importance of African American music as a model for their own artistic aims in shaping and sharing the African American experience. Plumbing the depth of the complexity of this experience, Toni Cade Bambara says in an interview with Beverly Guy-Sheftall that "music is probably the only mode we have used to speak of that complexity."[4] Likewise, Alice Walker has talked of her attempts at doing in literature what the music already has accomplished. "I am trying to arrive at that place where black music already is; to arrive at that unselfconscious sense of collective oneness, that naturalness, that (even when anguished) grace."[5] Toni Morrison has written that "For a long time, the art form that was healing for Black people was music."[6] Discussing the blues as a matrix or a network for African American literature, Houston A. Baker Jr. suggests that the blues is, in Derridean terms, "the always already" of African American culture.[7] For women healing women, too, the blues becomes a central maieutic instrument, which seems necessary for the healing processes at hand. Derived from the Greek word for midwife [*maia*], the maieutic can be seen as that force which acts or performs as an agent without becoming or being the subject. Repeatedly, the blues provokes the pregnant situation and, like a good midwife, allows the processes of change to conclude in healing and constructive ways. Often as in *The Color Purple* and *The Salt Eaters,* it strengthens the black women's sense of community and reminds them to reconsider the value of their traditional cultural forms.

The most recent novel by the 1993 Nobel laureate of literature, Toni Morrison's *Jazz* (1992),[8] a story in which the process of healing is mainly to learn to accept the wounds and the scars and the craziness of the past, is also suggesting that the process of healing involves learning to live with and love oneself such as one is, regrets and lost loves and all. In order to arrive at such a moment, the narrator suggests, one needs not only a room of one's own and

115

good company, but one must also have the music. *Jazz* begins with a woman named Violet who lets all her birds out of their cages after her husband kills the young woman who was his lover. At the end of the novel, Violet buys a new bird at a good price because the bird does not want to eat. She tries to feed it new kinds of bird seed and she talks to it, but the bird looks behind her and refuses its food. Violet feels that the bird was sad already when she bought it, so she does not think that it misses company. "So if neither food nor company nor its own shelter was important to it, Violet decided, and Joe agreed, nothing was left to love or need but music. They took the cage to the roof one Saturday, where the wind blew and so did the musicians in shirts billowing out behind them. From then on the bird was a pleasure to itself and to them."(224). Healing then, the narrator of *Jazz* suggests, comes about through the active interaction with the blues as a majestic and maieutic vehicle that heals the sadness and the badness of life.

The blues of Ursa Corregidora, blues singer and character in Gayl Jones's first novel *Corregidora* (1975), becomes the central vehicle through which she can confront the tension between what is possible and what is impossible to heal. Ursa Corregidora is a young blues singer in Happy's Cafe when one night her husband starts a fight about her singing in public, and she falls down the stairs behind the cafe. In the hospital it turns out that she was approximately one month pregnant and that the doctors find it necessary to perform a hysterectomy. Childless and barren, Ursa feels that the hurt is located well beyond her individual female body, since it affects the lives of all four generations of Corregidora women. Ursa Corregidora is the offspring of a Portuguese plantation and slave owner who fathered Ursa's grandmother, who was his own daughter by her great-grandmother, a slave of African descent. How many generations, Ursa wonders, will have "to bow to his genital fantasies?" (59). And when can the female generations feel more a part of the genealogy of the great-grandmother than children of a perverse and evil man? Ursa had always thought that she was different from her grandmother and her great-grandmother until she sees a photo of old Corregidora and realizes that she, too, has him in her. "I realized for the first time I had what all those women had. I'd always thought I was different. *Their* daughter, but somehow different. Maybe less Corregidora. I don't know. But when I saw that picture, I knew I had it. What my mother and my mother's mother before her had. The mulatto woman" (60). Even though the crimes of the past are written onto and into their own bodies, the Corregidora women have created an oral tradi-

116

tion of telling these crimes to each new generation so that there will be proof of what happened. When the slave system was abolished the owners of the plantation burned all the papers and documents about what had happened there, so the only remaining records are in the stories that are passed on from generation to generation. Ursa's frustrated rage at her barrenness stems from her inability to live up to her great-grandmother's and grandmother's wish for her to make new generations and to pass on the evidence.

Ursa remembers how her great-grandmother used to sit her in her lap on the rocking chair and tell her again and again the stories of a Portuguese sea captain who became the owner of a big plantation where he used the female slaves as prostitutes already when they were children and how her great-grandmother became his favorite, his "gold piece" (10). The necessity to repeat these stories intrigues Ursa. "It was as if the words were helping her, as if the words repeated again and again could be a substitute for memory, were somehow more than the memory. As if it were only the words that kept her anger" (11). As in Gayl Jones's second novel, *Eva's Man,* much of the creative power in *Corregidora* comes from an intense scrutiny of the difference between living and telling, between knowing in your own flesh and knowing in your mind only. In *Writing the Subject,* I have suggested that the exploration of "the gap between living and writing, between an event and the story about it" forms the central issue in *Eva's Man.*[9] The life crisis depicted in *Corregidora* complicates this issue by making Ursa's body the carrier of the evidence of the horrors of the slave system and by showing, in the end, how much knowledge she really carries in her flesh. And the maieutic vehicle which forces this realization is the blues.

For Ursa has inherited more than the stories from her great-grandmother; she has also learned from the repetitions and her great-grandmother's rocking body, from the ways in which these stories were told.

> Great Gram sat in the rocker. I was on her lap. She told the same story over and over again. She had her hands around my waist, and I had my back to her. While she talked, I'd stare down at her hands. She would fold them and then unfold them. She didn't need her hands around me to keep me in her lap, and sometimes I'd see the sweat in her palms. . . . Once when she was talking, she started rubbing my thighs with her hands, and I could feel the sweat on my legs. (11)

117

Ursa learns to sing the blues from the way the stories were told to her and its deep connection to bodily expression and experience. Her mother says that all songs that are not devoted to the Lord are of the devil and that Ursa is singing her own destruction, but Ursa tells her that she can only sing "as you talked it, your voice humming, sing about the Portuguese who fingered your genitals. *His* pussy. 'The Portuguese who bought slaves paid attention only to the genitals'" (53-54). Quoting the words of her great-grandmother Ursa nonetheless erases the boundaries of the Corregidora women, addressing them all with a collective "you." Ursa's way of singing the blues is intimately connected to the way her great-grandmother told the stories and so her singing the blues becomes a new, different way of bearing evidence against Corregidora. But, just as for the great-grandmother the repetition of the words seemed to become more than the memory, the blues becomes more than the evidence of past crimes. It becomes a maieutic vehicle in her healing process.

Through the blues Ursa can mourn the loss of her unborn child, her body's barrenness, and what she describes as the smell of old Corregidora in her own body. But the blues is also presented as a vehicle for desire and transformation. Ursa says: "I wanted a song that would touch me, touch my life *and* theirs. A Portuguese song, but not a Portuguese song. A new world song. A song branded with the new world" (59). Through the blues Ursa learns to apply her great-grandmother's lesson: she had said that when the slave owners burned all the documents they could not burn what they had put into the minds of the people who were enslaved. She told Ursa that the women themselves had to "burn out what they put in our minds, like you burn out a wound" and leave only the scar to bear witness. Ursa's singing the blues becomes analogous to that process, and it takes place parallel to the scarring over of the surgical wound on her stomach.

But why does the blues have this healing power? Ursa's answer seems to be that it is rooted in her life experience of how hate and desire can mix just like her great-grandmother's and grandmother's stories were rooted in their experiences of hate and desire of and for old Corregidora. Ursa's blues goes beyond regurgitating and reproducing stories from a distant past. In her dreams Ursa talks to her old husband, the man she hates and desires, about her mother, who would never tell her own life stories, but merely repeat the stories from the past. Ursa fills the gap around her mother's missing genuine experience with desire because, as she puts it, "I would have rather sung her memory if I'd had to sing any" (103). In her mind, Ursa equalizes her mother's and her own experiences with men with those of the older generations. The exploitation of four generations of women by first the slave owner and then the various men trying to gain a sense of self-respect and influence by oppressing their women leads Ursa to a moment where she can conceptualize a real intimacy between hate and desire, violence and love. After some twenty years of singing the blues and living alone, she is able to accept her old husband Mutt back again.

In *Corregidora* the blues is a cultural and metaphoric representation of African American women's experiences and bodies. Performing as a maieutic influence, it erases the distance between body and experience and thus brings the experience back to the body and the body back to the experience. It seems to suggest that healing must be a process during which one can return to one's blackness and history through the body. The blues then becomes the female genealogy that Ursa has asked for and the main key to the structure of the text. *Corregidora* is structured on the principles of black music, so the conflict between the music and the text appears to be minimal. In her extensive study on oral tradition in African American literature, *Liberating Voices,* Gayl Jones maintains that the cultural difference between African American and European American traditions "revolves around a problem of meaning."[10] She writes that

> it was easier for Western critics to appreciate the innovations when they were taken up by the European American artists themselves, as in the syntactical aberrations of postmodernist literature and the literary-artistic claims of improvisational technique of certain contemporary Western writers. Yet even here, what African American tradition means by improvisational, that is, something informed by tradition and mastery of its techniques which allows the improvisational riffs, and what European Americans generally mean by it, that is, something "thrown together" or "tossed off," are quite different matters. [ 91]

The blues structure of *Corregidora* illustrates this difference between traditions of cultural expression and representation and could therefore be described as a return to the African American tradition rather than as a modernist or a postmodernist experimental explosion. *Corregidora* provides one of the few examples where the blues structure and textual structure seem to be reconciled and merge into a progressive moment of personal and cultural healing.

119

*Corregidora* illustrates the thematic and structural struggle for self-representation in African American women's novels and uses the blues as a feminine and healing strategy. Likewise, in Alice Walker's *The Color Purple* (1982), the blues marks a return to a black female community and its healing powers as well as an alternative structure for self-representation. In her collection of essays, *Living by the Word*, Walker writes that there is "no story more moving to me personally than one in which one woman saves the life of another, and saves herself."[11] One reason the black female community has such a strong influence on Celie, the main character in the book, is because it sharpens the choice of self-representation Celie must make as a significant part of her healing. Because *The Color Purple* juxtaposes the epistolary mode (with its long-standing western tradition) with the blues, it intensifies the issue of cultural choice. Celie, who writes her letters to a God she envisions as a white man, becomes increasingly aware of her isolation from a black female community when she meets Shug Avery, the blues singer. The meeting between the outwardly docile, frigid Celie and the wild, sexy Avery produces one of the most heartwrenching healing processes in contemporary African American women's writings, and because it shows that healing can only begin when women share the tradition of black cultural representation thematically inscribed as the blues, it centralizes the issue of cultural representation.

With her mother dead, her sister gone, and her children taken away from her, Celie struggles on without a female community to help, protect, and guide her. Well aware of the nature of her illness she writes in her letters to God about her inability to feel anything at all. Sexually and physically abused by the man she believed was her father, Celie had two children whom he gave away without telling her where they went. She is finally married off to a man with four children, whose wife died. Celie is good to her husband's children, but she writes that she cannot feel anything for them at all (37). When her husband beats her, she feels nothing. She describes how she tried to find an outlet for the anger she felt, but she could not get angry at her mother and she dared not get angry at the man she believed was her father because it was against the Christian beliefs she was brought up with. Unable to find any other outlet for her feelings, Celie internalizes her anger and frustration. "Then after a while every time I got mad, or start to feel mad, I got sick. Felt like throwing up. Terrible feeling. Then I start to feel nothing at all" (47). Celie can describe her condition, but she is too lonesome and ignorant to know how to heal herself. This situation begins to change when her husband brings home Shug Avery, who has become ill.

Shug's arrival initiates a clash between two cultural systems of representing experience. Celie has struggled to express her life in a series of letters which, since her sister's disappearance, she addresses to God, while Shug expresses herself through the blues. Celie had been attracted to Shug before her husband brought her home and, since she does not like him, she is not jealous of Shug's presence. She feeds and cares for the singer until she becomes stronger. Shug, however, thinks that Celie is ugly and this does not change until she begins to understand the nature of Celie's life and Celie gives her a song. When Shug becomes stronger, Celie washes and cares for the other woman's hair, combing it as if Shug Avery was a doll or her own lost daughter or her dead mother. The process of combing and braiding the hair brings back a sense of community, especially since it is an experience that Shug shares. She says to Celie that it feels "like mama used to do. Or maybe not mama. Maybe grandma" (57). This moment of shared experience is marked, in the text, with the blues, which changes Shug's focus from her own illness to Celie's. While Celie is combing Shug's hair, the blues singer begins to hum a song.

> What that song? I ast. Sound low down dirty to me. Like what the preacher tell you its sin to hear. Not to mention sing.
> She hum a little more. Something come to me, she say. Something I made up. Something you helped scratch out my head. (57)

When Shug gets well and sings in Harpo's bar, she dedicates this song to Celie who, in the meantime, has become increasingly aware of her feelings of love for the other woman. "I look at Shug and I feel my heart begin to cramp. It hurt me so, I cover it with my hand" (74). At that moment, Celie feels many things. She feels ashamed of how she looks and how she is dressed. She is jealous of Shug's love for her husband, and she wishes that Shug would love her, too, in the same way, and she feels proud that Shug named a song for her.

What Felipe Smith has called Alice Walker's "redemptive art" is a healing process which is initiated and marked in the text through the maieutic influence of the blues.[12] This redemption or healing is made possible through the influence of women on other women to claim their own sense of being, to become subjects in their own right, instead of following their men's every order or whim. Shug makes Celie feel like a person and shows her how to stand up for herself. She also encourages Squeek or Mary Agnes, Harpo's new woman, to sing the blues. Mary Agnes starts by singing Shug's songs, but she soon begins to make her own songs. Listening to her, Shug formulates the intimate connection between the blues and the body, which was also part of Ursa Corregidora's experience, when she tells Mary Agnes that "listening to you sing, folks git to thinking about a good screw" and she tells her not to be "too shamefaced to put singing and dancing and fucking together" (111).

James C. Hall has argued persuasively that Walker shows how destructive the traditional patriarchal Christianity has been to the community of African American women.[13] He maintains that when Celie recovers her sister's letters, which her husband had hidden from her, it is a turning point in the novel which inscribes the recovery of the hidden female lineage. Since initially Celie thinks of the blues as the devil's music, the singing of the blues complements this paradigm of symbolic reversal of Christian tradition. Celie's changing views of the music follow her changing views of her own body and her sexuality. She cannot like herself until she learns to see herself in terms which are culturally and traditionally hers. Celie's response to Mary Agnes when she sings the blues is in this context significant because metaphorically it emphasizes the healing forces of the blues. Celie writes that Mary Agnes's blues puts her "in the mind of a gramophone. Sit in the corner a year silent as the grave. Then you put a record on it come to life" (96). Like a good midwife the blues assists at the birth of the African American woman and her community.

In the Foreword to her impressive essay on writerly blackness and whiteness, *Playing in the Dark: Whiteness and the Literary Imagination,* Toni Morrison discusses the processes of healing cultural *malaise* and the different relationship white and black cultures have to black music.[14] Morrison mentions how Marie Cardinal, who later wrote *The Words to Say It,* first understood that she was suffering a major breakdown during a concert with Louis Armstrong. Cardinal also connected her mental state to her experiences with colonization in Algeria. These experiences positioned Cardinal to view black and colored people as both threatening and liberating; in her text they become, in Morrison's words, "markers for the benevolent and the wicked, the spiritual . . . and the voluptuous" (ix). Morrison remarks that her situation as a black writer and reader "in the wholly racialized society that is the United States" (xii) differs fundamentally from Cardinal's. She questions the consequences of jazz on the young white girl and the fundamentally different consequences of jazz on her, a black woman and writer. In this context I would like to speculate that one such difference lies in the reaction to the black music which, in African American fiction, consistently has a healing and calming influence rather than the disruptive and maddening impulses Cardinal experienced.

The dichotomous rhythm of order and disorder, health and illness, well-being and pain, has curious consequences for the status of the text. In Toni Cade Bambara's *The Salt Eaters* (1981), for example, a battle is raging for the health of one black woman, Mrs. Velma Henry, and through her for the surrounding African American community. Frozen stiff physically and icily paralyzed mentally, Velma is in the hospital after a suicide attempt. Faced with her unresponsiveness, the traditional western physicians in the hospital regard themselves as helpless, so they have called in the local healer, Minnie Ransom. Minnie in turn receives know-how and advice from Old Wife, an ancestral spiritual conjure woman. The collective of past and present spiritual women eventually succeeds in reaching Velma, and it is suggested that she herself has the sensitivity to become one of them. Interwoven with the struggle for Velma's soul is an altogether and literally speaking fabulous panorama of the African American community during and after the civil rights movement. Velma's experiences of marching and community work are interlaced with the experiences of poets, doctors, street people, dancers, bus drivers, carnival participants, waiters, nurses, and workers at the local chemical plant. The collision of various experiences, dreams, visions, and nightmares focuses the attention on the struggle for meaning and cultural survival, which is the main theme of this book. In *The Salt Eaters* every word seems to be written against the extinction of a threatened culture, indeed, against death itself; yet, paradoxically, the exorcism of paralysis and stasis coincides with the end of the text.

In this novel, western systems of structuring and writing experience are scrutinized and discarded. Karla F.C. Holloway discusses the importance of cultural ritual in the healing experiences of the black woman and how an alien culture's texts cannot provoke beneficial changes. "Cultural ritual is directly oppositional to the doctor's ineffectual presence. As an emblem of Western values, the clinical psychologist can only hover around the edges of Velma's healing (and the text itself), waiting for her release from Minnie's first phase. At the novel's end he is totally disabled, an event that signifies the West's inability to heal cultural loss. Neither it nor he can address the dissonance of cultural pluralism. This is the territorial province of the Other."[15] Her suggestion is that the epistemology and ontology of the West differ in such profound and fundamental ways from those of other cultures that in processes of cultural healing, the western systems of knowledge are more harmful than helpful. To strengthen this point, the novel partakes in many parallel cases of questioning the structural inscriptions of the West. For example, somebody has erased all the information from the computer system at the local chemical plant where Velma works. The consequences of this erasure of information remain untold. Instead, there are several discussions about the loss itself and the empty space where one kind of knowledge and structure once was, but nobody seems particularly bothered by it. The loss is a matter of indifference or irrelevance to the black community. This confrontation with the significance of western epistemes provokes a crisis in the text, however, since it is certainly culturally indebted to what it struggles against. The contradiction between health and text illustrates this crisis and suggests that the novelistic structure of *The Salt Eaters,* with its Virginia Woolf-like modernist prose, its disrupted chronology, and displays of stream of consciousness also could be alien to the culture it describes. If that is so, then it too necessarily becomes a part of what must be discontinued if health is to be restored. Once again this struggle for cultural representation and survival is cast in musical terms. Minnie describes her art of healing as a meeting with the blues. She knows that the sick and crippled patients who seek her art wear their illness like a badge saying that they are different and special. Her job is to dismantle this "lie" and to make them "downright familiar with their bodies, minds, spirits to just sing, 'Blues, how do you do? Sit down, let's work it out'" (108). Throughout the novel, the return of Velma's health is anticipated when Minnie can get her on the same wavelength, so to speak, and make her listen to the rhythm of the music.

*The Salt Eaters* weaves an unusually complex pattern of musical phrases. Some are inside the hospital, others are outside on the street. Some belong to Minnie and Velma, others to the people around them. The music provides a sense of communication and dialogue between the hospital room and the community outside in the imagined town of Clayborne, Georgia, and its movement suggests that healing will occur when the distance between the outside and inside disappears and this dialogue is closed. Inside the room Minnie Ransom asks Velma: "Are you sure, sweetheart, that you want to be well?" (3) and hums a song for her, "unconcerned that any minute she might strike the very note that could shatter Velma's bones" (4) Velma tries to resist the pull of the music and the question and Minnie's presence: "her whole purpose was surface, to go smooth, be sealed and inviolate" (5). Velma's condition is similar to Celie's because she too has "down cold the art of being not there when the blow came" (4) and to withdraw "the self to a safe place where husband, lover, teacher, workers, no one could follow, probe" (5). Velma's condition puzzles Minnie and she discusses it with her spirit guide, Old Wife. She asks the spirit guide what is wrong with the new generation of women. "If they ain't sticking their head in ovens and opening up their veins like this gal, or jumping off roofs, drinking charcoal lighter, pumping rat poisons in their arms, and ramming cars into walls, they looking for some man to tear his head off" (43-44). In response to this madness, Minnie is looking for "some music to get it said" (46). "These crazy folks need some saying-it music" (47).

Minnie and the spirit guide set up some music for Velma to dance to, and the rest of their relationship is described in terms of resisting or following the music. In the first breakthrough during the healing session, for example, Minnie is still humming and Velma is still avoiding her frequency. "Velma's frequency was lowering as she danced away from the humming toward music of an earlier moment, the radio by the bed. . . . Velma's frequency sharper as she drifted back toward Minnie's humming. And they met somewhere in the air near the window, Minnie and Velma, pulling against each other and then together, then holding each other up out of the fall, holding each other stable on stools" (102-3). While Velma spins and sinks deeper into the music, she begins to listen to the talking drums.

During slavery, black music was mostly encouraged by the white slave owners with the exception of the "speaking" or "talking" drums, which were considered dangerous because they supposedly inspired insurrection. At the end of *The Salt Eaters* Velma is listening to some talking drums but, claiming ignorance, she is resisting their message: "I can't read drums, so how do I know they're saying 'barrier dropping'?" (250-51). The talking drums literally teach Velma to signify, to start naming things her own way and to claim both her heritage and her future. She names the giants "in their terrible musicalness" her teachers because they are "ready to speak the unpronounceable. On the stand with no luggage and no maps and ready to go anywhere in the universe together on just sheer holy boldness" (265). When Velma lets go of all the past bitterness, she frees herself and she experiences her rebirth as a kind of tabula rasa where the texts of personal as well as racial history have been erased and reclaimed in tunes that cannot and will not harm her.

The blues is probably the most striking and characteristic literary image for healing and self-healing among women in contemporary African American women's novels. It figures as the most powerful maieutic vehicle in the healing processes of all the female characters discussed. The image of the blues as a feminine and healing force suggests several things. First, it illustrates the historical depth behind most of the problems still facing African American women today. Second, it suggests that the African American women's community has survived thanks to the strength of their creativity and vision. But most importantly, it indicates the connection between cultural self-representation and cultural survival.

NOTES

1. Gayl Jones, *Corregidora* (Boston: Beacon Press, 1975). All subsequent references to this novel will be given in the text parenthetically.

2. Alice Walker, *The Color Purple* (New York: Washington Square, 1983). All subsequent references to this novel will be given in the text parenthetically.

3. Toni Cade Bambara, *The Salt Eaters* (New York: Random House, 1981). All subsequent references to this novel will be given in the text parenthetically.

4. Roseanne P. Bell, Bettye J. Parker, and Beverly Guy-Sheftall, eds., *Sturdy Black Bridges: Visions of Black Women in Literature* (New York: Anchor, 1979), 237.

5. John O'Brien, ed., *Interviews with Black Writers* (New York: Liveright, 1973), 204.

6. Mari Evans, *Black Women Writers 1950-1980* (New York: Anchor Books, 1984), 340. Toni Morrison, "Rootedness: The Ancestor as Foundation," 339-45.

7. Houston A. Baker Jr., *Blues, Ideology, and Afro-American Literature: A Vernacular Theory* (Chicago: Univ. of Chicago Press, 1984), 3-4.

8. Toni Morrison, *Jazz* (New York: Alfred A. Knopf, 1992). All subsequent references to this novel will be given in the text parenthetically.

9. Gunilla Theander Kester, *Writing the Subject:* Bildung *and the African American Text* (New York: Peter Lang, 1995), 84.

10. Gayl Jones, *Liberating Voices: Oral Tradition in African American Literature* (Cambridge, Mass.: Harvard Univ. Press, 1991), 91.

11. Alice Walker, *Living by the Word: Selected Writings, 1973-1987* (San Diego: Harcourt, 1988), 19.

12. Felipe Smith, "Alice Walker's Redemptive Art," *African American Review* 26 (3): 437-51.

13. James C. Hall, "Toward a Map of Mis(sed) Reading: The Presence of Absence in *The Color Purple*," *African American Review* 26 (1): 89-97.

14. Toni Morrison, *Playing in the Dark: Whiteness and the Literary Imagination* (New York: Random House, 1993). All subsequent references to this work will be given in the text parenthetically.

15. Karla F.C. Holloway, *Moorings and Metaphors: Figures of Culture and Gender in Black Women's Literature* (New Brunswick, N.J.: Rutgers Univ. Press, 1992), 125-26.

# Part 2

# THE EMERGENCE OF PROFESSIONALISM

# [ 7 ]

# WOMEN DOCTORS IN GREECE, ROME, AND THE BYZANTINE EMPIRE

HOLT N. PARKER

*Our sources for knowledge* about women doctors in antiquity are fragmentary: a few passing mentions in classical authors, some scattered references in the medical writers, nearly forty inscriptions.[1] We have no biographies, no details of their training, no specifics of their practice. Yet even from these fragments we can piece together some sort of picture, and the most important feature to emerge is simply that these women *existed.* The history of women as professionals in medicine does not begin in America in 1849 with Dr. Elizabeth Blackwell (1821-1910), the first woman to earn an M.D. in modern times; nor in Naples in 1422, with Costanza Calenda, the first woman we know of to receive a doctorate in medicine from a university;[2] nor in Naples in 1321, with Francesca de Romana, the earliest woman we currently know to have been licensed to practice medicine generally,[3] nor in Catania in 1276, with Virdimura, a Jew and wife of a Doctor Pasquale, who was licenced to practice on paupers,[4] but extends back to at least the fifth century B.C. in Greece.[5]

Second, the very nature of the evidence tells us something. There is no list of women doctors from antiquity, no direct comment on their existence as a class.[6] The very scattering of the facts shows that the Greeks and Romans did not consider the presence of women doctors to be in itself remarkable. Women physicians, though undoubtedly only a small percentage of the medical personnel, were an everyday part of the ancient world. This is shown clearly by the earliest source attesting to the existence of women doctors in Greece. Plato, in the *Republic,* whose fictional date is around 421 B.C.,[7] argues that for

131

the good of the state jobs should be assigned to people on the basis of natural aptitude. There may be physical differences between individuals, but they should be ignored if they are irrelevant to carrying out the proper functions. Thus a bald man and a long-haired man can be equally competent cobblers. The only important differences are those of the soul or mind. Plato then goes on to make a radical proposal: since the soul has no sex, in theory at least, some women may be found who would be suitable for most difficult job of all, that of the guardian who rules the state. To support his argument, he uses the following example (*Rep.* 454d2): οἶον ἰατρικὸν μὲν καὶ ἰατρικὴν τὴν ψυχὴν [ὄντα] τὴν αὐτὴν φύσιν ἔχειν ἐλέγομεν [So we meant that a man skilled in medicine (*iatrikos*) and a woman skilled in medicine (*iatrikê*)—in respect of their minds—have the same nature],[8] and a few paragraphs later (455e6-7): ἀλλ᾽ ἔστι γὰρ οἶμαι, ὡς φήσομεν, καὶ γυνή ἰατρική, ἡ δ᾽ οὔ, καὶ μουσική, ἡ δ᾽ ἄμουσος φύσει [As we said, one woman is skilled in medicine (*iatrikê*), another is not; one is skilled in music by nature, another is not]. It is important to note here that Plato is not arguing for the existence of women doctors, nor hoping to convince people that there *ought* to be women doctors. Rather, he is supporting his argument, almost in passing, for the role of women in the ideal state by pointing to something everyone could already see in the current state—that there were female doctors as well as male. Pomeroy summarizes (1978: 500) "Plato did not have to prove women's aptitude for the medical profession. On the contrary, his case rests on the actual existence of female physicians in the Athens of his own day, when the profession of physician was the only occupation available to women that was respectable and yet not banausic, and that required advanced formal education."

*Terminology*

Plato attests to female physicians as a matter of course for the end of the fifth century B.C., and our earliest inscription is not much later. The ordinary Greek term for midwife, that is, a woman whose practice was normally confined to aid in childbirth, is *maia* (μαῖα). Besides midwives, the Hippocratic writings refer to women helping at birth under the nonce formations of ἀκεστρίδες [healers] (Hp. 8.614.8) and ἡ ὀμφαλητόμος [umbilical cord cutter] (Hp. 8.106.7); we also find a woman described as ἰητρεύουσα [treating medically] (8.142.13; see Lloyd 1983: 60 n. 6, 76 n. 22). Beginning however, around the end of the fifth and during the fourth century, we find the Greeks making clear reference to female doctors and making the same distinction we do between midwives and doctors. Thus, the first woman doctor we know by name is Phanostrate (1; c. 350 B.C. from Acharnai in Attica), who is called on her gravestone "midwife and doctor" [μαῖα καὶ ἰατρός], simply using *iatros,* the regular Greek word for doctor. Phanostrate thus boasted that she was not merely a midwife but offered other medical services as well, services which entitled her to be called a doctor.[9]

The Greek language itself attests to the existence of women doctors. The regular word for a woman doctor in the inscriptions, papyri, and most literature is the specifically feminine ἰατρίνη (variously spelled), with a feminine nominal suffix, formed in the same way as the Italian *dottor-essa.* However, a number of grammarians argued that the only proper Attic form was simply ἡ ἰατρός (as attested by Phanostrate),[10] while the comic poet Alexis (c. 375-275 B.C.) used the form ἰάτρια (fr. 318). Therefore to translate ἰατρίνη as "midwife," "sage-femme," "Hebamme," or the like is prejudicial and misleading.[11] It is simply the feminine of ἰατρός and means "doctor, female." Between the midwife and the doctor was the ἰατρόμαια (*iatromea* in Latin), who appears to have been a midwife who had undergone some extra form of specialized training and education.[12]

For Rome the normal word for a midwife was *obstetrix,* literally "she who stands opposite/who faces."[13] The normal Latin word for "doctor" was *medicus* and it has a feminine form, *medica.*[14] Again, therefore, it is important to realize that a woman who called herself a *medica* was making a claim to offer more services than just midwifery.[15]

Roman literature also attests to women doctors as a matter of course. For example, Martial (c. A.D. 40–c. 104), on his way to make a dirty joke, mentions women doctors: The young wife of an old man claims that she is suffering from hysteria and needs the standard regimen, that is, intercourse.[16] And so, Martial writes (11.71.7), *protinus accedent medici medicaeque recedunt* [immediately the male doctors arrive and the female doctors depart].[17] Again, note that the existence of women doctors is taken for granted; they are simply part of the backdrop to the joke. Similarly in Apuleius (b. A.D. 123; *Met.* 5.10), one of Psyche's evil sisters complains that she has to deal with the smelly poultices and bandages of her old husband, playing the part of a *medica* not a wife; here, clearly a *medica* is not merely a midwife. The commentator Donatus (fourth century A.D.) says that in a scene of Terence (c. 190-159 B.C.; *And.*

481) one can see "the usual manner of a male or female doctor on coming out a patient's house."[18] Female doctors were clearly as much a part of daily life in the Roman Empire as they were for Greece.

### Status and Training

We can begin with one of the women doctors we know most about: Antiochis (3) of the city of Tlos, a moderate-sized town in Lycia. A statue base, dated to the first half of the first century B.C. reads: "Ἀντιοχὶς Διοδότο[υ] Τλωὶς μαρτυρηθεῖσα ὑπὸ τῆς Τλωέων βουλῆς καὶ τοῦ δήμου ἐπὶ τῇ περὶ τὴν ἰατρικὴν τέχνην ἐνπειρίᾳ ἔστησεν τὸν ἀνδριάντα ἑαυτῆς" [Antiochis of Tlos, daughter of Diodotus, commended by the council and the people of Tlos for her experience in the doctor's art, has set up this statue of herself]. Though brief, this inscription tells us a number of things. First, her father is almost certainly the Diodotus known from the *Materia Medica* of Dioscorides (first century A.D.; praef. 2), who cites him as an authority. Antiochis was therefore the daughter of a famous physician and like many learned women of the past probably received her first encouragement and education from her father. Second, Antiochis received high official honors from her city. Such awards were made only to those who had been recognized by a vote of the city as public benefactors. This honor and the general reference to the doctor's art probably indicates a citywide medical practice, not necessarily then confined to women, certainly not confined to childbirth.[19] Comparison to similar inscriptions shows that she might have held the office of city physician. Such doctors were appointed by the city, paid a regular fee, and given exemption from taxes and other public duties.[20] Third, she was rich. Such statues were usually allowed only to major civic benefactors, and the donor not infrequently specified the cost. In addition, we are lucky enough to know more about Antiochis from other sources. Galen (13.250, 13.341) cites Asclepiades of Bithynia (first century B.C.), who quotes her as an authority for treatment of diseases of the spleen, dropsy, sciatica, and arthritis. Galen also says (12.691) that the famous doctor Heracleides of Tarentum (first century B.C.) wrote a book on hemorrhages from the nose for Antiochis. We find Antiochis treated not merely as an equal by her fellow male doctors but as a recognized authority who was involved in the scholarship and practice of contemporary medicine at the highest levels.

Antiochis also demonstrates many features of the medical profession of antiquity, which differed in a number of ways from our modern system. One important factor is that the social standing of physicians varied greatly. While many were free, some coming even from the highest levels of society, others, especially in the Roman west, were slaves or former slaves.[21] The women of the earlier Greek and Hellenistic inscriptions were probably free, as most likely were all those cited as medical authorities. Antiochis (**3**) and Aurelia Alexandria Zosime (**7**), whose statues were erected, were probably wealthy. Metilia Donata (**32**), who paid for the construction of an important public building at Lyon, certainly was. Of the women we know from Roman imperial inscriptions, Asyllia Polia (**19**), (Vibia) Primilla (**25**), the unknown woman from Metz (**28**), Metilia Donata (**32**), and Scantia Redempta (**33**) were freeborn; Minucia Asste (**13**), Venuleia Sosis (**14**), Iulia Sophia (**16**), Restituta (**18**), and Iulia Sabina (**24**) were freedwomen; Sentia Elis (**15**), Sarmanna (**34**), Terentia Prima (**22**), Iulia Saturnina (**26**), Valeria Berecunda (**30**) and Valia Calliste (**31**) must have been free or freedwomen (more likely the latter, since none uses the formal filiation that indicates freeborn status); Iulia Pye (**20**) and Flavia Hedone (**23**) are uncertain but both are likely to have been imperial freedwomen; Melitene (**12**), Secunda (**17**), and the anonymous (**22**) were slaves; the status of the others is unknown.[22]

Second, there were no medical schools as such, no licensing body, no central authority. There was no standardized curriculum. Centers of medical education grew up in Cos, Cnidus, Alexandria, Rome, Pergamon, Smyrna, Ephesus, and elsewhere in proximity to the great libraries, but the primary form of education was an apprenticeship with other doctors, and the profession of medicine often descended in families.[23] Most inscriptions for (male) doctors say nothing about their training. For women doctors, however, besides Antiochis, we know that Restituta (**18**) was educated by her former owner, Claudius Alcimus, "doctor to Caesar." Pantheia (**5**) was the wife of a physician (whose father was a physician), as were Aurelia Alexandria Zosime (**7**), and Auguste (**41**). They may have received their training independently or from their husbands. As a mark of her learning, the funerary relief of Mousa (**2**) shows her with a scroll in her hand.

Though some form of education was required,[24] in practice doctors were those who called themselves doctors. More important, doctors were those acknowledged by their communities to be doctors.[25] This would have been in part informal, but in the Roman Empire, with the status of doctor went a number of civic honors and responsibilities. For example, Julius Caesar granted citizenship to all doctors practicing in Rome (46 B.C.; Suet. *Jul.* 42) and Vespasian (A.D. 75) granted them immunity from taxation. In practice this means that "it was still presumably up to the town council or the governor to declare who was a doctor" (Nutton 1977: 201). The public honors given to Antiochis (**3**) are an indication not only of her status as a doctor but as an exceptional doctor. Similarly, the statue erected to Aurelia Alexandria Zosime (**7**) "because of her medical knowledge," by her husband Asclepiades, undoubtedly also a doctor, points to high civic status. The highest status of all is accorded Auguste (**41**), who is praised "for having cured many who were sick in their bodies" and is called *arch-iatrinê* that is, "chief doctor," a title reserved for the highest rank of civic approved doctors. She shared that honor along with her husband, Aurelius Gaius, called *arch-iatros*.[26]

Later in the Byzantine Empire, we have clear evidence for women doctors with public responsibilities but in this case confined to practice on women (**42**). The twelfth-century *Typikon* [charter] for the great Pantocrator Hospital in Byzantium provides for a separate women's ward, supervised by two male doctors, who were aided by one female doctor [*iatraina*] and eight other women of lesser degrees within the medical guild: four women registered assistants, two women extra assistants, and two women servants. The woman doctor was subordinate to the two male doctors and paid only half their salary.

### Practice

It is likely, though we cannot know for certain, that the practice of many women doctors was primarily concerned with women's diseases and childbirth.[27] However, the examples of medieval and Renaissance Europe should warn us against too easy an assumption of a limited practice.[28] Phanostrate's (**1**) claim to be both doctor and midwife might point in this direction. For Rome, the tombstone of Iulia Saturnina, a *medica* (**26**), shows an infant in swaddling bands. The passages of Donatus and Martial discussed above also assume that a *medica* will be dealing mostly with women. Galen (8.414.8) speaks of *iatrinai* being consulted in cases of hysteria and examining the uterus digitally (8.425.1-2). Later, Leo the Physician (fourth century A.D.) speaks of male doctors using female doctors as intermediaries in vaginal examinations (*Consp. med.* 6.16.4); Palladius (fourth and fifth centuries A.D.;. *Historia Lausiaca* 68.3.5) speaks of a monk who helped a woman give birth as taking the place of an *iatrinê*; and Pseudo-Alexander of Aphrodisias (post fourth century A.D.; *Prob.* 2.64.8) speaks of an evil *iatrinê* attempting to hurt a woman who has just given birth. Finally, the law code of Justinian (*Cod.* 6.43.3.1; A.D. 531) considers *medicae* to be primarily *obstetrices*. In disputes over inheritance, slaves are to be evaluated but specially trained slaves have a higher price: *exceptis . . . medicis utriusque sexus . . . medicos autem et obstetrices sexaginta* [with the exception of . . . doctors of either sex. . . . Doctors and midwives (are to be evaluated) at 60 *solidi*].[29]

However, there are many indications of a wider practice. The civic honors accorded to Antiochis, Aurelia Alexandria Zosime, and Auguste, all point to a citywide practice.[30] The epitaph for Domnina (**6**) from her husband also points to a extensive practice: "No one of men will say that you died, but rather that the immortals snatched you away because you delivered your fatherland from disease." We do not know exactly what services Domnina provided,[31] but they appear to have extended to more than gynecology. Likewise, the tribute to Pantheia of Pergamum (**5**) from her doctor husband, Glycon, also seems to indicate a practice comparable to his: "You raised high our common fame in the art of medicine, and even though a woman, you did not fall short of my skill." Geminia (**29**) is called the "savior of all through her knowledge of medicine"; Iulia Saturnina is praised as "the best doctor"; and Scantia Redempta (**33**) is "outstanding in the discipline of medicine."

Also pointing to a wider medical practice is a large number of women whose writings are cited by other medical authorities. Five authors quote from the writings of women for therapies and drug recipes (and so give them their *termini ad quem*).[32] Here too the very nature of the evidence tells us something, for Pliny the Elder (A.D. 23/4–79), Galen, Pseudo-Galen, Aetius (c. A.D. 550), and Paul Aegineta (A.D. 625–90) quote the opinions and recipes of male and female doctors indiscriminately, moving from one to the other and back again. The women are not singled out, either for praise or blame, nor are their opinions privileged.[33] As with the male doctors, these encyclopedic works usually just give extracts from the authority's writing. There is seldom any information about biography or status. Pliny labels Salpe (**46**) and Sotira (**47**) as *obstetrices*, and their recipes seem to point to a level of practice closer to folk medicine. The rest, however, appear to be of the same status as the male physicians with whom and by whom they are quoted, and cover a similar range of preparations and complaints: panaceas, hematogogues, and abortifacients; diseases of the spleen and anus; dropsy, sciatica, arthritis, ulcers, suppuration, stomachache, impetigo, mange, as well as gynecological problems. Olympias (**45**) may perhaps have supplied her works with medical illustrations (the evidence, however, is very uncertain). Kleopatra[34] (**49**) is cited only for cosmetics (and a system of weights and measures), but cosmetics were an important and standard part of male medical practice and writing as well.[35] Most extensively quoted is Aspasia (**54**), by Aetius in his book on gynecology.[36] She is quoted as an authority on care during pregnancy, sickness during pregnancy, abortion, causes of difficult delivery, care after embryotomy, suppression of the menses, displacements of the uterus, and uterine ulcers. Even surgery, at least gynecological surgery, may not have been impossible for a woman to practice. Aspasia discusses venesection and surgery for hemorrhoids of the uterus, external edemous tutors of the labia, and for varicose hernia of the labia.[37]

### Metrodora

Besides these brief quotations, there has come down to us, in a single manuscript, the earliest surviving work by a woman doctor.[38] She is named Metrodora (**55**). Metrodora mentions no names, apart from saying that a cosmetic was used by "Berenike called Kleopatra" (a confused reference in the text), and cites no authorities. We can date the text only in the most general way to the span of the second to fourth centuries A.D. plus or minus a century on either side.[39] Medical language is uniform and of little aid in dating, but there is nothing in the text inconsistent with such a date.

Here I can provide only a sketch of this remarkable work.[40] The title, "From the Works of Metrodora," indicates a selection from a corpus of at least two books. Only one, however, has come down to us, headed "Concerning the Feminine Diseases of the Womb."[41] It contains sixty-three chapters and falls into seven basic sections, showing a well-planned organization—unlike their model, the Hippocratic works, which are fairly haphazard.

Metrodora begins with a general statement about the womb as the source of most of women's numerous diseases and treats hysteria and the movable womb, drawing in several places very closely on the Hippocratic *Diseases of Women*. She then deals with general conditions of the womb: first, a fairly lengthy theoretical and clinical chapter on inflammation; then suppuration, hardness, cancer, discharges, hemorrhages, prolapses, "coldness," and inflation of the womb. Next comes a section on diseases caused by excessive moisture: dropsy, cleansing of ulcers, and recipes to restore the appearance of virginity.[42] She then moves on to aids to conception (both generally and for female and male children), cures for sterility, and three recipes for contraception. These recipes contain some magical elements, though there are no spells or prayers. The original text may have had a section on drugs for abortion, but the text is damaged at this point. Then comes a brief section on childbirth, covering drug therapy with recipes to ease birth. There follows a group of magical recipes: various tests for fertility and virginity, aphrodisiacs and love potions, all of which were a standard part of medicine at the time. She next deals at greater length with diseases of the breasts. She includes cosmetics as a regular part of medicine and ends with recipes for incense, a common ingredient in many drug preparations.

It is important to note what Metrodora does not cover and what it implies about her status and practice. There is no mention of obstetrics, though there are a few recipes for drugs to ease childbirth. Her focus is entirely on pathology. Metrodora then was not confined to midwifery; indeed, she ignores it as apparently lying outside the range of medicine as she defined it. In this she follows Hippocrates and most of the doctors except for Soranus.[43] Instead, her writing covers the full area of medical practice, with the exception of surgery (for which see the comments on Aspasia [54] above).

Metrodora shares material and language with all her predecessors, including Soranus. She is, however, more than a mere anthologist in the style of Oribasius or an encyclopedist in the style of Aetius. She is an interesting figure in the history of medicine for reasons independent of her gender. Of particular importance is the fact that she does not depend on the growing secondary literature of the handbooks. Galen quotes from, comments on, and argues with Hippocrates throughout his works, but the later doctors—Oribasius, Aetius, Paulus, Alexander—though they know and have studied the Hippocratic writings, approach them, if at all, only through secondary sources. Metrodora, on the other hand, reaches directly back to Hippocrates, quoting, paraphrasing, looking for symptoms missed by other doctors.

Metrodora takes sides in several medical controversies over symptomatology and etiology. She formulates an individual classification of various vaginal discharges, a hotly debated topic. Besides an active engagement in the debates of her day, she makes several contributions to theory and etiology which are, as far as we know, original (for example, linking certain vaginal discharges to irritation of the adjoining rectum produced by intestinal worms). In therapy, though some of her compounds are shared with other authors and are part of the common stock of ancient medicine, the vast majority appear only in her work. All of these are indications of individual scholarship of a high level, backed by experience. In clinical practice Metrodora employs both digital examination and the vaginal speculum, providing a detailed description of pathology based on its use. In Metrodora's work we catch a glimpse of a remarkable woman: a practicing physician who was a scholar of the literature of her field and made original contributions to physiology, etiology, diagnosis, and treatment.

Beginning at least as early as the fifth century B.C. in Greece, women doctors have been part of the history of the western world. They had the same forms of training and education as male doctors. They called themselves doctors and were accepted as such by their communities. Their practice included gynecology and obstetrics but was not limited to these. Several achieved considerable social standing and high civic honors. Others wrote medical works which were used and cited by their male contemporaries. Even from such scattered evidence we can catch glimpses of a group of remarkable women: professional, literate, well educated, who were part of, and added to, the grand tradition of medicine.

## SOURCES

### Literary or Inscriptional Evidence for Individual Women

#### Greece and Asia Minor

1. Phanostrate, μαῖα καὶ ἰατρός. Achamai in Attica. c. 350 B.C. *IG* II².6873; Kaibel 1878: no. 45; Peek 1955: no. 342; Pleket 1969: 9 (no. 1); Conze 1893-1922: no. 340; Firatli and Robert 1964: 176; Berger 1970: 192, 410; Pomeroy 1977: 58-60, Pomeroy 1978: 499-500; Kampen 1981: 71 (fig. 63); Lefkowitz and Fant 1992: 266-67 (no. 376).
2. Mousa, *iatrinê*. Istanbul. II/I cent. B.C. Istanbul Museum no. 5029; Pfuhl and Möbius 1977: I, 151 (no. 467); Firatli and Robert 1964: 96-97, 175-8 (no. 139, pl.

XXXV). Daughter of Agathocles. Shown with a book-roll in her hand indicating her learning.

3. Antiochis. Tlos in Lycia. I cent. B.C. *TAM* II, 595; Firatli and Robert 1964: 175, 178; Pleket 1969: 27-28 (no. 12); Benedum 1974; Korpela 1987: 160 (no. 28); Lefkowitz and Fant 1992: 264 (no. 369). Daughter of Diodotus, who was "awarded special recognition by the council and the people of Tlos for her experience in the doctor's art" [ἐπὶ τῇ περὶ τὴν ἰατρικὴν τέχνην ἐνπειρίᾳ]. Cited by Galen 13.250, 13.341 for cures for diseases of the spleen, dropsy, sciatica, and arthritis; 12.691: Heracleides of Tarentum writes a book on hemorrhages from the nose for her. Dated to I cent. A.D. by Pleket (followed by Lefkowitz and Fant), but the citations by Asclepiades and Heracleides are decisive for a date in the first half of I cent. B.C.; see Benedum 1974.

4. Anonyma, *iatrinê*. Israel. I cent. A.D. Josephus, *Vita* 37; mentions a "Josephus, the (female) doctor's [ἰατρίνης] son."

5. Pantheia. Pergamum. II cent. A.D. Peek 1955: no. 2040; Fränkel 1895: no. 576; *IGRR* IV.507; Wilhelm 1932: 75, 84 = 1977: 100, 111; Firatli and Robert 1964: 175; Pleket 1969: 32-33 (no. 20); Lefkowitz and Fant 1992: 265 (no. 373). Her husband, Glycon, a doctor, set up an inscription for his father, Philadelphus, also a doctor, and for his wife; it reads in part: "You raised high our common fame in the art of medicine [καὶ κλέος ὕψωσας ξυνὸν ἰητορίας], and even though a woman, you did not fall short of my skill."

6. Do[mnina]. Neoclaudopolis in Asia Minor. II/III cent. A.D. Peek 1955: no. 1486; Wilhelm, 1932: 76-84 = 1977: 100-111 (who restored the name); Pleket 1969: 38-39 (no. 26); Firatli and Robert 1964: 175; Lefkowitz and Fant 1992: 265 (no. 373). Set up by her husband; reads in part: "No one of men will say that you died, but rather that the immortals snatched you away because you delivered your fatherland from disease" [πάτρην ῥυομένην νούσων].

7. Aurelia Alexandria Zosime. Adada in Pisidia (Karabaulo). Date uncertain. Sterrett 1888: 302-3 (no. 424); *IGRR* III.376; Firatli and Robert 1964: 175. Public statue set up by her husband Aurelius [Ponto]ni[a]nos Asclepiades, undoubtedly a doctor, "because of her medical knowledge" [ἀπὸ ἐπισ[τή]μης ἰατ[ρι]κ[ῆ]ς].

8. Anonyma, *iatrinê*. Oxyrhynchus, Egypt. III cent. A.D. *P. Oxy.* 1586.12: in a private letter to his wife, a man mentions that "the doctor [ἡ ἰατρίνη] sends you her greetings."

9. Treboulia, *iatrinê*, Ancyra in Galatia. Date uncertain. Mordtmann 1874: 21; Domaszewski 1885; 124 (no, 84); Firatli and Robert 1964: 178.

10. Anonymous, *iatrinê*. Tomis. Imperial epoch. Firatli and Robert 1964: 178; text (untranscribed) at Tocilescu 1887; 59 (no. 111).

11. Empeiria, *iatrinê*. Cios in Bythinia. Date uncertain. Husband Gaius Iulius Bettianus. Empeiria is a work name, meaning "experience." *CIG 3736;* Firatli and Robert 1964: 178.

## Rome and the Latin West

**12.** Melitene, *medica*. Rome. I cent. B.C./I cent. A.D. *CIL* VI. 6851; Gummerus 1932: 23 (no. 29); Korpela 1987: 163 (no. 42); Lefkowitz and Fant 1992: 265 (no. 372d). Slave of Apuleius.

**13.** Minucia Asste [Aste], *medica*. Rome. I cent. B.C./I cent. A.D. *CIL* VI.9615 (33812); Gummerus 1932: 36 (no. 112); Korpela 1987: 163 (no. 43); Lefkowitz and Fant 1992: 265 (no. 372b). Freedwoman of a woman.

**14.** Venuleia Sosis, *medica*. Rome. I cent. B.C./I cent. A.D. *CIL* VI. 9617; Gumemrus 1932; 36 (no. 114); Korpela 1987: 163 (no. 44); Lefkowitz and Fant 1992 1992: 265 (no. 372c). Freedwoman of a woman.

**15.** Sentia Elis, *medica*. Verona. I cent. B.C./I cent. A.D. *CIL* V.3461; Gummerus 1932: 73 (no. 273). Either free or a freedwoman, probably the latter. She entered the quasi-legal slave-marriage called *contubernium,* while one or both of the partners were still slaves (Treggiari 1991: 52-54). Her husband, C. Cornelius Meliboeus, also bears a typical freedman's name. Contra Le Gall 1970: 128 n. 4 who labels her free; listed as freedwoman by Kampen 1981: 116 n. 40.

**16.** Iulia Sophia, *medica*. Anacapri. Early I cent. A.D. *Epigraphica* 34 (1972) 141; *AEp.* 1972: 83; Rowland 1977: no. 437. Freedwoman of Isidorus, a freedman of Tiberius.

**17.** Secunda, *medica*. Rome. I cent. A.D. *CIL* VI. 8711; *ILS* 7803; Gummerus 1932: 26 (no. 42); Korpela 1987: 179 (no. 140). Husband, almost certainly, is the Titus Claudius Celer mentioned on the same tombstone. Slave of Livilla, the sister of the Emperor Claudius.

**18.** Restituta. Rome. I cent. A.D. *IG* XIV.1751; *CIG* 6604; *IGRR* I.283; *IGUR* 675; Gummerus 1932: 43 (no. 146); Korpela 1987: 166. Sets us a tombstone for Claudius Alcimus, "doctor to Caesar," "her patron and professor" [καθηγητής]. *CIL* and Gummerus rightly conclude that Restituta was Claudius' freedwoman and his pupil in medicine. Korpela doubts this, though it is difficult to see what else the text could possibly mean. She offers no argument nor any explanation of what καθηγητής would mean.

**19.** Asyllia Polia [Polla], *medica*. Carthage. I cent. A.D. (pre-Flavian). *CIL* VIII. 24679; Gummerus 1932: 82 (no. 316). Free; daughter of Lucius Pollus; buried in the necropolis devoted to imperial officials; her freedman, Euscius set up the monument.

**20.** Iulia Pye [Phye?], *medica*. Rome. Prob. late I cent. A.D. *CIL* VI.9614; Gummerus 1932: 36 (no. 111); Korpela 1987: 178 (no. 135); Lefkowitz and Fant 1992: 265 (no. 372a). Uncertain: possibly freeborn or imperial freedwoman: the name and the lack of filiation point to the latter; free or freed according to Günther 1987: 106; claimed as free by Le Gall 1970: 128 n. 4.

**21.** Anonyma, *medica*. Rome. I/II cent. A.D. *CIL* VI.8926; Gummerus 1932: 28

(no. 59); Korpela 1987: 185 (no. 176). Inscription is damaged; her name and that of her "husband" are missing. An imperial slave, "married" to another imperial slave or freedman; listed as *incerta* by Kampen 1981: 116 no. 40.

**22.** Terentia Prima, *medica*. Rome. I/II cent. A.D. (Flavian). *CIL* VI.9616; Gummerus 1932: 36 (no. 113); Korpela 1987: 190 (no. 203); Lefkowitz and Fant 1992: 264 (no. 371). Free or freedwoman. She has her own freedwoman; claimed as freedwoman by Le Gall 1970: 128 n. 3, Kampen 1981: 116 n. 40, Günther 1987: 105.

**23.** Flavia Hedone, *medica*. Nîmes. I/II cent. A.D. (Flavian). *CIL* XII.3343; Gummerus 1932: 88 (no. 343); Rémy 1984: 126 (no. 5). Probably an imperial freedwoman; claimed as free by Le Gall 1970: 128 n. 4.

**24.** Iulia Sabina, *medica*. Osimo (Auximum), Italy. I/II cent. A.D. *CIL* IX.5861; Gummerus 1932: 56 (no. 203). Freedwoman; husband, Q. Iulius Atimetus.

**25.** (Vibia) Primilla, *medica*. Rome. II cent. A.D. *CIL* VI.7581; *ILS* 7804; Gummerus 1932: 24 (no. 32); Korpela 1987: 200 (no. 256); Lefkowitz and Fant 1992: 264 (no. 370). Free. Daughter of L. Vibius Melito (unknown) and wife of L. Cocceius Apthorus (unknown); listed as *incerta* by Kampen 1981: 116 n. 40.

**26.** Iulia Saturnina, *medica*. Emerita, Spain. II cent. A.D.? *CIL* II.497; *ILS* 7802; Gummerus 1932: 84 (no. 323); Praised as *medicae optimae* [the best doctor]; husband, Cassius Phillipus. The tombstone shows an infant in swaddling bands. Free or freed; claimed as free by Le Gall 1970: 128 n. 4.

**27.** Anonyma, *ia]tromae(ae)*. Rome. II/III cent. A.D. *Bullettino della Commissione archeologica comunale di Roma* 90 (1985) 278 (no. 17); Korpela 1987: 203 (no. 267). Possibly a slave, but the inscription is too fragmentary to be certain.

**28.** Anonyma, *medica*. Metz, Germany. II/III cent. A.D. *CIL* XIII.4334; Gummerus 1932: 91 (no. 358); Kampen 1981: 157 (Catalogue III.52). Free; though damaged, the inscription preserves traces of a filiation.

**29.** Geminia. Avitta Bibba, N. Africa. c. III cent. A.D. *CIL* VIII.806; Gummerus 1932: 79 (no. 295); on a statue base. Called *salus omnium medicine* [*sic*] [savior of all through her knowledge of medicine]. Status uncertain.

**30.** Valeria Berecunda [Verecunda], *iatromaia*. Rome. III/IV cent. A.D. *CIL* VI.9477; *ILS* 7806; Gummerus 1932: 29 (no. 62); Korpela 1987: 205 (no. 280). Called, *iatromeae regionis suae primae* [the premier doctor-midwife of her region]. Free or freed: rightly Günther 1987: 105; claimed as free by Le Gall 1970: 128 n. 4. Husband, P. Gellius Bitalio [Vitalio] (unknown).

**31.** Valia [Valeria?] Calliste, *iatromea*. Rome. III/IV cent. A.D. *CIL* VI.9478; Gummerus 1932: 29-30 (no. 63); Korpela 1987: 205 (no. 281). Probably freedwoman: Günther 1987: 106 (free or freed); claimed as free by Le Gall 1970: 128 n. 4. Husband, Caecilius Lusimach{ich}us.

**32.** Metilia Donata, *medica*. Lyons; Date uncertain. *CIL* XIII.2019; (not in Gummerus); Rémy 1984: 138-39, no. 18; Rougé 1982; Jackson 1988: 191 n. 4. Large stone block for some important civic monument which she "put up at her own expense." Almost certainly free.

**33.** Scantia Redempta. Capua. IV cent. A.D. *CIL* X.3980 (cf. p. 976); *ILS* 7805; *ILC* 615; Gummerus 1932: 61 (no. 218). Praised as *antistis disciplin[ae in] medica* [outstanding in the discipline of medicine]. Free. Daughter of Flavius Terentius and Scantia Redempta; married, but her husband's name does not appear.

**34.** Sarmanna, *medica*. Gondorf, Germany. Early Christian? *Bonner Jahrbücher* 140/141 (1936) 456; *AEp.* 1937: 17; Rowland 1977: no. 410. Monument erected by her son, Pientius Pientinus, and daughter-in-law, Honorata.

**35.** Aemilia Hilaria. Bordeaux. Late IV cent. A.D. Aus. *Parent.* 6.6. Maternal aunt of the poet Ausonius (d. c. A.D. 395), who praises her as *more virum medicis artibus experiens* [trained in the medical arts as well as any man].

### Byzantine

**36.** Sôsanna, *iatrinê*. Athens. Byzantine period. *IG* III.2.3452 (p. 242); Bayet 1878: no. 6; Firatli and Robert 1964: 177; Mentzu-Meinaire 1982: 437 (no. 86).

**37.** Basilous, *iatrinê*. Korykos, Cilicia. Byzantine period. *CIG* IV.2.9164; *MAMA* III.269; Firatli and Robert 1964: 177; Mentzu-Meinaire 1982: 437 (no. 87).

**38.** Thekla, *iatrinê*. Seleuceia. Cilicia. Byzaqntine period. *CIG* IV.2.9209; Firatli and Robert 1964: 177; Mentzu-Meinaire 1982: 437 (no. 88).

**39.** Amazone, *iatrinê*. Byzantium. Byzantine period. Firatli and Robert 1964: 177. "Faithful servant of God, pleasing to God and man."

**40.** Stephanis, *iatromaia*. Korykos in Cilicia. Byzantine period. *MAMA* III.292; Firatli and Robert 1964: 176; Mentzu-Meinaire 1982: 437 (no. 89).

**41.** Auguste, *archiatrine*. Gdanmaa in Lyconia (Çesmeli Zebir). IV-VI cent. A.D. *MAMA* VII (1956) 566; Firatli and Robert 1964: 177; Nutton 1977: 198, 219 (no. 24). Chief civic doctor [ἀρχιειάτρηνα] along with her husband, Aur[elius] Gaius. She is praised for having "cured many who were sick in their bodies."

**42.** Anonyma, *iatrinê*. Byzantium. XII cent. A.D. Gautier 1974: 10, 11, 13; text: 85 (lines 942-3), 101 (lines 1198-99); see also Miller 1984: 60-61 (who mentions the woman assistants but not the woman doctor). The twelfth-century *Typikon* for the Pantocrator Hospital in Byzantium provides for a separate women's ward, supervised by two male doctors, who were aided by one female doctor [ἰάτραινα], four women registered assistants [ὑπούργισσαι ἔμβαθμοι], two women extra assistants [ὑπούργισσαι περισσαί], and two women servants [ὑπηρέτριαι]. The woman doctor was paid half the amount of the male doctors.

## Women cited as medical authorities

(3) Antiochis.

**43.** Elephantis: Pliny *NH* 28.81 (abortifacients; with Lais [44], as authority for book 28; Gal. 12.416 (cosmetics).

**44.** Lais: Pliny *NH* 28.81 (abortifacients; with Elephantis [43]), 28.82 (hydrophobia and malaria cured by amulet with menstrual blood; with Salpe), as authority for book 28.

**45.** Olympias of Thebes: Pliny *NH* 20.226 (abortifacient), 28.246 (pessary), 28.253 (sterility), cited as authority for books 20-28. She is perhaps the Olympias of Heraklea, credited in the MS of Soranus (Par. graec. 2153, 218v, *Pinax* 45) with sending a gynecological illustration to Cleopatra the Queen; see Burguière, Gourevitch, and Malinas 1988: lxii-lxiii; Hanson and Green 1994: 987.

**46.** Salpe, *obstetrix:* Pliny *NH* 28.38 (medical uses of saliva), 66 (medical uses of urine), 82 (see Lais [44], 262 (aphrodisiacs); 32.135 (hair removal; *obstetrix*), 140 (magic: preventing dogs from barking), as authority for book 28 and 32.

**47.** Sotira, *obstetrix:* Pliny *NH* 28.83 (menstrual blood for malaria), as authority for book 28.

**48.** Aquilia Secundilla: Gal. 13.976, 1031: A plaster called the *neopolitos* for various diseases.

**49.** Kleopatra (not the Egyptian queen; the name is a common one): Gal. 12.403-5 (*Cosmetics:* mange), 12.432-34 (*Cosmetics:* hair loss), 12.446 (her work coupled with that of Heracleides), 12.492-93 (*Cosmetics:* quote of recipes for dandruff and other diseases); Paul. 3.2 (οὐλοποία καὶ βάμματα τριχῶν ἐκ τῆς Κλεοπάτρας οὐλοποιῶν: a work on hairdressing); Aetius 8.6 (2.408.18-21 CMG: body lotion); *Anec. Oxon.* 3.164.14 (ἡ κομμωτικὴ Κλεοπάτρας τέχνη, perhaps a title); Ps.-Gal. 19.767-771 (= Hultsch, *Metrologicorum scriptorum reliquiae* 1864-6/1971: 233-36; Κοσμητικά: weights and measures). the late antique/medieval manuscript tradition of a Latin *gynaecea* attributed to the Egyptian Cleopatra, which I am in the process of editing, is unconnected to this tradition.

**50.** Eugerasia: Gal. 13.244 (pastille for spleen and dropsy).

**51.** Origeneia: Gal. 13.58 (recipe to cure ulcers and suppuration), 85 (hematogogue), 143 (pill for stomach ache).

**52.** Samithra: Gal. 13.310 (diseases of anus).

**53.** Xanite: Gal. 13.331 (impetigo and mange).

**54.** Aspasia: Aetius 16.12 (care during pregnancy), 15 (sickness during pregnancy), 18 (abortion), 22 (causes of difficult delivery), 25 (care after embryotomy), 50 (suppression of the menses: Aspasia and Rufus), 72 (displacements of the uterus), 104b (uterine ulcers), 109 (uterine hemorrhoids), 112 (edemous tumors), 114 (varicose hernia).

**55. Metrodora.** 1st-6th cent. A.D. MS: Florence, Laurenziana, Plut. 75.3, 4v-19r. Title: ἐκ τῶν Μητροδώρας· περὶ τῶsν γυναικϵίων παθῶν τῆς μήτρας [From the works of Metrodora: On the Feminine Diseases of the Womb].

### Dubia

**a. Hagnodice.** Preserved in Hyginus (prob. II cent. A.D.). Fabulae 274 is the story of Hagnodice (Agnodice in the MS), which begins "The ancients did not have midwives, and so women, led by their modesty, were dying. For the Athenians had been careful lest any slave or woman learn the art of medicine." It then relates how a certain Athenian girl named Agnodice, desiring to learn medicine, cut her hair, put on men's clothing, and apprenticed herself to Herophilus (Hierophilus in the MS). She would come in and expose her genitals to the women patients to prove she was a woman. She was eventually tried as a man and again exposed herself to the court. Instead she was found guilty of violating the law against women learning medicine. The Athenian women interceded for her and the law was changed. Athens never had such a law (contra von Staden 1988: 40, 61; Plato *Laws* 720a-e, 857c-d, sometimes adduced, does not describe the supposed situation; see Kudlien 1968 for the argument in favor and the bibliography cited by von Staden) and the statement that the ancients had no midwives is absurd (Pomeroy attempts to defend it by taking *obstetrices* to mean "women doctors"; see note 13, above). Despite these facts and folk tale elements (for which see King 1986), there may, however, be some remembrance here of a historical character, perhaps indeed an early woman doctor, who was associated in some way with the great physician and gynecologist, Herophilus (330/320-260/50 B.C.). However, the dubious source and fantastic setting make it unwise to place any reliance on the anecdote's veracity. See Pomeroy 1977, King 1986, von Staden 1988: 38-41, 53, 61.

**b. Maia?** Quoted by Gal. 13.840 for a remedy for condylomas. It is not clear if the word is supposed to be a proper name.

**c. The wife of Romulus?** [κυρία Ῥωμύλου]. Mentioned by Aetius 16.149 (171.6 Z) for an incense preparation. Her status and the medical use of the incense are unclear.

**d. Ammi(o)n.** Pleket 1969: 39 (no. 27); Robert 1964: 72 n. 6; Merkelbach 1971: 14; Robert and Robert 1972: 441. Epitaph for Ὄβριμον ἰητῆρα καὶ Ἄμμειν τὴν σώτειραν. Pleket called this an "Epitaph for Obrimos and his wife, both doctors." Merkelbach argued that the title σώτηρ (masc.) meant simply "doctor" and correspondingly the feminine ought to mean the same. However, while σώτηρ can be an epithet of a doctor, it is not a synonym. Without further reference, on contemporary inscriptions it more often refers to civic patrons. Robert points to the difference between Obrimos being called simply "doctor" and Ammion being called "a savior" (with the article): "le mot est ici un éloge, et non une function" (1977: 13). Were this in verse, I might be inclined to accept the epithet as a convenient poetic equivalent for "doctor." Robert rightly concludes (1966: 72 n. 6) that she "was associated with him in the art of medicine, possibly in the capacity of nurse," or more accurately, as assistant, without claiming the status of doctor.

## NOTES

Research for this article was aided by a fellowship from the National Endowment for the Humanities and by the Semple Fund of the University of Cincinnati. I have included in the Sources (numbered references in bold) all sources known to me; I believe the list to be substantially complete. However, this article is in part a request to the scholarly community for aid in finding other citations. Any additional references will be gratefully acknowledged.

1. See Appendix for the sources. Brief overviews, besides works mentioned in the notes, can be found in Kudlien 1979: 88-89, Gourevitch 1984: 223-26, Krug 1985: 195-97, Nickel 1988. Oehler 1909 provides a list of Greek inscriptional material, all of which is contained in Firatli and Robert 1964.

2. King 1991: 45; Kristeller 1980: 102-3; De Renzi 1857: cxxx (no. 388), 569.

3. King 1991: 44-45; Shahar 1983: 201; Ferrante 1980: 18.

4. Pierro (1964), cited from Green 1993: 132 and 1994: 322 n. 3.

5. Of previous surveys, Hurd-Mead (1983) is unfortunately completely unreliable through the Renaissance, as is the recent work of Bourdillon (1988) which repeats Hurd-Mead's errors.

6. As there is for women painters, for example: Pliny *NH* 35.40; Lefkowitz and Fant 1992: 216-17 (no. 307).

7. Allen 1944: 18-21.

8. The text is that of John Burnet's OCT (1902) as discussed by Pomeroy 1978. Note should be made of the emendation of George Luck (Pomeroy 1978: 498 n. 4).

9. Kudlien 1979: 89.

10. So Aelius Dionysius (II cent. A.D.), Alexander Cotyaeus (PW 95; II cent. A.D.), and Oros (PW 4; V cent. A.D.), cited by Eust. ad *Il.* 3.514 (244.15-20). Aelius Herodianus (II cent. A.D.; 3.1.333.13, 3.1.533.4, 3.2.13.27, 3.2.456.27) and the Byzantine encyclopedia, the *Suda* (I.64), also attest the word. Nickel 1988: 43 is wrong to call Phanostrate's usage "poetic."

11. On nomenclature, see Nickel 1979. Many texts are assembled by Van Brock (1961: 66-67), who, however, translates as "sage-femme."

12. So rightly Blümner (1911: 477 n. 6): "eine ärztlich geschulte Hebamme"; Van Brock (1961: 67 n. 2): "le composé ἰατρόμαια . . . doit impliquer plus de connaissances médicales que μαῖα"; Firatli and Robert 1964: 176-77. As Kudlien (1979: 89) points out, the distinction made between *iatromaia* and *iatrinê* implies that the woman was taken as a full colleague (or at least the functional equivalent) of the man.

13. Pomeroy (1977: 500) is incorrect to translate it as "woman physician," or (1978: 58-59) as "obstetrician," commenting "the career of obstetrician is to be distinguished from that of a midwife as requiring more formal education." It might be the case that an *obstetrix* in Rome had more training than a midwife in other cultures, but there is no other Latin term meaning merely "midwife" as distinct from *obstetrix*. See the comments of King 1986: 59.

14. So *TLL* s.v. *medicus* (553.7): *strictiore sensu de feminis in arte medicandi versatis, aegrotates curantibus* [in the strict sense, of women skilled in the medical arts, who cure the sick]. The sometimes cited passage: *obstetrices, id est medicae,* supposedly from Sen. *Ep.* 66 does not exist.

15. Rightly Le Gall 1970: 128. Accordingly, Gummerus (1932: 15) correctly includes *medicae* and *iatromaiae* in his list of doctors but excludes *obstetrices*.

16. For intercourse as the cure for hysteria, see, e.g., Hp. *Mul.* 1-7, 127, 137, *Nat.Mul.* 2, 3; Arist. *HA* 582b23-25; Gal. 13.319-20 (cf. 8.417, 420, 424, 432, 16.178); Aet. 16.87 (97.12-14 Z). See Veith 1965, Lefkowitz 1981, Manuli 1983: 189.

17. A similar joke at 11.60 also indirectly attests to the existence of women doctors; see Kay 1985: 202-3, 224.

18. *consuetudo medici vel medicae egredientis ex aegri domo.* Here the scene is the midwife (*obstetrix*) Lesbia leaving after a successful childbirth.

19. Kudlien 1979: 89.

20. See Nutton 1971, 1977, 1981: Jackson 1988: 57, Fischer 1979: 166; Kudlien 1986.

21. The question of the status of *the* doctors in antiquity (as if there were only one) is a vexed problem and there has been a tendency to overgeneralization. See Forbes 1955: 344; Cohn-Haft 1956: 4, 61-65; Kudlien 1968; Phillips 1973: 188-89, 194; Scarborough 1969: 27, 110-15; Kudlien 1979, 1986. On slaves in the later Empire, see Nutton 1984: 12 (and n. 111), with a proper warning on the dangers of generalization.

22. Earlier lists need some corrections. Le Gall (1970) unfortunately makes some errors of fact and is inclined to declare that someone was free because there is no evidence to the contrary. He fails to cite **18, 20, 22, 30,** and **33,** which are in *CIL* (though the last not in the index). Kampen 1981 is more cautious but overly certain on **15** and **23,** and errs on **22,** and **26** (also mistakenly lists *CIL* VI.9510, which is for a male veterinarian). She does not cite **20, 29, 30, 33** and **34** which are in *CIL*.

Günther 1987: 101 lists 9 *medicae* in her table: 3 slaves, 3 freedwomen, 2 free, 1 uncertain, but gives no documentation for this last (pp. 103-9); see also (**23**). Korpela 1987 also provides cautious assessment for those inscriptions from Rome, but see (**19**). Corrections for Jackson 1988: for p. 191 n. 4: *CIL* VI. 9619 is incorrect, XIII. 3343 should be XII; for n. 7: XII. 6851 should be VI; n. 11 is incorrect.

23. See Phillips 1973: 185-95; Jackson 1988: 19, 25-26, 58-59.

24. This would have varied greatly among times, places, and individuals. For example, Galen complains, with perhaps the exaggeration of anger, that most doctors of his time could not read very well (Gal. 19.9). On medical education in general, see Drabkin 1944, Phillips 1973: 182-96, Scarborough 1969: 122-33, esp. 125-28, Kollesch 1979. For Byzantium, see Duffy 1984: 21-22.

25. The point is made by Gourevitch 1984: 223-24, Gummerus 1932: 15, Phillips 1973: 190-91; King 1986: 59.

26. For the history of the term, see Nutton 1977.

27. Kampen 1981: 116, Günther 1987: 102-3.

28. See King 1991: 343, 347, 351.

29. Scott 1932: XIV, 53. Kampen 1981: 70 mistakes the passage (correctly at 117 n. 45). She also cites Iust. *Dig.* 50.13.1.2: "The obstetrix, Ulpian says, has the same status as a medicus or medica, and her status is not diminished by the fact that she works mainly with female patients." Rather, the passage merely says that midwives are allowed a kind of curtesy consideration, along with professors of the liberal arts and doctors: *quae utique medicinam exhibere videtur* [who seem to practice a sort of medicine] (so rightly Watson 1985: IV, 930; cf. Scott 1932: XI, 251). She also mistakes Pliny 28 [not 27].67: *obstetricum nobilitas* means merely "the best of the midwives."

30. Nickel 1979: 517, Gardner 1986: 240-41.

31. The language suggests perhaps service during a plague. A famous plague ravaged Asia Minor in 166 A.D. (Wilhelm 1932/1977: 108).

32. Pliny and others are drawing on a written, not an oral tradition; see Lloyd 1983: 60 n. 6.

33. Rightly Kampen 1981: 117. Pliny (*NH* 32.81) is the only one who speaks of women medical authorities with special disdain, and then only of Elephantis (**43**) and Lais (**44**) for being contradictory.

34. Not to be confused with the famous queen of Egypt. No source identifies her as such before Paulus Aegineta.

35. See Galen's discussion (12.434-35; cf. 12.450, 452 and 5.821-22). He cites Soranus' lost work on mange (12.416) and mentions books on cosmetics by Asclepiades, Herakleides of Tarentium (Gal. 12.445), Elephantis, and Moschion; also works by Archigenes of Apamaea (Gal. 12.445, 460), and Heras (Gal. 13.786). Andreas should perhaps be included (*Narthex,* [The Casket], the same title as Heras' work; see von Staden 1989: 473). The most famous were by Crito (physician to Trajan; Gal.

12.401, 435, 446-50: table of contents, etc.) and Kleopatra. Similar recipes can be found in Hippocrates, Dioscorides, Galen himself, Aetius, Paulus Aegineta and Oribasius. See Grillet 1975; Kudlien 1979: 104-11; also Scarborough 1984: 218, Faure 1987 (esp. 147-270), Jackson 1988: 54-55, von Staden 1988: 543. For the title, cf. Gal. 14.422.

36. Dean-Jones (1994: 33) is unduly skeptical: "However, when Aetius attributes several chapters on gynecological matters to Aspasia, the famous companion of Pericles in the fifth century BC, it is probable the attribution is apocryphal, though the work could be by a later Aspasia who was equated with Pericles' Aspasia because the latter was the only woman reknowned for her intelligence during the time of Hippocrates." Dean-Jones assumes Aetius must be thinking of the Aspasia best known to us. However, Aetius nowhere makes such an identification. Aspasia is quite a common name (as the masculine Aspasius), well attested from classical Greek into late Roman times (e.g., *SB* 14, 11717, IV c. A.D.) and there is no reason to assume that Aetius could only have been thinking of Pericles' Aspasia.

37. Her discussions need not imply actual practice, but it would be odd if Aetius chose her as the only source for these operations if she were merely excerpting other authorities.

38. Codex Pluteus 75.3 of the Biblioteca Laurentiana in Florence, 4v-19r.

39. The arguments are all necessarily imprecise. The lack of encyclopedic citation and the absence of any trace of Galenism argue for a date most likely before the fifth century.

40. The text was published by Kousis 1945 and Del Guerra 1953. Both are unfortunately rendered unusable by the numerous errors. I am currently preparing an edition, translation and commentary.

41. The earlier editors included under Metrodora's name fragments of four other works that follow in the MS: 1) three antidotes or theriacs, 2) six extracts from a *materia medica,* 3) the opening section of an alphabetically organized recipe book (thirty-one chapters from A-E), and 4) a series of extracts from Alexander of Tralles (numbered 62-105) rounded off by four miscellaneous recipes. The last is not by Metrodora and the others are very unlikely to be from her works.

42. Cf. Gal. 14.478, 486.

43. So Aetius 16.13 explicitly says that childbirth is woman's business and not a proper part of medicine.

## [8]

# THEY MET IN ZÜRICH
*Nineteenth-Century German
and Russian Women Physicians*

PAULETTE MEYER

*Not long after 1877,* when the first university-trained German women physicians opened a practice in Berlin, an anonymous complaint charged that they falsely advertised themselves as medical doctors on signs at their clinic. When Franziska Tiburtius went to answer the accusation, she displayed her diploma from the prestigious University of Zürich (Switzerland) to the young state official who, nevertheless, threatened to fine her the conventional three mark penalty for misrepresentation of credentials. The bureaucrat explained that by calling herself "Dr. med.," Tiburtius implied she had been certified by imperial German authorities to practice medicine; and, of course, women were not allowed to take the imperial certification examinations no matter what their education. To avoid future lawsuits, he concluded, she must have her sign repainted to show the foreign origin of her diploma: "Dr. med. der Universität Zürich Tiburtius."

As Dr. Tiburtius recalled in her memoirs: "The effect was completely other than one might think. In the next consultation hours, I was enthusiastically congratulated by various female patients: 'Ja, what had happened?' I must have become something special because now on the sign was written an especially long title!"[1] This telling vignette illustrates the ironic position of women physicians and their primarily female patients in Germany—a country renowned during the late nineteenth century for excellence in medical science and practice. Both women who sought medical training and women who chose medical treatment by female physicians were harassed and denigrated by medical men and others critical of women's ambitions, aspirations, and choices.

By legal definition, women in nineteenth-century Germany could not be certified physicians because they were not allowed to matriculate in German universities. Authorities responsible for admission to the state universities and bureaucrats controlling the imperial medical examinations categorically denied women access to formal medical education and accredited practice. Women doctors, no matter what their training or non-German education, were classed together with "irregular healers" including magnetopaths, hydropaths, or other alternative medical practitioners likely to be labeled *Kurpfuscher* (quacks).[2] The Prussian Commercial Code of 1869 recognized that poor and rural populations probably would not have access to the costly services of university-trained physicians, and thus the code made provision for allowing informal health-care providers to work as long as they did not misrepresent themselves as *Praktischer Arzt* (practicing or general physician).

Until the turn of the century, German women who wanted to graduate from university medical schools were compelled to study abroad. In order to practice medicine upon their return, women physicians constructed careers for themselves within the confines of the commercial code and despite the opposition of male physicians who shut them out of professional associations and often excluded them from hospital and other consulting privileges. In the popular press, former Zürich professors like Victor Böhmert defended the abilities of women students against criticisms of their aspirations. An exceptional German physician, Franz Winckel, allowed Zürich women graduates to gain practical experience working as voluntary assistants in his women's clinics in Dresden and Munich. Dr. Winckel had travelled to many countries to observe medical practices in his specialty of obstetrics and gynecology. Perhaps his trips to Russia where women physicians were at work convinced him to train German women. He also instituted a lecture series on the history of women in medicine for students at his clinics. Despite the efforts of such energetic individual professionals, Imperial Germany was the last western European nation to allow women (in 1899) to take examinations that would certify them as physicians.

Under formal legal strictures and informal social constraints, Dr. Franziska Tiburtius and Dr. Emilie Lehmus operated the Berlin Clinic of Women Doctors, where they sometimes treated forty patients a day at a usual charge of 10 pfennigs per visit—for those who could pay at all. In comparison, Dr. Tiburtius reported that famous male physicians of the era collected 50 marks for one house call.[3] These men were often the very influential doctors who worried that an influx of women into their profession might oversupply German cities with medical care.

The fact that in neighboring Czarist Russia, women physicians were more accepted, and even honored for their service during the Russo-Turkish War of 1877, did not, for the most part, sway male opposition in Germany. Russia was so large and backward in health care, went one argument advanced at German medical society meetings, that even women were necessary auxiliaries to practice medicine in rural *zemstvos* (village communities) or on the frontiers as medical missionaries to subject nationalities. A woman doctor might be better than none at all. In Germany, however, asserted professor of medicine Franz Penzoldt, there was no shortage of doctors; and women who wanted to be involved with medical care should devote themselves to subsidiary careers in dentistry, pharmacy, or nursing.[4]

Russian women physicians had faced many of the same discouragements as their German colleagues; nevertheless, after 1867 numerous Russian women practiced medicine both as employees of government agencies and as private physicians. One reason for their relative success was the historical development of Russian women's work in medicine as it evolved from midwifery and other subordinate occupations to that of full-fledged physician. Even when women were not allowed to matriculate at Russian universities, not all physicians' training was withheld from them. The course of incremental education and accreditation followed by the czarist medical establishment made it possible for more than six hundred women to gain medical degrees in St. Petersburg by 1887.[5] Numbers of other women studied at schools for rural midwives, which eventually added further training to qualify women as *feldschers* (Russian: *fel'dsher,* physicians' assistants or paraprofessional medics). Finally, the largest contingent of foreign students in many continental medical universities came from Russia; and at the University of Zürich, it was a Russian, Nadezhda Suslova, who became the first woman to matriculate for medical studies.

Contrasting socioeconomic conditions partly explain these varying successes of ambitious women medical workers. Cultural and religious differences also defined limits which individual women sought to overcome in both Germany and Russia. Interestingly, many of the women medical students wrote autobiographies and life-stories that recall meetings with foreign students during their university days in Zürich, Switzerland. From a macroscopic point of view, the differing familial and class backgrounds of the German and Russian women medical students shed light on contrasts between the new Prussian-dominated German empire and the ambitious yet aging multicultural Russian state. The types of medical careers open to the Zürich graduates in each country highlight the ironic situation of German women who lived in a nation honored for scientific enlightenment even as it excluded female physicians. Czarist Russia, on the other hand, allowed many women to work in medical professions. Even in modern times, Soviet Russia and the successor states have some of the highest percentages of female physicians. The following comparisons of individual women's accomplishments in medical careers draw upon personal recollections of pioneering female medical students and political writings by their feminist advocates which provide clues to differing cultural constraints limiting behaviors and roles viewed as respectable and feminine in Russia and in Germany.

## The First Woman Medical Graduate of the University of Zürich

Nadezhda Suslova graduated from the University of Zürich in 1867 during a decade noteworthy in Russia for national reforms prompted by a shocking military defeat at Crimea. These Great Reforms went beyond a compensated emancipation of Russian serfs in 1861. Women, too, accelerated their resistance to traditional subordination in legal, financial, and educational status. Auditors at university courses included ambitious women like Suslova, the daughter of an emancipated serf; however, in 1863 czarist decrees once again closed courses to women. Suslova and others left Russia to audit university courses in Switzerland and other foreign locales even before women were permitted to matriculate or register for studies leading to degrees in most European universities.

At the relatively new University of Zürich, founded in 1833, liberal political aspirations united émigrés from many nations, including expatriate medical professors who had left Germany after the failed political revolutions of 1848. Swiss authorities allowed these professors to lecture to coeducational audiences of laypersons interested in science, as had been customary in German salon circles. When Suslova eventually was allowed to matriculate and defend her dissertation in a public forum, Professor Edmund Rose, himself an émigré from Berlin, awarded the degree and spoke in favor of women in medicine.[6]

Whether Suslova could work in Russia was a question debated by czarist officials. Published articles and letters supported her; and after passing a special examination at the St. Petersburg Medical Surgical Academy, Suslova opened a private practice in that city. Her Swiss husband, Dr. Friedrich Erismann, joined her in 1869 to research hygienic conditions in urban workers' slums. Dr. Nadezhda Suslova-Erismann concentrated on teaching mothers preventative health measures. By 1873, 153 men and 103 women from Russia were attending the University of Zürich when the czarist government banned new enrollments because of the influence of *niliski* (nihilist) agitators in Switzerland, who were supposedly subverting education—particularly that of young women.[7]

During these turbulent 1870s, Franziska Tiburtius and a Bavarian-German pastor's daughter, Emilie Lehmus, met Russian women in medical courses. Looking back in her 1923 "memoirs of an eighty-year-old," Dr. Tiburtius composed a description of the times and constructed an apology for the motivations of the Russian girls who had welcomed her upon her arrival in the unfamiliar environs of Zürich. She was most impressed with the Russian students' fanatical altruism out of sympathy with "the people or common folk" and with their readiness to sacrifice religion, family sentiments, and social approval in pursuit of their ideals.[8]

### Remembering the Russian Women Medical Students

From the point of view of the Prussian-German Franziska Tiburtius, Russian women students could be divided into three types: first, the gentry, who did not take part in political activities and drew a line between themselves and their countrywomen, whom they regarded as inferior in class and backward in behavior. Feelings of *noblesse oblige* and also compassion for the suffering poor motivated some of these aristocratic women to study medicine in order to better care for retainers and peasants working their family properties.

The second type of Russian medical student Tiburtius described as talented and well-intentioned, but not very thoroughly educated. By continuing academic studies, they found expression for their idealism in the profession of medicine, rather than in fruitless political disorders. This "middle-class" type included women physicians who later practiced in Russia—Drs. Grujewska, Jacowliea, and Putajata. The majority of Russian Jewish women students, such as Fanny Berlinerblau,[9] were idealists of this type, Tiburtius averred.[10]

The Russian Jewish women medical students appeared more conventionally polite and carefully dressed than the disruptive nihilists who usually studied in the humanities faculty. Other students had named this last or third type of Russian women "the Cossack Ponies." Their insolent public behavior prompted condemnatory news reports, such as one by a Professor Scherr who criticized the girls' short hair, blue-lensed eyeglasses, and short, plain black dresses sewn of shiny, "umbrella-like" fabrics.

The nihilists wore no jewelry, but sported round sailor caps. Smoking cigarettes and wandering the streets *en masse,* these "Cossack Ponies" inspired tirades and pictorial caricatures against women university students. Both their personal grooming and their politics appeared frightfully revolutionary. Cartoons in the German press of the 1870s warned of the bad habits respectable German women might learn from associating with such foreigners from Kiev or even from wayward American women who also studied medicine in Zürich.[11]

The American press, too, carried reports of the women students at Zürich. Student Susan Dimock wrote to the *Boston Medical and Surgical Journal* in December 1870 when the Swiss general government, "being instructed in regard to the wishes of the Swiss physicians, passed by a large majority an act admitting a woman, 'not only for the especial case, but as a principle,' to the State medical examinations." Dimock added wistfully: "thus opening to her [the Swiss woman physician] every medical society, giving her the possibility of attaining instructors' chairs, and rendering incumbent upon her every duty which a physician owes the State. The Swiss government has thus removed every official obstacle to the practice of medicine in Switzerland by a woman—obstacles from private prejudice will be few, since she is allowed to study with the young men who will be her fellow practitioners, and so has the opportunity to make them her friends."[12] Dimock turned out to be overly optimistic about the end of private prejudices: the first woman professor at Zürich, Hedwig Frey, did not occupy her chair in anatomy until the eve of World War I; and one of the first two women physicians practicing in Zürich, Dr. Caroline Farner, was hounded by specious lawsuits and jailed in solitary confinement at the turn of the century.

## German Feminists Counter Arguments that Women Are Incapable of Scientific Work

Eighteen years after Susan Dimock's report from Zürich, in 1888, a spokes-woman for the middle-class German women's movement, Mathilde Weber, wrote pamphlets to advocate continuing efforts to certify women physicians in Imperial Germany and to support women medical students at Zürich. Weber was a professor's wife whose interest in medicine was prompted by ill-nesses in friends and family and by volunteer medical work for the public. During the Franco-Prussian War of 1871, she had organized nursing and relief work among war casualties. In commenting upon the pioneering Russian women students, Mathilde Weber was sympathetic to their political and social difficulties.

In her defense of the Russians' reputations, Weber's analysis echoed a social Darwinist argument about the relative stages of civilization in differing nations: she concluded that the Russian students at Zürich in the 1870s ap-peared to be at a different cultural stage than west Europeans. They were self-conscious about being the first to oppose barriers to study; and they found themselves in unfamiliar surroundings in Zürich, where the usual morals and forms of society did not support their unusual path to employment. If one thinks about their situation objectively, continued Weber's logic, one can imagine the exceptional courage it took for the Russian girls to fight against long-rooted views and to master medicine as a possible profession for women at a time when it was believed that only men could do scientific work.

For the women students of 1888, the right to study was built upon a firm base of twenty years' past experience; women had learned that co-equal edu-cation with men should teach them more than how to take on male values and mannish attire. The greatest heights of spiritual strivings, science, and learning were completely within the realm of normal femininity. Most stu-dents in 1888 understood that medicine contributes to women's welfare and answers the *Frauenfrage* (women's question) as to what women are capable of accomplishing. According to Mathilde Weber, it was a matter of honor for female students to demonstrate feminine behavior and morality.[13]

These arguments were intended as a response to assertions that women were unsuited to study science and unfit to practice medicine. Throughout the nineteenth century, many male physicians attempted to justify the exclusion of women practitioners from medical professions. Educational and career paths by which women became practicing physicians during the nineteenth century account, in part, for differing success rates in Germany and Russia. The apprenticeship system of learning medicine by accompanying an experienced practitioner was gradually supplanted by formal training courses. Physicians and, eventually, surgeons began their studies in science and medicine in male-dominated university courses. The exclusion of women from German universities automatically denied them the opportunity for medical study. In Russia, the government permitted women to attain certificates as "learned midwives," a step up the medical professional hierarchy. For a time, Russian women could also study more general medicine at the St. Petersburg military medical and surgical academy. When political decisions eliminated this route, many female medical students went abroad in order to complete degrees. Continuing the trend toward permitting them gradually to achieve more status in the medical profession, Russian women were allowed to work as physicians in far-flung territories of the czarist empire.

In Germany, control by the new medical professional organizations over certifications and medical practices more stringently limited attempts by women to work up from midwives, medical assistants, or apothecaries to fully accredited physicians. Only a university degree and the right to take and pass state administered certification examinations were required qualifications for medical practice. The provision in the Prussian commercial code of 1869 for "irregular practitioners" provided health care for poor and rural patients. Before 1900, German women who graduated from Zürich and other foreign universities were able to construct careers under this "liberal" market-oriented proviso. However, the prejudices against women in medicine were reinforced regularly by pseudo-scientific interpretations of data gathered by many prominent medical men.

The most infamous German statement of opposition to women's employment in medicine was published in 1872. Professor Theodor Bischoff insisted that women would damage their reproductive tracts by inappropriate mental exertions if they studied medicine beyond nursing or midwifery. He came to these conclusions after his research on female dogs, from which he drew an analogy to female human sexuality to conclude that upper-class adolescent girls should be kept quietly at home, conserving their bodily energy for the sake of future childbearing functions.[14]

During her visit to the women students in Zürich, Mathilde Weber observed that none of the young women displayed the "unsexed characteristics" which Professor Bischoff predicted would result from female education; namely, extravagant and unfeminine deportment linked to nervous hysteria caused by unaccustomed mental efforts which could only drive them to a gruesome and frightful androgynous existence.[15] Weber concluded her eye-witness report on German women students with statistics about the successful practice of Swiss physician Marie Heim-Vögtlin, who in fifteen years had delivered 750 babies and performed 450 operations, losing only three patients in childbirth because they had waited too long before calling in the doctor. Just once in those years was it necessary to call on her female colleague (probably Dr. Caroline Farner) to assist in treating a patient. For Mathilde Weber, Dr. Heim-Vögtlin was the very model of a successful woman physician who had married a university professor and raised two beautiful children while running an exemplary medical practice. A parallel model for German women physicians might be the Brandenburg native Fräulein Dr. Anna Kuhnow, who graduated from Zürich and went on to do research in America (and to serve until 1890 as professor of microbiology among other duties at the Medical College of the New York Infirmary for Women and Children).[16]

Women writers who countered theoretical arguments against women's practice of medicine repeatedly pointed to practical evidence that they were, in fact, already doing medical work in midwifery, apothecary dispensing, and nursing—both informally for families at home and formally as paid attendants or charitable volunteers. In countries like Russia and Switzerland, women also practiced as certified physicians. Publications for and against German women in medicine were especially crucial in 1888. Crown Prince Frederick, son of Kaiser William I, who had ruled a unified German empire since 1871, was believed ready to institute important political and social reforms upon ascending the throne. The Crown Prince was married to the Princess Royal of Britain, Queen Victoria's eldest daughter, "Vicky," who was friendly with liberal reformers in education seeking to improve employment opportunities for women. Just before her marriage and move to Berlin, she had met with Florence Nightingale in England to discuss nursing and military hospital arrangements. In Germany, the Crown Princess, with her children, became patients of a pioneering woman dentist, Dr. Henriette Tiburtius-Hirschfeld.

By 1887, however, a regime sympathetic to the cause of women's education could no longer be anticipated since Crown Prince Frederick was suffering from terminal throat cancer. Petitions were circulated to show public support for women teachers in girls' schools and for opening universities to women students of medicine and philosophy.[17] In March 1888, Kaiser William I died; but in the ninety-nine days of reign by the dying Kaiser Frederick, little could be accomplished in the way of educational reform from above. Under the rule of the third emperor of 1888, Kaiser William II, women's movement leaders became more dependent on publications and organized campaigns to sway imperial government agencies toward reform. The largest show of support came in a petition for the opportunity to choose "female physicians for women's diseases." Forty thousand German women and fifteen thousand German men signed this appeal to the imperial parliament by 1891.[18]

Theoretical arguments against women physicians continued to be raised for more than ten years after Mathilde Weber's visit to the Zürich students. Further, it took twenty years of recommendations by reformers and requests by women before the Prussian state government agreed to open its universities to female degree candidates. In 1908, women could finally study medicine in Berlin, though some adamant professors still kept their courses closed to all women.

### Russian Reformers Attempt to Educate Medical Women in Their Own Country

In St. Petersburg, too, the women students at the special courses taught for them in the Russian Military Medical-Surgical Academy faced limitation and periodic closings of opportunities during the late nineteenth century. In 1873, Zürich had been declared off-limits to Russian students; however, in 1872 new women's medical courses in Russia had opened under the sponsorship of the War Ministry and with the financial support of a wealthy woman donor. For ten years, women students studied separately but in the same facility as men. Sympathetic professors ignored the supposed limitations of the women's courses to pediatrics and gynecology, teaching female students the full range of topics included in the five-year Russian medical curriculum.[19] Professors and supportive women raised funds for students through the Society for Aiding Women Students at the Medical and Pedagogical Courses.

Ten years of teaching and fundraising ended with a conservative backlash against the universities following the assassination of Czar Alexander II. After 1882, the Women's Medical Courses could admit no new students. The last women's class graduated in 1887; it was another ten years before new courses for women medical students opened. In the meantime, Russians again went abroad to audit or matriculate in Swiss or French universities. Still, the situation of women physicians in Russia was far better than that in Germany. During the decade of the 1870s, women doctors had become an accepted part of Russian medicine.

Most spectacular was the service of the entire first class of the St. Petersburg Women's Medical Courses, who volunteered their help in the Russo-Turkish War of 1877. The Ministry of War accepted them as medical students; but refused to allow a graduated woman, Dr. Varvara Kashevarova, to accompany them to the front. As a full-fledged physician, Dr. Kashevarova might be considered equal with other male military doctors, entitled to rank and bureaucratic privileges. A graduate of Swiss medical courses, Dr. Marie Siebold (Russian, Mariya Sibold) went to Serbia in order to serve with Russian allies since the czarist government would not employ her, either. In the Balkans, she organized a military hospital where she could practice her surgical specialty.[20]

Less qualified female students who had not yet received diplomas did not pose the same bureaucratic problems over entitlements to military rank. These young women were attached to Red Cross units or served under the direction of Military Inspector Nicholas Pirogov, who had been impressed by the battlefield work of the 163 Russian Sisters of Mercy in Crimea. From that time on, Dr. Pirogov advocated women's work in medicine even as he fought for improved health care in the rural Russian *zemstvo* villages (communal settlements). In time, the Pirogov Society (named in his honor) became a base for political agitation to reform and improve Russian medicine, education, and health care.

On the Turkish front, Inspector Pirogov permitted women medical students to perform surgery as independent operators. He watched them minister to victims of cholera and typhus, and recommended battle honors for the twenty-five women students. Newspapers praised their heroism and self-sacrifice. Eventually, the women received special gold medals on the ribbon of the Order of St. George and were given graduation documents. However, these were not medical diplomas, only certificates stating that they had passed all the diploma examinations and were qualified to treat women and children. Finally, in 1880 Czar Alexander II bestowed on them the title *zhenskii vrach* (woman doctor) and gave them special insignias.

161

Anxieties over allowing women public honors, military rank, bureaucratic status and possible pension rights were not unique to Russia. The public recognition and official honors awarded Russian women physicians were exceptional, however, even though this acclaim was hedged by bureaucratic distinctions and limitations. In effect, the years 1877-1880 were a turning point in distinguishing opportunities for Russian women in medicine from German women healthcare workers. Gradual acknowledgments of women physicians' talents and status by czarist bureaucrats and by the general public after the Russo-Turkish War were only part of the change in status for women physicians.

Another part of the process in expanding professional opportunities for women doctors resulted from alterations in the system of health care for the Russian countryside: there, peasant populations rejected the hierarchy of medical workers envisioned for them by government bureaucrats, which boxed women medical advisors into confining special practices. Pressures from the rural populace in the form of *zemstvo* resistance to hiring or consulting specialized "learned midwives" persuaded czarist officials to permit women students to take combined courses in midwifery and general paramedical training to become *fel'dsheritsa-akusherka* (medic-midwives).[21] Further, these women paramedics were then often encouraged, at some point, to complete full medical degrees, sometimes with the financial support of rural governments. This step-wise accreditation for women medical workers was not acceptable in nineteenth-century Imperial Germany,[22] where state governments trained only midwives. During the years when the women's medical courses to train physicians were closed, female enrollments in the Russian paraprofessional combined training continued.

### Russian Medic-Midwives and Feldschers *Open Career Paths for Women Doctors*

In the midst of campaigns to improve both childbirth practices, which were traditionally the responsibility of a local women healer (*povitukha* or midwife combined with post-partum nurse), and general medical care, which might be provided by a *znakharka* (medicine woman),[23] the burning issue behind the consolation awards given to heroic women medical veterans of the Russo-Turkish War came to the fore. In that year of 1883, the minister of the interior responded positively to petitions from the Czarist Medical Council, hospitals, and provincial officials asking that women be permitted to practice medicine and surgery in the face of an overwhelming need for health care: the czarist government agreed that women physicians could finally be listed for employment in the medical register of physicians as entitled to treat *all* patients; however, they were yet excluded from concomitant rights to bureaucratic rank and state service credit.[24] Women physicians were simply to be placed outside the societal ranking of other state servants as a way of avoiding conflicts over their elevated professional status.

Nevertheless, with new titles for the women physicians and broader training for female paramedics, Russian medical women went to work in the countryside and urban slums. They delivered babies, performed surgeries, and fought epidemics of smallpox and cholera. In a *zemstvo* village thirty miles outside of Moscow, Dr. Aleksandra Arkhangelskaia planned and built a new hospital in 1885, where three women physicians worked in the expanded facility by 1902 assisted by women *feldschers* who administered anesthesia and practiced new methods of asepsis and antiseptic care. Arkhangelskaia was renowned as an abdominal surgeon and hospital administrator; she wrote an acclaimed pamphlet to educate the lay public, *Why Doctors Operate* (1902).[25]

In both urban and rural locales, women doctors attempted to accomplish a task assigned them by the czarist War Ministry—specifically, to battle the spread of venereal diseases that followed market trade routes, the track of telegraph and railroad networks, and paths of rural wet nurses who delivered infected urban orphans to country foster homes.[26] Dr. Mariya Pokrovskaia made statistical surveys of rural living conditions to guide these public health campaigns. She used comparative studies of western European countries to project models for sanitary boards and reform techniques. Military efforts to control syphilis, for example, had centered on state regulation of prostitution.[27] When her plan was duly noted and then ignored by health authorities, Pokrovskaia turned to fiction as a means to social critique through a story of a woman doctor in *How I Was a City Doctor for the Poor* (1903). The narrative illustrated how women doctors were not truly supported in reform efforts by a society which remained indifferent to the appalling living conditions of impoverished families in city and countryside.[28]

Still, Russian governments were more generous with opportunities for women physicians than nearby nations. In 1897, courses in a new Woman's Medical Institute reopened possibilities for medical degrees without study in foreign universities. The following year, Russian women physicians were given complete equality with men similarly employed by governmental agencies as far as pensions and compensations. But the customary honors and uniforms were still denied women, for such external signs of rank as representations of women's place in the social order were most threatening to equality of employment with men.

## Women Physicians Confront Oppressions in Capitalism and Patriarchy

Conflicts between popular requests for women physicians and the reluctance of czarist officials to compromise bureaucratic prerogatives were highlighted in debates over women employed to investigate working conditions in Russian factories. Workers who migrated from rural *zemstvo* communities for employment at city factory sites maintained connections with home villages by frequent trips back to country relatives and by living in urban *artels* (communal quarters) with other emigrants from home regions. *Zemstvo* councils even hired their own inspectors or physicians to visit migrants at factory work sites to check on health and other conditions of employment. Women physicians working for the villagers reported back on women factory workers' lives. Female workers were described as surprised at the women doctors' "respectful treatment of them." As Rose Glickman concluded, "The main arguments for a female inspectorate were that women workers had problems that male inspectors could neither understand nor cope with, and that, in any case, women workers were too shy with male inspectors to discuss their problems with them."[29] Nevertheless, despite requests by the women workers and their village councils, the czarist government never employed women in the imperial factory inspectorate, rejecting a *Duma* (parliament) committee compromise that "since by law women were not entitled to rank in the civil service, women inspectors would not be entitled to receive medals, honors, personal or hereditary nobility, and other kinds of rewards reserved for men."[30] The specter of a woman, even without external social rewards, given authority to criticize male factory operatives or to judge the adequacy of capitalistic paternalism toward women workers was too far removed from tolerable female behavior. In Russia, women physicians might serve governmental agencies and give advice to councils, but women medical inspectors acting as agents of governmental authority in a regulatory capacity over male factory management was an unimaginable departure from gender hierarchies of power.

While appeals by factory women for female inspectors were dismissed, the sensibilities of Muslim patriarchs in border regions of the expanding czarist empire required that harem women be tended by female physicians only. Male authorities in the Russian imperial government acknowledged such patriarchal prerogatives for Muslim chieftans to choose women doctors when they allowed Varvara Kashevarova to train for medical service on the Bashkir frontier. Kashevarona was a Jewish orphan befriended by teachers and medical workers. With their help and inspiration, and the financial support of a husband arranged for her to marry, she began to study midwifery. A stipend from the Bashkir trial patriarch, advocacy by War Minister Miliutin, and appeals from the military governor of the Orenburg province won permission for Kashevarona to continue with her medical degree studies. After graduation, the paradoxical problems with czarist bureaucracy prevented her from serving the frontier Muslim women, since the only hospitals open in Orenburg were military; therefore, the first woman to earn her medical degree in Russia could not serve her sponsors because a physician's work in a military hospital was attached to bureaucratic rank, which women could not hold.[31]

The issue of female authority and governmental service continued to frustrate Kashevarona after she successfully earned the doctor of medicine diploma in 1878.[32] She declared that she pursued this advanced degree in order to qualify as an instructor in the Women's Medical Courses; yet this employment was denied her. If rank for women physicians was a problem, even more prestigious professorships were unimaginable.[33] Women could not instruct or exercise authority over men in the bureaucratic civil service, nor instruct other women if that authority in a female chain of command usurped male entitlements to status and salary.

The female impetus to state service was most acceptable when it coincided with czarist imperialist expansionism. Many of the first women medical students saw themselves as cultural missionaries to subject nationalities and to women segregated by Muslim cultural practices. Nadezhda Suslova thought that practicing medicine among Muslim subjects would give her access to the population for political agitation toward social reform. Sofia Kovalevskaia, reared in a military family, "had at first intended to become a doctor for the political exiles in Siberia and had planned to study her beloved mathematics only in her spare time."[34] Women who felt oppressed by their own reactionary social system sought training to serve those even more subordinated than themselves. Suslova planned to assist tribal women controlled by a patriarchy she viewed as more confining than that which she experienced in European Russia.

Some Russian women medical students decided to place social revolutionary goals above education or medical practice. Vera Figner left her medical diploma course in Switzerland one term before graduation to join the populist movement of *niliski* and other students who travelled to the Russian countryside in the summer of 1874. Among the Russian peasantry and factory workers, student reformers and social revolutionaries hoped to organize cadres for changing social conditions and political dominations. Figner had come to the conclusion that true revolutionaries studied medicine "in order to have in our hands *weapons for social activism.*"[35] "A *zemstvo* doctor might seem like just another master, remote from the people—but what about a paramedic [*feldsher*]?[36]

## Women Physicians as Agents for Social Change

At Zürich, politically active Russians labelled the German women students "narrow Philistines" for doggedly pursuing academic training.[37] The German-Russian student Marie Siebold of St. Petersburg was excluded from a communal library organized by radical Zürich students because "she had come to Zürich to study medicine and nothing more."[38] Franziska Tiburtius remembered that the Russian women believed themselves to possess a "larger" nature in that they were more concerned with social reform and artistic life beyond the university. One reason for the limited political involvement of German women students might be attributed to their reluctance to be identified with radical reformers like the *niliski*. Women physicians who hoped to practice at all in German territory were careful of their public reputations; and under imperial German laws, women were debarred from involvement in political organizations.

Mathilde Weber specifically warned Zürich women students to avoid questions of social issues or even of the *Frauenfrage* (women's question) in general. In this way, they might live down the distrust of women's organizations stemming from the earlier circles of *niliski* Russian students. Weber hoped that misunderstandings and prejudices about the respectability of women university students could be dispelled through meetings sponsored by a women's union between the better circles of Zürich society and women students. Such social gatherings and salon discussions on general cultural subjects could also improve the prospective woman physicians' *Bildung* (general education).[39]

Many of the German medical students were considered members of the *Bildungsbürgertum* (educated middle classes). The women's movement in Germany had advocated their higher education so that women might have more control over the education of girls and over the medical care of women and children in particular. In Germany, feminism or advocacy of female progress was based less on the claims of egalitarian rights that buttressed Anglo-American reform demands. German feminism, in contrast, was essentially maternalist in that many reformers accepted the concept of a separate sphere of women's influence over other women and successive generations of girls. The influence of women over unrelated females was considered *geistliche Mütterlichkeit* (spiritual motherhood) while coordinated campaigns for reform were termed *organisierte Mütterlichkeit* (organized motherhood).[40]

Franziska Tiburtius noted with some amusement that despite vigorous arguments by leading *Frauenrechtlerinnen* (women's rights advocates) for women's opportunity to choose women physicians, many socially prominent ladies were cautious about visiting the Clinic of the Women Doctors. Apparently, the entire *Frauenwelt* (world of women) was not waiting breathlessly for this first experiment in women's medical practice, Tiburtius declared. Instead, the rich and important families first sent employees like maids and cooks to the women physicians; and if that experience worked out well, then the *gnädige Frau selbst* (gracious lady herself) appeared at the clinic. Or perhaps she sent her children accompanied by a governess. The Berlin clinic also served many elderly women factory workers who invited the women doctors to visit working-class homes while becoming close friends and supporters of the medical practice.[41]

It was difficult in Germany for women to operate an uncertified practice and compete for private patients against male physicians who could work as salaried doctors in the state-sponsored medical insurance system for workers. Tiburtius reported that women physicians were later useful in administering private life insurance examinations to women workers who preferred female doctors.[42] In the early years, however, the Clinic of Women Doctors was fortunate to be hired by the privately-run Lette Association to care for women training at the school.[43] Other German girls' schools would have employed women physicians if they had been available, according to educator Helene

167

Lange. In neighboring Austria, a woman doctor in 1895 did begin her career teaching hygiene in a girls' school.[44]

Once women physicians began to work in Germany, they "found much interest and good-will among the public," as Tiburtius put it.[45] Abstract discussions reviewed by Tiburtius in her memoir might well have been useful in informing potential patients of the merits of women physicians, yet the decades-long delay in actually allowing women to study and work in certified medical practices resulted in very few German physicians to serve the poorer classes[46] or to meet the needs of any women who preferred women doctors before the twentieth century.

### Advocates and Supporters of Women's Medical Practices

In Russia, women physicians and *feldschers* proved through a type of field testing during war and in *zemstvo* service that women could practice general medicine, including surgery. Russian women also benefitted from a base of support by colleagues in the Pirogov Society.[47] Furthermore, the medical professors who taught in the Women's Medical Courses became allies in the struggle to broaden educational opportunities for women students. In governmental bureaucracies, some czarist officials became advocates for women's rights to work in medical practices for military purposes or to care for the poor in *zemstvo* health systems or in urban workers' clinics. Finally, the financial and social support of wealthy women benefactors in Russia undergirded the founding of separate medical training for women, which enabled them to enter the profession decades before German universities became resigned to medical co-education.

One factor slowing the course of higher education for girls could well have been that, as Tiburtius implies, German women generally did not control large private fortunes which might be spent funding women's causes.[48] Support for the first Berlin Women's Polyclinic came through fundraising efforts of women who organized many concerts, bazaars, and other charity functions to earn money. The most important contribution of a building for the clinic was arranged by persuading a wealthy industrialist to donate space rent-free in a workers' neighborhood. Luckily, his wife was a patient of dentist Henriette Tiburtius-Hirschfeld. Franziska Tiburtius explained that her sister-in-law's usual dental patients were women and children. However, Frau

Bötzow convinced her husband to consult with "Frau Doktor Henny" about his bothersome teeth. Once the wealthy gentleman was in the chair with his mouth full of dental gum for bite impressions, Tiburtius-Hirschfeld pleaded the case of the women physicians and the need for a working women's medical clinic. The donor, unable to argue against the petitioners,[49] responded to their pleas positively. Yet, clever and successful though this strategy for soliciting funds was, the incident shows how even wealthy women of good intentions necessarily relied on men in their families to decide on the disposition of charitable donations. Financial dependence was a fact of life for German women that reinforced their social subordination.

In contrast, Russian Law Codes of 1836 allowed both married and single women to possess private property, to inherit from their fathers, and to claim one-fourth of a husband's moveable estate and one-seventh of real estate.[50] After the industrialization era and the wars of German unification in the mid-nineteenth century, a disproportionate number of dependent single women attached to German families led to what Franziska Tiburtius remembered as the "Revolution of Aunts."[51] In other words, single women in extended households were no longer employed in the traditional support activities of sewing for family needs or of educating young relatives after the mechanization of needle-work and the establishment of community schools.[52] The necessity of self-support for even middle and some upper class single women was a driving motivation to seek further education for a variety of respectable careers.

Objections were rarely raised to the fact that lower-class women—married or single—had to work outside family homes. Women of the "leisured classes" could not be employed in the same occupations as poorer women and keep a higher social status. Paid medical attendants—including nurses and midwives—were often doomed to loss of reputation and respectability until Florence Nightingale reformed the training and practice of laywomen in medicine. Religious orders of women who nursed the sick, or women attending family members, were more exempt from that social degradation associated with women who dealt with the bodily problems of strangers. However, nurses and women physicians throughout the Western world faced various degrees of condemnation for their exposure to unseemly corporeal situations.

Most middle-class German women were introduced to respected professional careers in religious or scientific endeavors through family connections. Franziska Tiburtius' brother was a military doctor and Emilie Lehmus was the daughter of a Protestant pastor. In Germany, service to the state could be through both military and religious institutions. Women might gain respectability by linking their service aspirations to social arbitrators and institutional authorities in religion, science, or the governmental and military bureaucracies.

In czarist Russia, too, many students of medicine came from the families of priests, with their connections to social service ideals. Since Orthodox priests were not all well reimbursed for their work, their families were sometimes in precarious financial situations. The daughters often married other young priests, but those women who rejected such alternatives were compelled to think about supporting themselves—possibly by midwifery or advanced medical careers.

In Russian Jewish families, medical practices were commonly shared among family members or by successive generations as a household occupation. The Russian universities set quotas on Jewish students: their numbers were limited to 2.5 percent of the enrollment, reported Franziska Tiburtius, in explaining why so many Russian Jewish medical students came to Zürich.[53] Furthermore, medical or midwifery training gave Jewish Russians the opportunity to live outside the Pale of Settlement, that region open to Jewish inhabitants. During the 1880s, increasing antifeminism and antisemitism were expressed in official prejudices against Jewish women physicians. For example, Dr. Varvara Kashevarova was not only refused her post with the Bashkir tribe, but also rejected by *zemstvos* that advertised for physicians. She established a private practice in rural Russia near Kharkov where she wrote a book to inform women of preventive medical practices, *Popular Hygiene of the Female Organism* (1884).[54]

Jewish women like Kashevarova may have anticipated insecurities in planning for their futures given the cycles of antisemitism throughout European history. In addition, with the economic changes accompanying industrialization and in Russia, the emancipation of the serf labor force, more propertied women of the middle, gentry, and even aristocratic classes faced the prospects of loss of land or of financial support from the men in their families. Members of the Russian *intelligentsiya* (intellectual circles) attempted to ignore marks of social status so prominent in czarist society in order to counter the dominant traditional culture. Physicians were regarded as heralds of new ways of thinking scientifically and as alternatives to traditional authority figures in religious and czarist governmental bureaucracies. With the self-conscious egalitarianism of the intelligentsia as a model, doctors of varying social origins, of differing religious backgrounds, and of both genders were more accepted in many Russian social circles.[55]

## Cultural Constructs Influencing Popular Acceptance of Women Physicians

In Imperial Germany, sciences and especially new theories of evolution as to natural hierarchies were interpreted by many professors and other experts as providing modern reasons to fix women in a subordinate sphere of existence. Previously, German romantics like Schiller and Goethe had elevated women to an idealized separation from men. Goethe asserted that the eternal feminine leads men to strive for accomplishments. Schiller's paean to femininity, "Honor the women, they braid and weave heavenly roses in this earthly life," was quoted to buttress, for example, Professor Rydigier's assertion that women should not join men in medical practices inappropriate to their inspirational roles.[56] Thus, civilized women were not to sully themselves in occupations competing with men, but to limit feminine activities to those complementing male endeavors. New anthropological studies of the nineteenth century concluded that a hallmark of more primitive cultures was the rough equality of male and female roles—the strong figures of women among working classes, peasants, and backward peoples did not grace an advanced civilization as did those leisured ladies of the educated classes in modern Germany.

In contrast, the popular culture of Russia defined as desirable strong women with powerful maternal qualities: "The Russian people firmly believe in the power of a mother's blessing and a mother's curse."[57] After the Crimean War, Russian women wrote in journals and letters to the press requesting, in particular, improvements in education.[58] The end result, at the turn of century, was that the czarist government fully funded women's medical studies. This was, however, the only course of female higher education completely paid for out of public funds.

On the eve of World War I, which marked the demise of both Imperial Germany and Czarist Russia, Russian women comprised 10 percent of the medical profession. In 1892, before Czar Nicholas II funded the new women's training courses, women physicians in Russia were 4 percent of the profession (equal to the percentage of American women physicians at the same time, coincidentally). Fifty years after the 1917 revolution, 70 percent of Russian physicians were women. The comparable statistic in Western Germany was 20 percent in 1965.[59] Financial support for women medical students, whether from private donations or through public funds, was crucial to increasing the percentage of women physicians. Also important to bolstering the aspirations of women toward medical practice were public perceptions of women's abilities. The Russian women studying in Switzerland confounded traditional expectations by their behavior and attitudes. Germans were confused when women students threatened their sense of social order by being assertive and undominated by male paternalism.

Such cultural misunderstandings might have contributed to a tragic encounter when a German male student in Leipzig reportedly committed suicide after his attentions were spurned by a Russian woman auditing classes at the university. The German Minister of Education responded to this sensational event by banning all women from classrooms, so that females would not attend lectures and distract the university fellows.[60] Women auditors were blamed for the university students' lack of attention to their studies. Feminine presence in the public sphere could not be allowed to divert German men from their courses of achievement.

Since the 1860s, the German empire had been unified by winning expansionist wars in Central Europe. The German fatherland was strengthened through militaristic nationalism. Imperial Russia, in contrast, suffered more reverses in military campaigns in the nineteenth century. Losing wars made national leaders more open to changes in social arrangements—including those for women. In popular parlance, "Mother Russia" was a land where women were expected to sacrifice and serve national causes in maternal and caretaking roles. Women physicians were able to enter that national service in Russia, while in Germany they remained adjuncts to male efforts to prove national superiority through the struggles between empires that culminated in World War I.

For those last battles, the German army did accept women nurses' services in war zones, but rejected the recently certified women doctors because women medical officers would be entitled to military rank and "a German man can never be responsible to a woman. That would endanger discipline."[61] A former opponent of women in medicine, Dr. Herman Fehling, did admit that during the Great War, "For the first time I used the services of women assistants, and I can offer the best recommendation of their clinical obstetrical activity . . . and their assistance in operations."[62] Battlefield testing of surgical assistants and practical work in obstetrics finally allowed German women to prove their abilities as Russian women physicians had done forty years earlier during the Russo-Turkish War of 1877.

Franziska Tiburtius had told an audience in 1909, the year after women were allowed to matriculate in Prussian universities, that a Low German proverb promised: *"Wer slöppt and flink löppt, kümmt ook noch mit"* [People who sleep long but run quickly, may still arrive in time].[63] She went on to explain that German reluctance to accept women physicians lay "in the whole order of things" that led "in the German character to a tendency to conservatism and respect for everything of historical growth."[64] Despite the social revolutions in both Russia and Germany which followed the end of World War I, women in German medicine did not catch up to Russian physicians in either numbers or responsibilities. As late as 1977, for example, 100 percent of *assistants* to German pharmacists, doctors and dentists were female; but far fewer women practiced as independent professionals in these medical disciplines.[65] One explanation for this gender division in medicine was that "there were many men in medicine and law who, while having no objection to women studying *per se,* were not prepared to see female doctors, judges and lawyers practicing their profession, whatever the circumstances. They did accept the notion, however, that women could be medical and legal *assistants.* While it was quite clear that these men feared professional competition, there were many academics who were at least as anxious about the effect female involvement would have on the reputation of their field."[66] The greatest hinderances to the practice of medicine by women physicians were male insecurities, including both fear of economic and social competition with women in the medical professions and fear that professional women might upset traditional social order and gender rankings.

NOTES

Translations and paraphrases from the German originals are mine. I would like to thank our editor, Lilian Furst, for her patience, for careful reading of this submission, and for her many invaluable suggestions for improving the text.

1. Franziska Tiburtius, *Erinnerungen einer Achtzigjährigen* [Memoirs of an Eighty-Year-Old] (Berlin: C.A. Schwetsche & Sohn, 1923), 153-4.

2. Ibid.

3. Ibid., 155.

4. Sandra L. Chaff, et al., *Women in Medicine: A Bibliography of the Literature on Women Physicians* (Metuchen, N.J.: Scarecrow Press, 1977), 665-66. This useful collection includes translated abstracts of foreign language publications.

5. Jeanette E. Tuve, *The First Russian Women Physicians* (Newtonville, Mass.: Oriental Research Partners, 1984), 107. Valuable source of translated biographical information.

6. Ibid., 21.

7. Ibid., 24.

8. Tiburtius, *Erinnerungen,* 103.

9. Fanny Berlinerblau later practiced medicine in the United States as Dr. Berliner, chief surgeon at the New England Hospital for Women and Children founded by Berlin émigré, Dr. Marie Zakrzewska.

10. Tiburtius, *Erinnerungen,* 104.

11. *Fliegende Blätter* (March 8, 1873): 85 reprinted in James C. Albisetti, *Schooling German Girls and Women* (Princeton, N.J.: Princeton Univ. Press, 1988), 133.

12. *Boston Medical and Surgical Journal* 84 (1871): 50.

13. Mathilde Weber, *Ein Besuch in Zürich bei den weiblichen Studierenden der Medizin* [A Visit in Zürich to the Women Students of Medicine] (Tübingen: Franz Fues, 1888), 5.

14. Bonnie G. Smith, *Changing Lives: Women in European History Since 1700* (Lexington: D.C. Heath, 1989), 205, 324.

15. Weber, *Ein Besuch,* 4.

16. Ibid., 13, n.1.

17. James C. Albisetti, *Schooling German Girls and Women* (Princeton, N.J.: Princeton Univ. Press, 1988), 160. For a comprehensive survey of bureaucratic schooling decisions.

18. James C. Albisetti, "The Fight for Female Physicians in Imperial Germany," *Central European History* 15 (1982): 108-9.

19. Student Anna Shabnova remembered an incident "when a high official unexpectedly visited a physiology lecture in which the professor was lecturing about the nerves of the heart. The girls stood up and bowed to the visitor and the lecturer quickly shifted to the physiology of pregnancy, but reverted to his lecture on the nerves of the heart when the visitor left." Quoted in Tuve, *Russian Women Physicians,* 62.

20. Werner Dettlelbacher, "Dr. med. Marie Siebold," *Münchener Medizinische Wochenschrift* 115 (1973): 2052.

21. Samuel C. Ramer, "Childbirth and Culture: Midwifery in the Nineteenth-Century Russian Countryside," in *The Family in Imperial Russia,* ed. David L. Ransel (Urbana: Univ. of Illinois Press, 1978), 233.

22. Two distant German relatives of Dr. Marie Siebold received special doctor of obstetrics degrees from the University of Giessen in Germany: Josepha von Siebold in 1815 and her daughter Charlotte Heidenreich-von Siebold in 1817. The University of Marburg awarded French midwife, Marie-Anne Victorine Boivin, an honorary doctor of medicine degree for a book dedicated to the university in 1827. These were exceptional accomplishments; and in 1852, the head midwifery instructor in the Prussian Charité Hospital of Berlin, Marie Zakrzewska, found it necessary to emigrate to the United States in order to study for her M.D. degree.

23. Ramer, "Childbirth and Culture," 229.

24. Tuve, *Russian Women Physicians,* 67.

25. Ibid., 85.

26. David L. Ransel, *Mothers of Misery: Child Abandonment in Russia* (Princeton, N.J.: Princeton Univ. Press, 1988) details the spread of syphilis through wet nursing.

27. In 1889, Dr. Pokrovskaia estimated that 17,603 prostitutes were registered by Russian police. At Kalinkinsky Hospital, case studies of 103 infected women led the doctor to recommend eighteen steps to eliminate prostitution, since state regulation had not proved effective in limiting disease. Furthermore, the regulatory strategy had been abandoned by many other countries as both demeaning to women and ineffectual for disease prevention. Tuve, *Russian Women Physicians,* 95-97.

28. Tuve, *Russian Women Physicians,* 98.

29. Rose L. Glickman, *Russian Factory Women: Workplace and Society, 1880-1914* (Berkeley: Univ. of California Press, 1984), 143-45, 266.

30. Ibid., 270.

31. Tuve, *Russian Women Physicians,* 51.

32. "I insisted on defending my dissertation because I wanted to be an instructor in the Women's Medical Courses. I had everything required: a degree as doctor of medicine, scientific works, and proven lecture ability." Varvara Kashevarova quoted in ibid., 52.

33. Ibid., 32 n. 29.

34. Ann Hibner Koblitz, "Science, Women, and the Russian Intelligentsia: The Generation of the Sixties," *Isis* 79 (1988): 219.

35. Ibid.

36. Barbara Alpern Engel and Clifford N. Rosenthal, eds. and trans., *Five Sisters: Women against the Czar* (New York: Alfred A. Knopf, 1975), 27, 35. Translations of memoirs by Vera Figner and other female revolutionaries in nineteenth-century Russia.

37. Tiburtius, *Erinnerungen,* 104.

38. Richard Stites, *The Women's Liberation Movement in Russia* (Princeton: Princeton Univ. Press, 1978), 86.

39. Weber, *Ein Besuch,* 6.

40. Ann Taylor Allen, *Feminism and Motherhood in Germany, 1880-1914* (New Brunswick, N.J.: Rutgers Univ. Press, 1991). This history of maternal feminism focuses on the kindergarten movement.

41. Tiburtius, *Erinnerungen,* 160.

42. Franziska Tiburtius, "The Development of the Study of Medicine for Women in Germany, and Present Status," *The Canadian Practitioner and Review* 34 (1909): 496.

43. Tiburtius, *Erinnerungen,* 165.

44. Chaff et al., *Women in Medicine,* 123.

45. Tiburtius, "Study of Medicine for Women," 495.

46. Reinhard Spree, *Health and Social Class in Imperial Germany: A Social History of Mortality, Morbidity, and Inequality,* trans. Stuart McKinnon-Evans (Oxford: Berg Press, 1988). This statistical and analytic study gives evidence for "the impact of class formation and stratification on chances of survival."

47. Nancy Mandel Frieden, *Russian Physicians in an Era of Reform and Revolution* (Princeton, N.J.: Princeton Univ. Press, 1981). The analysis of professionalization stresses the importance of the Pirogov Society for improving *zemstvo* medicine.

48. Tiburtius, "Study of Medicine for Women," 493.

49. Tiburtius, *Erinnerungen,* 151-52.

50. Stites, *Women's Liberation,* 7-8.

51. Tiburtius, "Study of Medicine for Women," 493.

52. Ruth-Ellen B. Joeres and Mary Jo Maynes, eds., *German Women in the Eighteenth and Nineteenth Centuries: A Social and Literary History* (Bloomington: Indiana Univ. Press, 1986). This collection includes examples of changing occupations and employments for women of various classes.

53. Tiburtius, *Erinnerungen,* 101.

54. Tuve, *Russian Women Physicians,* 54.

55. Observers of the universities in both Germany and Russia commented, for example, that in Russia women students were basically treated as equal comrades by the men studying with them. "Fraternity is never seen to better advantage than in the student colonies," insisted Russian sociologist A.S. Rappoport. "One girl's family lives in Russia and leaves her to do as she pleases . . . there is not flirtation with her male comrades. And what a difference between America and Russia! In Russia, the men do not *look up* to women; they are equals, comrades, nothing more. In Russian universities, where the two sexes are separated, there is just the same solidarity between them . . . the women were side by side with the men . . . they wish to share the burden of those who are heavy-laden. They are the romanticists of philanthrophy and intellectuality." A[ngelo] S. Rappoport, *Home Life in Russia* (London: Methuen, 1913), 244. The testimony of Russian-German physician Elsa Winokurow supports these impressions: "Looking back on my professional life, I must say that an educated woman was

176

shown more comradeship and courtesy in Russia than in Germany. I would like to emphasize here how grateful I am to Professor Valentin for his decision to accept me, a woman, as his colleague [in Russia]." Quoted in Leone McGregor Hellstedt, *Women Physicians of the World* (New York: McGraw-Hill, 1978), 15.

56. Professor Rydigier, "Zur Frage der Zulassung der Frauen zum Medicin-Studium" [In Regard to the Question Concerning Permission for Women to Study Medicine], *Wiener Klinische Wochenschrift* 15 (1896): 275-78.

57. Rappoport, *Home Life in Russia,* 84.

58. Ibid., 33.

59. Statistics from John B. Parrish, "Women in Medicine: What Can International Comparisons Tell Us?" *The Woman Physician* 26 (1971).

60. Albisetti, *Schooling German Girls and Women,* 128.

61. Quoted in Thomas Neville Bonner, *To the Ends of the Earth: Women's Search for Education in Medicine* (Cambridge, Mass.: Harvard Univ. Press, 1992), 118.

62. Ibid.

63. Tiburtius, "Study of Medicine for Women," 492.

64. Ibid., 494.

65. Ute Frevert, *Women in German History: From Bourgeois Emancipation to Sexual Liberation,* trans. Stuart Mc-Kinnon-Evans et al. (New York: Berg Press, 1988), 276.

66. Ibid., 124.

# [ 9 ]

# THE MAKING OF A WOMAN SURGEON
*How Mary Dixon Jones Made a Name for Herself in*
*Nineteenth-Century Gynecology*

REGINA MORANTZ-SANCHEZ

*In much of my work* on the history of women physicians I have tried
to explore historically the intersection of gender and professional values. I have
rejected essentializing notions regarding women's behavior as physicians and
have argued instead that women doctors—as citizens, as professionals, as clinicians, as participants in politics, and as the shapers of cultural and medical discourse—demonstrate a considerable range of views and behaviors. In spite of
their differences, however, I have found that most pioneer women doctors
stated publicly, and likely believed, that they belonged in the medical profession by virtue of their natural gifts as healers and nurturers. They defended
their role in the nineteenth-century medical profession by arguing that women
would bring cooperation, selflessness, nurturing, purity and social concern to
their work. They saw these special qualities as the strongest possible justification they could muster for the continued existence of the woman physician.[1]

I have further suggested that women physicians shared a certain social
positioning. Somewhat estranged from the larger social milieu by their decision to become professionals, while segregated within the medical profession
by their separate identity as women, they often viewed the emergence of late
nineteenth-century medical professionalism from a different and more critical
vantage point than the majority of their male colleagues. As the Blackwell sisters urged at the beginning of their campaign to train women in medicine, the
primary task of the "medical movement amongst women in America," was
"for the purpose of occupying positions which men cannot fully occupy, and
exercising an influence which men cannot wield at all."[2] Many female physi-

cians, while quite conversant with changing therapeutic modalities, were slower to respond in their clinical behavior to the emerging "modern" professional ethos, which discarded traditional holistic methods of care in favor of more technocratic approaches.

While at mid-century women physicians readily characterized themselves in their public statements as a "connecting link" between the science of the medical profession and the everyday life of women, the medical science they had in mind still privileged the physician-patient encounter, emphasized the importance of knowledge gained through experience at the bedside, and stressed the exercise of keen judgment in meeting each sick individual's idiosyncratic needs. They built institutions—hospitals and medical schools—which attempted to give voice to these particular approaches to patient care.[3]

But in the last third of the nineteenth century, with the emergence of bacteriology and a new epistemology dependent as much on observation in the laboratory as at the sickbed, older conceptions of the good practitioner were challenged. The germ theory offered the paradigm of experimental science to practitioners who had long since come to doubt the efficacy of heroic methods of treatment, which included copious bleeding, purging and puking. The new ideology of science in medicine replaced a belief in illness as a disequilibrium of the entire body with an acceptance of specific etiology, the identification of various pathogenic organisms, the promotion of specialization, and a growing willingness to resort to evidence produced in the laboratory. The result was in some cases to deemphasize and in most cases to transform physician-patient interaction at the bedside. According to the new science, less attention needed to be paid to the patient's social and physical environment, while prior dependence on his or her narrative identification of bodily signs and symptoms gave way to a concentration on specific parts or functions and a new reliance on objective evidence and tests, such as the reading of a thermometer or the determination of the chloride level in urine.[4]

Some women physicians were highly suspicious of this novel approach to illness, in part because they believed that women's particular strength as physicians lay in their abilities to treat the patient holistically, invoking what Elizabeth Blackwell, a prolific writer on the subject, had labelled "the spiritual power of maternity." This complex of qualities informed not only Blackwell's notions of the doctor's moral responsibility, but her formulations of what constituted good science. These she described as "the subordination of self to the welfare of others; the recognition of the claim which helplessness and ignorance make upon the stronger and more intelligent; the joy of creation and bestowal of life; the pity and sympathy which tend to make every woman the born foe of cruelty and injustice; and hope—which foresees the adult in the infant, the future in the present." Though she believed women physicians derived their moral insights from the social practice of mothering, Blackwell argued that all physicians, male and female alike, could be taught "the spiritual power of maternity."[5]

I have argued elsewhere that Blackwell's invocation of culturally available gender symbols to criticize laboratory medicine represented a contestation of changing power relationships among practitioners. While her association of nurturing and empathic expertise with femininity was something new in medical discourse, an older concept of professionalism, advocated by and potentially accessible to both sexes, maintained a place for intuition and sympathy and stressed the therapeutic powers of moral and social concerns. Indeed, Blackwell was joined in her opposition to the new science by highly respected clinicians, many of whom, like Austin Flint and Alfred Stille, both past presidents of the American Medical Association, also viewed the shift of focus to the laboratory as a conspiracy to ignore the particular needs of individual patients. "There is an art of medicine," Stille opined, "[that] completely eludes, or flatly contradicts science, by means of empirical facts, and gives the palm to sagacity and common sense over laws formulated by experiment." "Clinical experience," he noted, "is the only true safe test of the virtues of medicines." But, whereas Stille and Flint struggled to preserve a particular style of behavior for all clinicians, Blackwell re-gendered it as a female characteristic, one that arose, not out of woman's "nature," but from social conditioning.[6]

Although they may not have articulated their *raison d'être* with the same sophistication as Elizabeth Blackwell, many women physicians continued to subscribe to an ideology which promoted their uniqueness in the profession and critiqued the reductionist tendencies of the new medical science. As late as 1925, Eliza Mosher, a past president of the American Medical Women's Association, regretted the loss of "the sympathetic relation which formerly existed between doctors and their patients," and warned her colleagues to beware of "narrowing and concentrating their vision upon the purely physical to the exclusion of the psychic and human."[7] Indeed, even today, women physicians are believed to be more partial than men to holistic approaches to care.[8]

This emphasis on women's special qualifications and the privileging of the "art" of caring has been a strong tradition among women physicians in both the nineteenth and the twentieth centuries. Of course, such arguments always carry with them the risk of marginalization. But these ideas have clearly given cultural meaning to women physicians' work and have provided individuals with crucial self-understanding and valuable agendas that have helped shape personal goals within the larger profession. Especially notable in this regard was the disproportionate interest of women physicians in preventive care, public health and social medicine in the period between 1870 and 1930.[9]

But there were those women at the end of the century who were powerfully drawn to the new science and less animated by the idioms of domesticity and metaphors of mothering publicly appropriated by the women's medical movement. Some were less troubled by perceived tensions between caring and curing; moreover, their enthusiasm for laboratory medicine and the insights it could provide at the bedside was palpable. For them the transformation of medical practice proved a special challenge. They needed access to new knowledge being generated by centers of medical research at home and abroad. This task demanded a willingness to pursue informal postgraduate training from groups of male medical elites not interested in the needs of the woman doctor or particularly concerned with her professional advancement. For a few women this meant moving away from the female networks that offered nurture, education, support and employment to women physicians, and going it alone in the world of men.

One such individual was Mary Dixon Jones, a pioneer gynecological surgeon who, through extraordinary effort, gained entree into the small, transnational group of self-proclaimed elite physicians consciously attempting to shape the direction of the specialty of gynecology. In exploring her career, I hope to describe, not only some of the less-known options for career-building open to courageous and determined women, but also the ways in which some both articulated and challenged accepted cultural meanings attached to the woman physician. Dixon Jones spent almost thirty years negotiating a professional identity at a time when boundaries, behaviors and ideologies of practice were in flux. Her career was at once typical and quite extraordinary. Especially notable in her story is a discernible careerism that drew her away from comfortable female networks and led her to the newly-forming community of male gynecologists and surgeons who, in the last third of the nineteenth century, were themselves vulnerable to criticism from traditional practitioners and the public because they advocated specialization and new approaches to treatment. It will be argued that Dixon Jones participated in creating the specialty of gynecology, but she did so, as we shall see, at the sufferance of her male colleagues, who treated her as a not-always-welcome guest.

A graduate of the Woman's Medical College of Pennsylvania in 1873 at the age of 45, and only seven years younger than Elizabeth Blackwell, Dixon Jones's path to professional prominence was a familiar one for women physicians of her generation. She began as a teacher, taught physiology and literary subjects at various female seminaries, and read medicine with a well known Maryland physician, Dr. Thomas Bond. In the 1860s she received a sectarian medical degree from a coeducational hydropathic college in New York, at a time when no orthodox medical college was accepting women on a regular basis and the first women's medical college, The Woman's Medical College of Pennsylvania, had opened its doors only several years before.[10]

Like several women physicians in those years who attended sectarian institutions because no regular medical school would accept them, Dixon Jones found herself drawn back into medical study later in her career, this time at an orthodox institution. She spent three years in the early 1870s matriculating in Philadelphia at the Woman's Medical College, displaying a particular interest in laboratory science—microscopy and pathology—and in surgery. Here Dixon Jones came into contact with the new science of bacteriology. She also attended surgical clinics at Blockley Hospital, and she engaged Benjamin B. Wilson, the school's professor of the principles and practice of surgery, as a private tutor. In 1873 she passed a three-month preceptorship in New York with Mary Putnam Jacobi, a highly respected Paris-trained woman physician, who herself was passionately devoted to the new medical research. Dixon Jones then reestablished her medical practice in Brooklyn, where she had resided before her move to Philadelphia. Subsequently, she took courses in gynecological surgery at the New York Postgraduate Medical School.[11]

The work in surgery was crucial to her subsequent career, for one of the earliest by-products of the new experimental science occurred in the operating room. While the gradual use of anesthesia after mid-century had lessened the pain of surgery, Lister's adaptation of the germ theory in his principles of antisepsis guaranteed the relatively safe surgical invasion of the body for a variety of hitherto incurable complaints. Many of these were gynecological, and by far the largest proportion of abdominal operations between 1860 and the end of the 1890s were performed on women.[12]

Patients presented with a variety of complaints, including chronic pelvic pain, usually accompanied by excessive bleeding during or between periods, tenderness or swelling in the ovarian region, and a host of menstrual irregularities. In addition, there were women with huge ovarian cysts and other types of abdominal tumors, whose distended abdomens, excruciating pain, and emaciated bodies caused unspeakable suffering. A small group of bold surgeons in America and abroad rejected the palliative measures of traditional gynecological therapy—namely, draining cysts through the use of a sharp instrument called a trocar, prescribing rest, massage, pessaries and changes in diet—in favor of operative solutions. Although risk was initially high, they believed they offered the possibility of complete cure, and often patients themselves preferred surgery to enduring what some regarded as an indefinite living death.

Especially controversial were the removal of "normal" ovaries, often called oophorectomy or ovariotomy, an operation first introduced by Robert Battey of Rome, Georgia, a founding member of the American Gynecological Society, one of the most prestigious of the new specialty associations. Battey argued that even ovaries displaying no demonstrably gross pathology could, in some instances, do such damage to the nervous system of certain unfortunate patients that their removal was justified.[13]

Although Battey viewed this treatment as a *"dernier resort"* for desperate cases, "Battey's operation," as his procedure came to be called, helped open up a new era in operative gynecology in the 1870s and 1880s, as surgeons became increasingly willing to try laparotomy (opening the abdomen for a variety of procedures), in cases that were not life-threatening. Some historians have been particularly critical of physicians involved in gynecological surgery during this era, urging cultural interpretations that represent doctors' enthusiasm for it as an attack by men on women's bodies arising from a desire to control women increasingly viewed by social critics as restless, discontented, and disorderly.[14] But although it is useful to question the motivation of physicians and to recognize that they did indeed learn abdominal surgery by way of surgical gynecology, such an interpretation misses the complexity of developments in nineteenth-century medicine.[15] There is no question that there was much irresponsible decision-making, as an element of impatience crept into case reports in the last two decades of the nineteenth century. Surgeons and patients alike seemed more willing to proceed at the earliest signs of pain or disease, and many an overeager young surgeon performed oophorectomy for questionable indications.[16] By this time, practitioners had perfected technique and reduced mortality to such an extent that they had become comfortable even with exploratory operations for diagnostic purposes. But this gradual expansion of accepted indications for surgery, together with the conviction among many leading surgeons that early operations were preferable to traditional treatment, created controversy even among gynecologists themselves. In the United States they tended to divide into two groups, labeled "radical" and "conservative," and the debates among them were heated. It was at this juncture in the development of the specialty that Mary Dixon Jones began her surgical work, identifying herself most readily with the radicals. In 1881, she became the chief medical officer of the Women's Dispensary and Hospital of the city of Brooklyn, a charitable institution whose "Board of Lady Managers" boasted some of the most prominent matrons in the city. Heightening discord with the hospital's trustees, however, probably over Dixon Jones's increasing interest in ovariotomy, led to a severing of that relationship in January, 1884, and the establishment a few months later of her own gynecological hospital, an institution that allowed her complete autonomy and flexibility in medical decision-making, since she dominated its board of trustees. The new attending staff consisted of Dixon Jones, her son Charles, a recent graduate of Long Island College Hospital, and another woman physician, Eliza J. Chapin Minard.

In the beginning, the hospital was called the J. Marion Sims Hospital and Dispensary, though its name was soon changed to the Woman's Hospital of Brooklyn. The original name is revealing of Dixon Jones's apparent desire to identify herself with the recently deceased pioneer gynecological surgeon of New York City, who had successfully presided over a revolution in gynecological surgery with the founding of the New York Woman's Hospital in the 1850s.[17]

Increasingly in the nineteenth century, hospitals began to play a crucial role in training doctors as well as in treating the sick.[18] Moreover, the rise of specialty hospitals was an important chapter in the development of gynecology in this period. In England, the typical founder of a special hospital was a practitioner who couldn't secure a coveted elite position at a general hospital, either because he didn't have the proper social connections with prestigious members of the profession or he was not wealthy enough to influence the vote of lay governors. Specialty hospitals were often established at a distance from elite, highly competitive London, and provided a venue for a number of prominent surgeons from the provinces to rise to the top. In this way entre-preneurship rivaled patronage as a means of getting ahead.[19]

Though the more flexible class system in the United States provided a leavening element among ambitious young doctors, specialty hospitals were also used here as a means of providing those practitioners who had uncertain social connections with a field of endeavor in which to make a mark. Running her own hospital provided Dixon Jones with the clinical opportunities to pursue gynecological surgery. As a woman, of course, her interest in surgery could not have been successfully satisfied at any of the existing hospitals, except those few in Boston, New York, Philadelphia and Chicago affiliated with a woman's medical school, and Dixon Jones seems to have consciously rejected such connections.[20] As for a coveted position at a male-run institution, the situation in New York was typical. Though the Board of Lady Managers at Sims's New York Hospital had stipulated that he appoint a woman assistant, Sims neglected to do so, and it was well into the twentieth century before a woman surgeon operated at the hospital he founded.[21]

Once she had established her own hospital, Dixon Jones both performed operations and meticulously went about the task of constructing a professional identity in gynecological surgery and pathology. In the spring of 1884 she attempted her first laparotomy, removing a diseased ovary and its appendages from a woman she diagnosed as a classic case of "hystero-epilepsy due to reflex irritation."[22] Four cases of ovariotomy followed the next year and seven the year after that. In the ensuing decade, Dixon Jones performed between one hundred and three hundred laparotomies.[23] In the beginning, she often sought the advice and assistance of other experienced practitioners in New York and Brooklyn. Several of these men, themselves in the process of building careers, attended her operations. Moreover, she continued to attend operations at the New York Woman's Hospital and at Bellevue, where she undoubtedly met Lawson Tait, the renowned English ovariotomist, and saw him operate during his trip to the United States in 1884.[24]

In 1886, Dixon Jones made an extended visit to Europe, studying in various hospitals and visiting the clinics of some of the most skilled surgeons, including Tait, Theodore Bilroth, August Martin, Carl Shroeder and Jules Pean. Upon her return the following year she completed the first total hysterectomy for fibroid tumor ever attempted in the United States.[25]

Along with her surgical accomplishments, Dixon Jones continued the interest in pathology she had developed in medical school, carefully studying with a microscope tumors and tissue removed from the bodies of her patients. She developed an intimate acquaintance with Dr. Carl Heitzman, a Hungarian immigrant who was known as an expert microcopist and a specialist in skin diseases. He aided her in making slides and preparing specimens and she accomplished much of her scientific work under his guidance. She became a member of the New York Pathological Society and frequently brought in specimens to meetings for discussion. She began publishing pathological findings and clinical case reports in leading journals like the *American Journal of Obstetrics, The Medical Record,* and the *British Gynaecological Journal* beginning in 1884, calling attention to herself both as a technical virtuoso in the operating room and a careful scientist in the laboratory. During her lifetime Dixon Jones published more than forty papers in gynecology and surgery. Indeed, the *Dictionary of American Medical Biography* credits her, not only with being the first U.S. surgeon to perform total hysterectomy for uterine myoma (growths, usually fibroid), but also with describing and identifying two diseases—endothelioma, cancer of the lining of the uterus, and gyroma, a cancerous tumor of the ovary.[26]

Dixon Jones had learned to operate by taking advantage of the generosity of male colleagues in Brooklyn and especially in New York who were willing to consult with her, have her attend their operations, and occasionally assist at hers. She was aggressive in penetrating these informal networks, and she was not hesitant to attempt ovariotomy, as the men themselves had done, when it became necessary to move from observation to performance. With similar determination, she used publishing to construct an international professional identity as a gynecological surgeon. Her articles found their way into leading specialty journals at home and abroad, and she worked hard to make her achievements known.

One gains some insight into her gift for self-promotion by looking carefully at these articles, which she used successfully to convince readers that she was indeed a member of a relatively small group of elite practitioners who were pioneering in operative approaches to women's diseases. Her first article, for example, entitled "A Case of Tait's Operation," was a rather audacious attempt to associate her work with the world-renowned ovariotomist from Birmingham, Lawson Tait. She not only references him over and over again in subsequent publications, but corresponded with him as well, excerpting one of his letters to her in a footnote to one article and telling her readers in another that her son, Charles, had operated with him during their grand European tour in 1886. She eventually attracted Tait's attention sufficiently to prompt him to refer to her with effusive praise in one of his own publications.[27]

Indeed, given the controversies raging among "radical" and "conservative" practitioners over the legitimacy of ovariotomy, Tait, a radical, appeared delighted to have a woman surgeon on his side. Responding to critics who decried the sterility resulting from "Tait's Operation," as the removal of diseased ovaries and appendages was often called, he offered Dixon Jones's argument (also his own) that it was disease, and not the operation to cure it, that caused sterility in the first place. Prefacing his reprinting of her comments with the remark "I have great belief in the opinions of women upon all matters concerning their own sex. Here is the opinion of a very clever woman on this subject, Dr. Mary Dixon Jones of Brooklyn," he used Dixon Jones to take a swipe at his rival, Sir Spencer Wells. "He will see," Tait observed of Wells, directing him to one of Dixon Jones's published articles, "how a woman can understand, recognize, and successfully treat the troubles of these out-of-the-way organs when [they are] the subject of irreparable disease."[28]

It was not only with Tait that Dixon Jones persistently identified in her published work. She also mentions connections, conversations and consultations with prominent gynecological surgeons in New York, Boston and Philadelphia, and demonstrates familiarity with the work of most ovariotomists who published in the respected journals. Indeed, her articles are characterized by incessant name-dropping, coupled with continuous self-referencing to her other articles, and frequent claims to being "the first" to discover a particular cell formation or to try a certain procedure. In terms of her self-presentation, Dixon Jones was a person who had made it in the world of gynecological surgery and whose expertise in the new science was manifest in her publications in surgical pathology. By 1889, Dixon Jones had launched a promising career in gynecological surgery without connection or aid from any of the networks of female physicians. Certainly she was not the only woman doctor interested in ovariotomy, nor was she the first to perform it. Emmeline Cleveland and Anna Fullerton did abdominal surgery at the Woman's Hospital of Philadelphia, as did Elizabeth Keller and Mary Smith at the New England Hospital for Women and Children. In New York, Emily Blackwell, who had passed a preceptorship with Sir James Y. Simpson in Edinburgh, was also reputed to be a skilled surgeon, as was Elizabeth Cushier, also at the New York Infirmary for Women and Children. Mary Thompson and Marie Mergler both had active hospital practices in Chicago. In 1880, an ovariotomy in private practice was performed in Rhode Island by Anita E. Tyng, the first woman to be admitted to the Rhode Island Medical Society. Tyng, like Dixon Jones a graduate of the Woman's Medical College of Pennsylvania, was assisted by no less than four other women physicians, all of them fellow graduates of the school, who travelled to Providence especially for the event.[29] But none of these women sought out the recognition and approval of their male colleagues with the persistence and energy of Dixon Jones. While they may have privately regretted and publicly protested their constricted opportunities, their reference groups were formed primarily out of female communities linked to the various women's institutions.[30]

Dixon Jones's carefully crafted professional identity reached well beyond the more typical achievements of nineteenth-century women physicians and, in the end, the aggressiveness with which she orchestrated her own success probably hastened her downfall. Wishing to advertize her hospital, she invited the *Brooklyn Eagle* newspaper to feature it as a charitable institution. But her energetic surgery, her penchant for name-dropping, and her assertive personality had offended local practitioners, many of whom were more conservative in the treatment of women's diseases and sensitive regarding Brooklyn's reputation as less up-to-date than New York. In the course of investigating her career the *Eagle* reporter met with a host of detractors who questioned her "character," including members of the King's County Medical Association. The *Eagle* eventually produced a series of unflattering articles about Dixon Jones that touched off an avalanche of public criticism against her surgery and resulted in two manslaughter charges and eight malpractice suits against her. The newspaper painted a portrait of an ambitious social climber, a knife-happy, irresponsible surgeon who forced unnecessary operations on innocent and unsuspecting women and used the specimens gleaned from them to advance her reputation in diagnosis and pathology.

Malpractice suits had become an increasing problem, especially for surgeons doing advanced and risky surgery, but Dixon Jones was not prepared for the negative allegations in the *Eagle*'s attack.[31] Although the legal charges were eventually dropped, she attempted to restore her reputation by charging the *Eagle* with libel.[32]

Jones's lawyers sought $300,000 in damages, claiming that their client had been victimized by the newspaper, aided by certain disreputable members of Brooklyn's medical establishment. The trial involved some of the most prestigious physicians in New York and Brooklyn and proved to be a legal spectacle of major proportion. Testimony took almost two months; roughly three hundred witnesses were called, including former patients with babies in their arms. Jars full of specimens and surgical mannequins became common sights in the courtroom.

The *Brooklyn Medical Journal* claimed the event involved the "honor and reputation" of its medical establishment, and even the *Journal of the American Medical Association* commented on the verdict. The popular press, already entering the age of "yellow journalism," gave it abundant play. The *New York Tribune* dubbed the inquiry "by far the most important ever tried in this city." The *Brooklyn Citizen*, the *Brooklyn Times*, the *New York Times*, and the *New York World* highlighted the story. The *Eagle* covered the proceedings daily and printed much of the court testimony *verbatim*. The *Philadelphia Ledger*, undoubtedly reacting to the keen public interest which filled the courtroom with curious spectators of all stripes, hailed the case as "the most important . . . since the Beecher" scandal, a reference to the lurid Beecher-Tilton adultery trial that had riveted citizens in the New York area in the early 1870s.[33]

When Dixon Jones lost her case, the state and city withdrew public funds from her hospital and its charter was revoked. The deprivation of an operating theater effectively ended her surgical career. Relocating to New York City, she became an editor of the *Woman's Medical Journal* and passed the decade and a half before her death publishing articles on pathology, utilizing over and over again the specimens and slides collected from the hundred-odd operations she had performed in the previous decade. On occasion, she continued to be recognized for her work by male practitioners; in 1898 the president of the British Gynaecological Society cited her achievements in his presidential address.[34] But her surgical career was cut short, and her promise as a voice in shaping the direction of the specialty of gynecology abruptly terminated before it could be fulfilled.

How do we evaluate this narrative of success and failure? The trial testimony gives us some interesting clues. Reading the transcripts published by the *Brooklyn Eagle*, one learns much about Dixon Jones's status with the Brooklyn medical community, the subtext of her relationship with the self-created group of elite gynecological surgeons in New York City and elsewhere, the tensions over specialization seething within the profession at large and the ways in which representations of gender were imbedded in the construction of new professional identities. I will touch briefly on each of these subjects in turn.

In retrospect, it is clear that Dixon Jones's blatant pursuit of her own professional goals and her somewhat aggressive personality were tolerated best by colleagues with whom she came into contact only occasionally. Her immediate professional community in Brooklyn took clear offense at her behavior. In the spring of 1884, for example, her application for membership to the King's County Medical Society was tabled on the grounds that there was too much opposition to her candidacy. In contrast, her son, Charles, her surgical assistant, was accepted by the society in 1886 and remained a member in good standing until 1892.[35]

Nor were Dixon Jones's medical detractors all men. Several women physicians deplored her behavior and testified regarding her poor medical reputation. Caroline S. Pease claimed to have worked briefly as Dixon Jones's assistant in 1886 and complained of "a very marked discrimination" in favor of surgical cases.[36] Eliza Mosher and her partner Lucy Hall Brown, both members of the County Medical Society, joined Pease in expressing reservations regarding Dixon Jones's character on the witness stand. Moreover, in a letter to her friend and mentor, Elizabeth Blackwell, written the week Dixon Jones's first case report appeared in the *American Journal of Obstetrics,* Mosher announced, no doubt referring to Jones: "There are several regularly graduated women who are already members of the Kings Co. Med. Socy. There is one who, judging from her paper read before the Pathological Socy not long since, is rather an able woman, but her manners are beyond description—we could not identify our selves [*sic*] with her safely and she is an element of evil because of her coarseness."[37]

One can only guess at what offended Mosher about Dixon Jones. But she was not the only one to record reservations about her behavior. Howard Kelly and Walter Burrage, the authors of the *Dictionary of American Medical Biography,* remark on Dixon Jones's reputation for giving offense. They note that she was "peculiar in person" and "flashy and tawdry in appearance." A younger contemporary of hers, Kelly speculates that "lack of judgment and of intimate contact with the better members of the profession may have been responsible for a certain mental obliquity with which she is accredited."[38]

Witnesses for the *Eagle* similarly drew a portrait of a strong willed and outspoken woman who was not above tongue-lashing uncooperative colleagues and laypeople. A.J.C. Skene, a prominent senior gynecologist in Brooklyn with a dignified reputation in the field, confessed at the trial that Dixon Jones threatened him when he ceased consulting with her, warning that "she had a tongue and would use it." Indeed, the *Eagle* reported that during her testimony the trial judge had to request several times that she stick to answering the questions.[39]

It is possible that their use of words like "coarse" and "tawdry" demonstrates that these witnesses lacked a vocabulary to describe Dixon Jones's assertiveness, a quality unconventional and unacceptable in a woman at the time. But at least some of this professional hostility came from traditional physicians whose overt disapproval of her surgical solutions to pelvic ailments represented a larger suspicion of the changes taking place in medicine which her medical work represented. Her critics, all of whom practiced in Brooklyn, focused primarily on the uncertain validity of her therapeutics. The testimony of A.J.C. Skene was typical. Known to be a staunch conservative on the subject of ovariotomy, Skene was professor of gynecology at the Long Island College Hospital. He acknowledged that he had known Dixon Jones for fifteen or sixteen years, that she had operated on two of his patients against his recommendation, and that he no longer consulted with her. When her lawyer tried to characterize him as a member of the "conservative" as opposed to the "radical" school of gynecology, Skene demurred, commenting that with good surgeons "surgery was never resorted to except in cases where life would be in danger if no operation should be performed."[40]

But here Skene was being disingenuous. There were plenty of surgeons by 1892 who believed in operating well before pathological conditions became immediately life-threatening, while others agreed with Lawson Tait that in many cases exploratory surgery was indicated. Skene's remarks rather suggest disapproval of the manner in which doctors specializing in surgical gynecology went about creating a place for themselves in the profession. Young, and definitely on the make, surgical enthusiasts were orchestrating a decided power shift in the medical hierarchy. Their ambitious and entrepreneurial approach to professional disputes prompted more traditional physicians like Skene to fear the passing of an older, gentlemanly image. Suspicion of the new professional style fueled outcries against too much specialization and raised anxieties regarding the proper relationship between laboratory science and bedside practice.

In defense of Dixon Jones came an array of prominent young surgeons from New York City and Philadelphia. A.M. Phelps, W. Gill Wylie and J. Marion Sims each confirmed that they had done hundreds of laparotomies of the type performed by Dixon Jones and that they had consulted with her

191

on numerous occasions.[41] It is important to note that none of these practitioners was personally friendly with Dixon Jones. Nor were they particularly committed to opening up opportunities for women in medicine. What brought them across the Brooklyn Bridge to give evidence on behalf of a woman was the realization that it was not simply Dixon Jones's career in gynecological surgery that was on trial, but their own.

In addition, gender tensions can be detected in the debates between expert witnesses, especially around the subject of the relationship of physicians to patients. Dixon Jones was accused of misusing her professional power to manipulate and harm patients, all of whom were women. Though her lawyers employed the matter of her sex in her defense, urging that she embraced the "best in femininity" in her work, detractors found her particularly heinous because she was a woman. They emphasized her poor communication with patients and their families, though A.M. Phelps explained that it was not usual for physicians to explain to ignorant patients the nature of imminent operations. Confident of the value of their surgical solutions, Gill Wylie observed that because laparotomies had become routine, "much less ceremony was observed than there used to be about obtaining consents."[42]

The disagreements voiced by various practitioners in the trial testimony represent the reluctance of Dixon Jones's Brooklyn colleagues to accept the experimental, active and manipulative stance toward gynecological problems that she and her supporters espoused. Indeed, if we remember that the prevailing image of the woman physician was nurturing and sympathetic, the fact that Dixon Jones was a woman may have actually heightened existing anxieties about the meaning of her various activities for the future of medical practice. Was she not performing aggressive scientific experiments on patients? Using pathological specimens in the name of science to advance her career? Refusing to inform patients properly of her intentions? Surely her conduct was inappropriate for a woman, but lurking beneath the surface of that conviction was distress over how representative she was of the profession at large. For if a woman was tempted to behave in this manner, what kind of insensitivity might the public expect from men?

In point of fact, the worriers might have been comforted at least partially by the knowledge that Mary Dixon Jones's career was not representative of the majority of her female colleagues. Most of them were pushed to the margins of medical practice, or carved out niches for themselves in family practice, treating primarily women and children, and in public health and preventive medicine. They ran their own institutions and functioned within a series of professional networks which provided mutual support and a positive professional identity within a larger, masculine world.

But Dixon Jones was clearly not satisfied with the professional pathways carved out by the first generations of women physicians, nor was she willing to act out the gender scripts they had developed for insuring comfortable relations with male colleagues. Shunning the female medical community, she set out very much on her own to make it in a world dominated by medical men on the make. One can only speculate on her motivations. Evidence from the trial suggests that she was imperious, strong, and forceful. One has little trouble believing that she rejected marginality because she was used to wielding power and authority. Moreover, her love of scientific investigation comes through in her published work. Science, and more specifically surgery, was in the process of putting medicine on the map, especially in the public imagination. In a larger cultural sense, Dixon Jones came of age during a period of medical expansionism represented by a gradual shift from art to science, from general practice to specialization, and from medical to surgical solutions. "A gynecologist of the future, without surgical attainments," argued T. Gaillard Thomas in 1879, "will be as impossible as an opthamologist without them is today."[43] The normal pathways of professional life pursued by most women physicians were primarily clinical, and did not involve keeping up with the latest surgical or scientific developments. Dixon Jones was not satisfied with this state of affairs. Her values were clearly those of the surgeon, she believed operations cured most serious gynecological complaints, and she treated patients accordingly.

The newness of gynecology as a specialty meant that boundaries of entry were just flexible enough for an ambitious and determined women to exploit to her advantage. Her acceptance by male peers also reflected a willingness by leaders in the field to welcome all comers who promoted the work and who could demonstrate ability and skill. After all, Dixon Jones played an important role by adding the imprimatur of a woman physician to complicated and controversial surgical procedures whose efficacy was still being tested. As long as gynecology struggled for acceptance, increasing the ranks of the converted was strategically desirable, even if it meant muting traditional gender antagonisms in the interests of professional solidarity.

The accessibility to her chosen specialty Dixon Jones experienced, however, was only temporary. It declined for others as maturation and enhanced status, represented by the institutionalization of formalized courses of study, internship and residency programs, and the emergence of gatekeeping specialty societies, gradually limited opportunities in gynecology for women. But for a unique moment at the end of the nineteenth century, one bold individual stepped out of line, and for her trouble Mary Dixon Jones remains to this day the only nineteenth-century woman surgeon whose name crops up repeatedly in classic textbooks on the history of gynecology.[44]

NOTES

1. Regina Morantz-Sanchez, *Sympathy and Science: Women Physicians in American Medicine* (New York: Oxford Univ. Press, 1985); Morantz-Sanchez, ed., *In Her Own Words: Oral Histories of Women Physicians* (New Haven: Yale Univ. Press, 1985).

2. See Elizabeth Blackwell, "On the Education of Women Physicians" [1860], Elizabeth Blackwell Papers, Box 59, Library of Congress; and her *Medicine as a Profession for Women* (New York, 1860), 10-11.

3. See Blackwell, *Medicine as a Profession for Women,* 10-11; Regina Morantz and Sue Zschoche, "Professionalism, Feminism and Gender Roles: A Comparative Study of Nineteenth-Century Medical Therapeutics," *Journal of American History* 67 (Dec. 1980): 568-88; Virginia Drachman, *Hospital with a Heart* (Ithaca: Cornell Univ. Press, 1984).

4. See John Harley Warner, *The Therapeutic Perspective: Medical Practice, Knowledge, and Identity in America* (Cambridge, Mass.: Harvard Univ. Press, 1986), "The Fall and Rise of Professional Mystery: Epistemology, Authority and the Emergence of Laboratory Medicine in 19th-Century America," in Andrew Cunningham and Perry Williams, eds., *The Laboratory Revolution in Medicine* (Cambridge: Cambridge Univ. Press, 1992), 110-41, and "Ideals of Science and Their Discontents in Late Nineteenth-Century American Medicine," *Isis* (1991): 454-78.

5. Elizabeth Blackwell, "The Influence of Women in the Profession of Medicine," in *Essays in Medical Sociology* (1902; New York: Arno Reprint, 1972), 9-10.

6. See Regina Morantz-Sanchez, "Feminist Theory and Historical Practice: Rereading Elizabeth Blackwell," *History and Theory,* Beiheft 31 (Dec. 1992): 51-69. Stille is quoted in Warner, "Ideals of Science and Their Discontents," 463.

7. Eliza Mosher, "The Human in Medicine, Surgery and Nursing," *Woman's Medical Journal* 32 (May 1925): 117-19.

8. For a discussion of how these attitudes emerged, see Regina Morantz-Sanchez, "The Gendering of Empathic Expertise: How Women Physicians Became More Empathic than Men," in Ellen S. More and Maureen A. Milligan, eds., *The Empathic*

*Practitioner, Empathy, Gender, and Medicine* (New Brunswick, N.J.: Rutgers Univ. Press, 1994), 4-58.

9. See Morantz-Sanchez, *Sympathy and Science,* especially chapter 10.

10. Details of Dixon Jones's life and career have been gleaned from the following sources: the *Brooklyn Eagle,* February 4 & 5, 1892; biographical sketches in Howard A. Kelly and Walter L. Burrage, eds., *Dictionary of American Medical Biography* (1920; Boston: Milford House, 1971) 677, and Irving A. Watson, *Physicians and Surgeons of America* (Concord, N.H.: Republican Press Association, 1896), 808-10; *Catalogue of the Officers and Students of the Wesleyan Female Collegiate Institute of Wilmington, Delaware, 1838-1849* (Wilmington: Evans and Vernon, 1848) 1, 13, 17, 23, 26.

11. Dixon Jones's reminiscences of her experience at the college are published in "College Memories," *Transactions of the Alumnae Association of the Woman's Medical College of Pennsylvania* (1897): 60-63.

12. Helpful histories of these developments can be found in James V. Ricci, *The Development of Gynecological Surgery and Instruments* (Philadelphia: Blakiston, 1949); Jane Eliot Sewell, "Bountiful Bodies: Spencer Wells, Lawson Tait, and the Birth of British Gynaecology" (Ph.D. diss., Johns Hopkins University, 1991); Ornella Moscucci, *The Science of Woman: Gynecology and Gender in England, 1800-1929* (Cambridge: Cambridge Univ. Press, 1990); John Duffy, *The Healers* (Urbana: Univ. of Illinois Press, 1979): 247-59; Gert Brieger, "American Surgery and the Germ Theory of Disease," *Bulletin of the History of Medicine* 40 (1966): 135-45.

13. On Battey's operation see Lawrence Longo, "The Rise and Fall of Battey's Operation: A Fashion in Surgery," *Bulletin of the History of Medicine* 53 (Summer 1979): 244-67.

14. This interpretative tradition to nineteenth-century gynecology has a long history. See especially G.J. Barker-Benfield, *The Horrors of the Half-Known Life: Male Attitudes toward Women and Sexuality in Nineteenth-Century America* (New York: Harper & row, 1976) and Ann Douglas Wood, "'The Fashionable Disease': Women's Complaints and Their Treatment in Nineteenth-Century America," *Journal of Interdisciplinary History* 4 (summer 1973): 25-52. For more sophisticated versions of this approach see Elaine Showalter, *The Female Malady: Women, Madness and English Culture, 1830-1980* (New York: Random House, 1985), and Mary Poovey, "'Scenes of an Indelicate Character': The Medical Treatment of Victorian Women," *Representations* 14. (spring 1986): 137-68. For helpful historiographical discussions of these issues see Judith M. Roy, "Surgical Gynecology," and Regina Morantz-Sanchez, "Physicians," in Rima D. Apple, ed., *Women, Health, and Medicine in America: A Historical Handbook* (New York: Garland Press, 1990).

15. For a more balanced view see Moscucci, *The Science of Woman,* and Wendy Mitchinson, *The Nature of Their Bodies: Women and Their Doctors in Victorian Canada* (Toronto: Univ. of Toronto Press, 1991).

16. Given prevailing notions about women's bodies, shared by doctor and patient alike, patients were often complicit, and occasionally enthusiastic, about the decision to operate. See Morantz-Sanchez, *Sympathy and Science,* 215, and Nancy Theriot, "Women's Voices in Nineteenth-Century Medical Discourse: A Step toward Deconstructing Science," *Signs* 19 (Autumn 1993): 1-31.

17. Deborah Kuhn McGregor, *Sexual Surgery and the Origins of Gynecology: J. Marion Sims, His Hospital and His Patients* (New York: Garland Publishing, 1989).

18. See Charles Rosenberg, *The Care of Strangers* (New York: Basic Books, 1987), especially chapters 7 and 8.

19. See Moscucci, *The Science of Woman,* especially 75-101. Also helpful is Sewell, "Bountiful Bodies."

20. She turned down an offer to join the faculty of the Woman's Medical College of Pennsylvania after she graduated in 1873.

21. See Article XVI of the Woman's Hospital Constitution in *First Anniversary of the Woman's Hospital* (New York: Miller and Holman, 1856), 29; Mary Putnam Jacobi, "Woman in Medicine," in Annie Nathan Meyer, ed., *Woman's Work in America* (New York: Henry Holt, 1891), 154-55; Agnes Vietor, ed., *A Woman's Quest: The Life of Marie E. Zakrzewska* (New York: D. Appleton, 1924), 224-27.

22. Mary Dixon Jones, "A Case of Tait's Operation," *American Journal of Obstetrics* 17 (Nov. 1884): 1154-61. Reflex theory argues that all parts of the body are connected, and disease in particularly vulnerable organs, like the uterus, ovaries and tubes, can produce hysterical symptoms. The physician cures those symptoms by treating the source of the infection, in this case the ovaries and tubes.

23. See *Brooklyn Eagle,* Feb. 4, 1892; Mary Dixon Jones, "Personal Experiences in Laparotomy," *Medical Record* 52 (Aug. 1897): 182-92.

24. Mary Dixon Jones, "Removal of the Uterine Appendages—Nine Consecutive Cases," *Medical Record* 30 (Aug. 1886): 198-208; see footnote p. 206.

25. Dixon Jones, "Personal Experiences in Laparotomy," 191.

26. Kelly and Burrage, *Dictionary of American Medical Biography,* 677.

27. See Dixon Jones, "Oophorectomy and Diseases of the Nervous System," *Women's Medical Journal* 4 (Jan. 1895): 1-11, 5; "Removal of the Uterine Appendages—Recovery," *Medical Record* 27 (Apr. 1885): 400. For Tait's reference to Dixon Jones, see "A Discussion of the General Principles Involved in the Operation of Removal of the Uterine Appendages," *New York Medical Journal* 44 (Nov. 1886): 562-67.

28. Tait, *op. cit.*

29. Audrey D. Stevens, *America's Pioneers in Abdominal Surgery* (Melrose, Mass.: The American Society of Abdominal Surgeons, 1968, 12. Stevens cites the *Transactions of the Rhode Island Medical Society* 2 (1880): 265-74.

30. See Morantz-Sanchez, *Sympathy and Science,* 90-103.

31. For information on malpractice, see Kenneth Allen De Ville, *Medical Malpractice in Nineteenth-Century America, Origins and Legacy* (New York: New York Univ. Press, 1990), and James C. Mohr, *Doctors and the Law: Medical Jurisprudence in Nineteenth-Century America* (New York: Oxford Univ. Press, 1993).

32. The *Eagle's* articles on Dixon Jones ran almost daily from April 24 to May 31, 1889. For coverage of the libel trial see *Brooklyn Eagle,* February 1 to March 17, 1892.

33. See *Brooklyn Medical Journal* 6 (May 1892): 302; *JAMA* 18 (Apr. 1892): 431-32; *Brooklyn Eagle Almanac,* Mar. 15, 1892, for coverage by several presses; "Dr. Raymond Horsewhipped," *New York Times,* May 3, 1892; for other *Times* coverage, see Feb. 2, 4, Mar. 12, 13, 15, 17, May 10, and Dec. 30, 1892; the *Brooklyn Citizen* covered the trial almost daily from February 1 through March 14; *New York Daily Tribune,* Feb. 2, 4, 9, 10, 11, 16, 18, 24, Mar. 12, 14; for the *Philadelphia Ledger's* comments regarding the Beecher-Tilton scandal, see the *Eagle Almanac,* Mar. 15, 1892.

34. H. MacNaughton Jones, "Presidential Address: The Position of Gynaecology Today," *British Gynaecological Journal* 14 (May 1898): 8-30. See also *American Journal of Surgery and Gynecology* 12 (Jan. 1899): 148.

35. Council Minutes, Kings County Medical Society Archives, April 9, May 14, 1884. A spokesperson for the Society allegedly told the *Eagle* in 1889 that Dixon Jones's application had been rejected four times for "unprofessional conduct." *Brooklyn Eagle,* May 4, 1889. There is no evidence of this in the minutes.

36. Pease to Dean Clara Marshall of the Woman's Medical College of Pennsylvania, Jan. 18, 1892, Marshall MSS, MCP; *Brooklyn Eagle,* Feb. 9, 1892.

37. Mosher to Blackwell, Nov. 3, 1883. Mosher MSS, Bentley Library, University of Michigan.

38. *Dictionary of American Medical Biography,* 677. Kelly was a distinguished surgeon at Johns Hopkins Medical School.

39. *Eagle,* Feb. 9, 1892. See also the *Eagle's* comments regarding Dixon Jones's unruliness as a witness, her habit of making comments under her breath, and the testimony of Cornelia Plummer, Feb. 4 and 6.

40. *Brooklyn Eagle,* Feb. 19, 1892.

41. *Brooklyn Eagle,* Mar. 8, 9, Feb. 27, 1892.

42. *Brooklyn Eagle,* Mar. 8, 9, Feb. 27, 1892. The profession was only just beginning to develop a concept of informed consent, and it would be well into the twentieth century before procedures for obtaining patient permission were carefully worked out.

43. See Thomas, "The Gynecology of the Future and Its Relation to Surgery," Presidential Address before the American Gynecological Society, *Transactions* 4 (1879): 25-44.

44. See especially Ricci, *One Hundred Years of Surgery and Gynaecology.*

# [ 10 ]

# SEPARATIST HEALTH
### Changing Meanings of Women's Hospitals in Australia and England, c. 1870-1920

ALISON BASHFORD

*In the Queen's Jubilee* year of 1897, women doctors in the Australian colony of Victoria together with philanthropic ladies and feminists launched a major fundraising enterprise to establish the Queen Victoria Hospital for Women, an institution to be staffed entirely by women doctors. Women throughout the colony were invited to contribute one shilling towards the proposed hospital, which was to be modelled on the New Hospital for Women in London. In the appeal for this Shilling Fund, the organizers enumerated the reasons why Victorian women should contribute. First, "to provide a place where women would be free to secure the privilege of detailing their symptoms to women doctors, and freedom from the painful ordeal (inevitable in every other hospital) of examination in the presence of male students." Second, women should contribute because Queen Victoria herself held sympathy with the "sufferings of poor and helpless women" and would get considerable "personal gratification" from the establishment of such a hospital. And third, the organizers argued that this Shilling Fund and the hospital itself would unite women in Victoria "of all parties and all classes. . . . It is a practical step towards the federation of all women."[1]

This chapter examines three women-only institutions which were modelled explicitly on each other, the New Hospital in London established in 1872, the Queen Victoria Hospital in Melbourne (1899), and the Rachel Forster Hospital in Sydney (1922). Each became a major health-care institution in the first half of the twentieth century, and each has subsequently been dismantled, reduced or incorporated into other institutions, losing its women-

198

only status in the 1960s. Like the arguments put forward by the Victorian women for the Shilling Fund, these hospitals often represented seemingly radical and conservative sympathies simultaneously, and it is this tension of meaning I am most interested in exploring in this essay. Each of these hospitals had to negotiate the difference between being a women's institution on the one hand and a medical institution on the other, the demands and political meanings of which were never quite reconcilable. They also had to negotiate the difference between being a women-only institution and a feminist institution; the latter sometimes explicitly and at other times implicitly, in the sense that any effort to establish a hospital run by women is a criticism of male medicine at some level. Institutional and cultural separateness of the sexes is an inherently difficult issue, both theoretically and in practice. However, I am less interested in the issue of separatism versus integration—a central problematic for Virginia Drachman in her study of the New England Hospital for Women[2]—than in teasing out the range of meanings contained within separatism itself in these specific contexts.

I have isolated four discourses at work, through which sense was made of the idea of women's health and of separate female institutions. First I examine a feminist discourse around the critique of men and of male medicine, which functioned most strongly in the late nineteenth century and which by the 1920s had become more or less unavailable as a reasoning for women's institutional health care to be delivered by women. Second, I look at the way in which these hospitals were defined within a philanthropic framework. This strong tradition of women's benevolent work for other women fostered a sense, for middle-class women at least, of women's collectivity. In many ways a product of this sense of collectivity was a set of progressivist ideas about social reform in general and women's advancement in particular, examination of which forms the next section. And finally I look at a maternalist discourse, which is central also to Penny Russell's interesting study of the first generation of women doctors in Victoria.[3] This discourse saw women and women's health primarily in terms of eugenic reproductive health, in terms of maternal and infant welfare, and became the dominant but not exclusive understanding of such institutions by the 1920s. This chapter will explore how each of these ways of defining health care by and for women worked in the different hospitals at different times, but also how often these institutions managed to mean all of these things simultaneously, sometimes with minimal contradiction, sometimes with considerable tension.

## The Hospitals

The New Hospital for Women opened as a very small institution in 1872, having operated as St. Mary's Dispensary, an outpatient medical service for poor women in London since 1866. Both the dispensary and the subsequent hospital centered very much on Elizabeth Garrett, who had recently qualified as a doctor amidst much controversy and publicity. The venture was also closely linked to the mid-nineteenth-century women's movement, the general committee including, nominally at least, such figures as Helen Taylor, John Stuart Mill, Frances Power Cobbe, and Henry Fawcett.[4] Working-class women responded immediately to the opportunity of consulting a female doctor, and the hospital expanded rapidly. A whole range of women practitioners sought clinical experience there, from deaconesses to missionary women to the increasing number of female medical students. In 1875, with the establishment of the London School of Medicine for Women, the New Hospital became a place for unofficial clinical instruction, but because of its small size and the regulations of the General Medical Council, it was never officially recognized.[5] Like all of these hospitals it provided crucial opportunities for women doctors to gain appointments as resident medical officers and as honorary medical officers or specialist-consultants. Indeed, most late nineteenth-century women doctors in Britain and many from places like Australia had some experience at the New Hospital in London.

The Australian doctor Constance Stone was one of these women. Stone and several other Melbourne women who had links with the New Hospital, notably the suffragist Annette Bear Crawford, were the prime movers to create a similar institution in Melbourne. It was only from the early 1890s that small numbers of women each year had been graduating from Melbourne University Medical Faculty. In 1896, after considerable opposition, the large general Melbourne Hospital accepted two women residents.[6] However, rather than continue within general medicine, which required the treatment of men, and within a male professional hierarchy, nearly all of the women doctors in Melbourne opted for involvement in the new venture, which was opened in 1897 as a dispensary and in 1899 as a small inpatient hospital. These women doctors, then, unlike those who had inaugurated similar institutions in America and in England, had the option of work in general hospitals, albeit an option still fraught with personal and structural discrimination. As Monika Wells has noted, the Queen Victoria Hospital was not established as a result of exclusion, as was the case in London and in some American institutions, but from a positive conception of the idea of women's health care delivered by women.[7]

Like the New Hospital, the Queen Victoria Hospital in Melbourne was a charitable institution treating poor women and children for a nominal fee. All of its staff were female, including doctors, nurses, honorary dentists, dispensers, and honorary masseuses. It also grew very rapidly, attracting women from throughout Melbourne and even from quite isolated parts of the colony. Women doctors educated in the neighboring colonies/states of New South Wales and South Australia gained considerable experience at the Queen Victoria Hospital, and some, in turn, were involved in establishing the third institution in question, the Rachel Forster Hospital in Sydney.

Although Dr. Constance Stone had some experience of American women's hospitals, having graduated from the Women's Medical College of Pennsylvania, the New Hospital in London was the model for the Melbourne women. Firmly located within an imperial context, the organizers in Melbourne were as eager to associate their hospital with the by now famous and respected Elizabeth Garrett Anderson, who had toured Australia in 1885, as they were reluctant to associate it too closely with American initiatives. In both England and Australia, the figure of the American woman doctor was much caricatured. Particularly in the male medical world, there was some antipathy towards the perceived radicalism and stridency of such women, and indeed of the American women's movement generally, an antipathy more strongly held by the previous generation, but nonetheless still quite current in the late nineteenth century.[8] Mission work was also an important part of the identities and experiences of both metropolitan and colonial women doctors. Hence, many sought to define their project in terms of colonialism/imperialism rather than drawing attention to an international feminism.

For many years, Sydney women doctors encountered far more stringent opposition both to their medical training and to their hospital appointments, than their colleagues in Melbourne. Despite the outright refusal of the two major Sydney hospitals to appoint women until around 1906, and the personal connections of some of these women doctors with Elizabeth Garrett Anderson and the New Hospital in London, there was no move to establish an all-women's hospital in Sydney until well into the twentieth century.[9] By 1922, when the Rachel Forster Hospital opened (initially also called the New Hospital for Women and Children), there were many other options available to these professional women in terms of medical practice and employment.

Men were involved in all of these hospitals at some level. Most often, this was a relatively nominal involvement in management committees. At other times they exerted more significant influence. In the early years of the New Hospital in London, men were asked intermittently to assist clinically, for example, in the administration of chloroform while Elizabeth Garrett Anderson operated.[10] In 1888, when there was some question over Garrett Anderson's surgical skill, several prominent male surgeons were asked to attend her operations.[11] On the other hand, when one of the women doctors in Melbourne sought the advice of a male colleague who subsequently performed an operation at the hospital, the committee expressed its disapproval in the strongest terms, and emphasized its policy that men "take no active part in the work of the Hospital, but . . . act as Consultants or advisers."[12] Magnanimously it would seem, each hospital had a policy of inviting a range of male specialists to act as consultants, suggesting, as the governor's wife did, when she opened the hospital, that sex is not to be an absolute barrier where extra opinions and advice are necessary. "There are no sex in brains."[13] Of course, at every turn, these hospitals were about sexual difference, as the editor of the British *Sanitary Record* realized when he playfully corrected an article originally published in the *Lancet*:

> The idea of a hospital for women to be worked by women (men) seems to us neither a sound idea nor a liberal one. . . . We can imagine nothing more injurious to poor women than to create hospitals for them from which (fe)male intellect and skill are to be excluded. . . . It is very doubtful indeed whether ordinary midwifery practice is suitable for women (men); but that (wo)men should be excluded from a hospital for the treatment of diseases of women is a suggestion of the narrowest and most injurious import.[14]

### A Critique of Male Medicine

Criticism of male doctors was a particularly strong strand in the British mid-nineteenth-century debate on women's medical education and medical practice, and this has all been well documented.[15] A general unease about the growing specialty of "women's diseases" was given focus by the Contagious

Diseases Act agitation, the vivisection debates and, in particular, by Frances Power Cobbe's and Josephine Butler's scathing pronouncements against the profession. Throughout these decades Elizabeth Blackwell also sustained important critical public comment on male doctors and their treatment of women, and on the type of medicine that women should be practicing.[16] Elizabeth Garrett Anderson generally distanced herself from these particular feminist campaigns, and even aligned herself with the mainstream medical camp in favor of the Contagious Diseases Acts. There was, of course, no single coherent position for feminists and women doctors to assume with regard to the male medical profession. However, this very public critique of doctors and the linking of male medical practice to male sexual practice through the idea of the "instrumental rape" of women was a quite dominant concern of British feminism over these years. Like Elizabeth Garrett herself, the New Hospital as an institution had to reckon with, and by and large, distance itself from such radicalism. There was often a considerable gap between the feminist theorizing about male medicine on the part of Butler, Cobbe, Blackwell and others, and the ways in which the New Hospital (which still must be seen as a product of nineteenth-century feminism) related to mainstream medicine.

Differences between women over this critique of male medicine every now and then upset the otherwise fairly smooth philanthropic workings of these institutions, which will be examined. There was a world of difference between advocacy for women doctors on the grounds of a benevolent sympathy among women, and advocacy on the grounds of wanting to practice a different type of medicine. The nature and frequency of surgery, for example, were sometimes at issue. Not surprisingly, many women doctors placed considerable weight on proving their proficiency through surgery, seen to be a particularly masculine and, increasingly, a high-status aspect of medical practice. Moreover, at this time of new surgical and anesthetic developments, particularly in gynecology, hospitals themselves gained status by displaying the successful surgery undertaken—the more complicated and risky, the better. In 1879 the committee of the New Hospital declared in their annual report that two ovariotomies had been successfully performed that year: "The Committee are not aware of this formidable operation having been ever before, in Europe at least, performed successfully by a woman."[17] Ovariotomies were a fast route to mainstream medical and public acceptance.

Elizabeth Blackwell, who was for some years a consulting physician for the New Hospital, was very critical of such procedures and practice. Blackwell was an influential proponent of a feminine, moral, and preventive medicine, which, amongst other things, meant a practice based less on surgery. She was highly critical of what she saw as an "epidemic" of ovariotomies. In an interview called "Human Vivisection" she said: "The danger lies mainly in the substitution of surgery for medicine in the treatment of disease." . . . The interviewer asked her: "Do you consider that women practitioners are less liable to this 'operative madness' than men?"—she answered, "I have no hesitation in saying that *at present* my own sex is suffering from the epidemic, but it is imparted to them by their surroundings. You see it is very contagious. They learn from men, and live in the atmosphere of surgery. They are overanxious to do as men do, and so their reverence of creation and their sympathy for the poor and suffering is in abeyance."[18] In portraying this "operative madness" as "contagious," Blackwell offers an interesting pathologizing of male medical behavior—a pleasing reversal of the more usual pathologizing of feminine behaviors.

By and large the New Hospital pursued medicine and surgery like any other hospital. Voices of protest such as Blackwell's, while they carried on in other social locations, became more and more isolated in the context of women's hospitals run by and for women. Blackwell belonged very much to the mid-nineteenth-century generation of feminist women doctors. As will be seen, by the 1920s women doctors' investment in women's health was less defined by this critique of men in medicine and far more defined by emerging maternalist discourses and eugenic concerns.

An important way in which the women and men involved in the New Hospital in London and the Queen Victoria Hospital in Melbourne could distance their institution from controversial feminist critiques of doctors was by emphasizing its philanthropic role. Yet even those seeking to define such ventures in the most respectable and acceptable terms had to articulate some sort of justification for women doctors. Sometimes the issue of the fundamental impropriety of men examining women was focused upon, sometimes the sympathy among women, but often it was the issue of harassing male medical students. In public discourse on both the London and the Melbourne hospitals the issue of male medical students and their treatment of working-class women in hospitals was accorded great weight. Indeed it became almost commonplace to explain the need for women's hospitals in these terms. The following two accounts are fairly typical. The first describes the New Hospital: "it is not difficult to imagine the pain that a woman must suffer when, sup-

204

posing her to be a victim to one of those terrible internal maladies, peculiar to the sex, she is aware that she is the object of demonstration to the young male students, and can hear the none too delicate remarks that they may pass."[19] And at the opening of the Queen Victoria Hospital in Melbourne a woman journalist wrote,

> It is not generally known how repellent is the ordeal through which poor women have to pass in obtaining treatment at an ordinary hospital, where they have to . . . be exhibited as "cases" for the instruction of groups of male medical students. Nor is it known how frequently women of the poorer and more helpless classes, rather than undergo this ordeal, postpone application to the hospitals. . . . These things, unnoticed or unconsidered by the general public, struck some of the women doctors of Melbourne with painful force.[20]

The frequency with which the issue of male students arose attests to the seriousness of this problem for working-class women. At every turn there are accounts of women with gynecological illnesses refusing to seek medical treatment from men. And this is surely why women traveled such long distances at such expense to consult women doctors, and why, indeed, all of these hospitals were successes. But there is never any suggestion that it might be possible to modify the behavior of the students. The story of loutish medical students is repeated with such ease, that one must ask what the wider function of this relentless focus was. It worked to contain criticism of doctors within fairly limited parameters. That is to say, in texts written by proponents of the women's hospitals this critique of the behavior of male students rarely became linked with a wider feminist critique of male medicine or of male sexual culture. One might well argue that feminist criticism of male doctors was taken and recast as a problem about students and working-class women in hospitals. Not only did the emphasis on medical students in a sense let the "real" doctors off the hook; any mention of students immediately located the issue within a hospital context, and the specific context of working-class women's medical care. It kept the rationale for women's medical practice within the bounds of philanthropic work for working-class women, problematizing relations between students and working-class women in hospitals, rather than relations between women and male doctors generally.

205

## Women's Philanthropy

Like all nineteenth-century hospitals, both the New Hospital and the Queen Victoria Hospital for Women were charitable institutions. They were run as philanthropic ventures by upper- and middle-class voluntary committees for sick working-class women. Upper- and middle-class women themselves, of course, received their health care in their own homes, and ventured into hospitals only as doctors, as nurses, as committee members or as lady visitors. The hospitals were also considered charitable institutions in the sense that the services of the doctors, excluding the few paid resident medical staff, were voluntary. It was crucial to the development of the professional lives of medical women that they be able to secure such honorary positions, and they were highly unlikely to do so in other hospitals.

The fundamental social and cultural framework for these institutions was philanthropic rather than narrowly medical. In both England and Australia there was a very strong tradition of women's philanthropic work for other women, and these hospitals fit squarely into this tradition. For all their links with prevailing feminism and even with criticism of male medicine, such women's hospitals were usually perceived as entirely respectable, laudable ventures. As a measure of the establishment status which these hospitals could acquire, in London the Archbishop of Canterbury was invited and happily agreed to open new wards of the hospital on several occasions.[21] In Melbourne, the venture was so firmly located within this respectable discourse of women's philanthropic work that the wife of the governor of the colony, traditionally the first lady of philanthropy, was able to assume a substantial role in its publicity, and was called upon officially to open it.[22] And in Sydney the governor-general's wife, Rachel Forster, gave her name to the hospital. Given that the women doctors and committee members sought not only public recognition, but all-important public subscriptions, this link to eminence and respectability is not surprising. In many ways these were entirely mainstream institutions.

In the public display of these hospitals, respectability often rested on the portrayal of the helplessness, the degradation and the vulnerability of sick working-class women: our "afflicted and helpless sisters" as Melbourne women were described, or as the British feminist journal *Work and Leisure* wrote of London women, our "suffering sisters . . . the most suffering of all the suffering classes."[23] It was crucial for the viability of the hospitals, not least in finan-

206

cial terms, that they be conceptualized and presented in a philanthropic framework, in some way as assisting a group "less fortunate." Of course the whole notion of philanthropy, while it is about contact between classes, functions fundamentally to reaffirm the distance and the power differential between them. In the last analysis philanthropy is about defining the middle- and upper-class status and social authority of those who undertake philanthropic work, a class relationship symbolized by the committee of ladies who would screen each potential patient for suitable poverty and respectability. While on the one hand none of these institutions meant *only* this, on the other, this philanthropic meaning was always there, and was often deployed, sometimes entirely strategically, to justify and legitimate all-female hospitals. Amongst other things, it worked well to draw attention away from the fundamental subversiveness of all-woman or women-only enterprises.

It was also crucial that the whole idea of women medical practitioners could be constructed well within this model of benevolence.[24] All of these women's hospitals functioned importantly as places where women's medical education and practice was legitimated, rendered socially viable and respectable, connecting the image of the women doctor intimately with her suffering sisters. The debate about British women medical practitioners treating Indian women was crucial in a similar way. The need for medically trained women to treat Hindu and Muslim women in India became an issue fraught with the significance of gaining access to the "darkest" innermost sanctum of Indian culture.[25] This was a very central aspect of the experience of early women doctors, as many British and Australian medical women did work as medical missionaries. It was an entirely workable way to resolve the contradictory demands of femininity (self-sacrifice and moral goodness) on the one hand, with a yearning for independence and interesting professional work on the other. To premise the need for medical women on the figure of the helpless working-class woman or on the Indian woman caught in the dark and closed physical and spiritual space of her zenana, appropriated powerful cultural codes of philanthropy and colonialism, both of which had significant room for the play of women's moral authority. This is one example of the way in which the feminism of this period worked from and through class and racial difference; both philanthropic and colonial discourses provided the possibility for women's activism, for a sense of female solidarity and for the development of a women's movement.

The female nature of the hospitals could either be harnessed to a feminism, or could be used to give a feminine, moral and seemingly benign edge to their philanthropic function. It is interesting that those who most sought to present such women's hospitals as respectable and uncontroversial—usually the fundraisers—often did so by emphasizing the femaleness, the femininity of the ventures. Sometimes, of course, this emphasis on feminine attributes reduced the hospitals to being represented as little more than a harmless, domestic world. An article in an 1892 issue of *The Christian World*, for example, described the New Hospital as "Bright, Beautiful and Homelike. . . . the cheerful open fires, the bright blossoming plants, the dapper nurses in their pink striped gowns and dainty white lace caps, and the quiet unprofessional-like doctors."[26] At other times this emphasis on the femininity of the hospitals was far more ambiguous. In a public letter seeking funds in the 1880s, the chairman of the New Hospital committee, Rev. Llewellyn Davies, wrote of that double-edged sword, "woman's sphere of work":

> this is an age at once enlarged of activity on the part of women, and of increased interest in the conditions of women and girls. It is admitted to be becoming and reasonable that the action of women should turn itself especially into the channel of doing what is wanted by persons of their own sex. We have women Guardians, who look after women and girls in our workhouses; women on School Boards, who give special attention to the girls in the schools. . . . Any need or disadvantage in the circumstance of a young girl appeals with peculiar force to what is womanly in the heart of a woman.[27]

Louise Creighton, wife of the Bishop of London and at this stage still firmly antisuffragist, presided over the annual meeting of the New Hospital in 1897. In a similarly ambiguous way, Creighton presented an image of the New Hospital which was fundamentally domestic, but which suggested the power that many women attributed to this domesticity. She said that women were "naturally fitted for hospital control, both by possession of the charitable qualities essential to philanthropic work and by their home training in household economy and management." While Creighton also wished to speak of the hospital as a place of science, in the final analysis, she even ascribed a special feminine meaning to this. The hospital, she said, "is the centre of the movement for opening the medical profession to women, and its medical and surgical staff includes many lady doctors of eminence, who are successfully following the antiseptic treatment initiated by Sir James Paget and Lord Lister, a method for which their own ideas of cleanliness give them especial sympathy."[28]

In Melbourne, women involved in managing and raising funds for the Queen Victoria Hospital similarly strove to present it as a quintessentially feminine enterprise. An important and very effective part of the strategy was to invoke the spirit of the Queen at every opportunity. This strategy not only rendered it ultimately respectable, it also located the hospital in an all-important imperial framework. Victorian women were asked to contribute to the hospital in memory of "our late beloved and lamented Queen—whose heart was always gladdened by every movement which helped or elevated her own sex. . . . Let us now see what women will make of it, for the love of women and womanly tenderness."[29] Because of the philanthropic construction of both hospitals and the ability to code these institutions so effectively as feminine and even domestic, there was minimal outright opposition to them, even though there was considerable opposition to women doctors per se.

## Women's Advancement and Social Reform

Alongside this philanthropic meaning of the hospitals there was also a sense in which they were about social reform and progress in general, and women's advancement in particular. At the most simple level, each of these hospitals was concerned with the promotion of different areas of employment for women. The New Hospital committee in the 1870s through the 90s saw part of its role as dispersing information on women's medical education in Britain. In most annual reports until around the turn of the century, a special "progress report on the education of women in medicine" outlined which universities were open to women, which hospitals allowed clinical practice or residencies to women, and, increasingly, the number of women's hospitals being established through the country run by women doctors. Annual reports also regularly included a list of female medical practitioners in Britain. Additionally, many women worked as dispensers or pharmacists,[30] as masseuses and electrical therapists,[31] and as dentists.[32] Others gained experience as paid secretaries and administrators, occupations which were increasingly common amongst women in the 1920s, but which were unusual when the New Hospital and the Queen Victoria Hospital were established.

209

For many women involved in women-only hospitals, any distinction between women's philanthropic work for other women, social reform in the interests of women and children, and the idea of the advancement of their sex was far from clear. Often, all of these discourses were complementary and could be written together easily, as in the following from an 1875 annual report of the New Hospital:

> The philanthropic will help the New Hospital for women, because the sick and suffering here find relief, and none the less willingly, it is hoped, because that relief is administered by women's hands; those who gladly welcome women to a larger share in the work of the world will help, because the Hospital is a new field of labour thrown open to women, and because they will see in it an appropriate way in which edu- cated women may minister to other women, and soften many of the most painful features of sickness.[33]

As was the case for late nineteenth-century feminism generally, what emerged from the philanthropic justifications of these hospitals was a distinct sense of female collectivity. The Queen Victoria Hospital was envisaged as an important, large scale enterprise which would link women throughout the colony by virtue of their sex: "It is the largest endeavour which has yet been made by Victorian women, combining women of all parties and all classes, in one united effort throughout the Colony . . . a step towards the federation of all women."[34] And here it is important to note that this notion of collectivity was clearly one defined by middle-class women. Their understanding of "all women," for example, excluded Aboriginal women. Nonetheless, this belief that women could be united was one of the extraordinary aspects of small colonial societies such as Victoria, and of women's politics within them. It was certainly never an ambition of those involved in the New Hospital in London to unite the women of England.

The success with which (most) women in Victoria were drawn together over the Queen Victoria Hospital, in terms of contributions to the enor- mously successful Shilling Fund as well as use of the new medical facilities, is surely a significant precursor to the efforts to unite women, to "federate" them into an explicitly political grouping. Vida Goldstein, leader of the Women's Political Association in Victoria, a non-party organization aiming (unsuccessfully) to elect women to Parliament on women's issues, was an early committee member of the Queen Victoria Hospital. She was also a political protégée of Annette Bear Crawford, the central organizing figure of the Shilling Fund and the early years of the hospital.[35] Bear Crawford, who travelled with some regularity between Melbourne and London, was an important link between the women's movements of the two countries. Involved with the New Hospital in voluntary social welfare work, Bear Crawford was also extremely active in the National Vigilance Association in Britain and established the Victorian Vigilance Society. She was a crucial figure in Victorian suffrage organization and agitation, bringing together separate groups under the United Council for Women's Suffrage.[36] It was very much Annette Bear Crawford who broadened the picture which the women doctors held of the hospital, envisaging it as an enterprise involving women throughout the colony, and coordinating the Shilling Fund via the branches of the Women's Christian Temperance Union.

Many women prominent in turn-of-the-century Melbourne feminism, then, were involved in the Queen Victoria Hospital, and most of the original doctors had strong connections with the women's movement. The committee was made up of women equally involved in charities like the Melbourne Benevolent Society, the Melbourne District Nursing Society, the Maternity Aid Society on the one hand, and in organizations with social reform and feminist agendas on the other: the Women's Social and Political Reform League, the Victorian Women's Franchise League, the United Council for Women's Suffrage.[37] It was clearly consistent for many of these women to be, simultaneously, philanthropists, advocates of women's health care by and for women, and suffragists. However, it is perhaps more telling of the complexity of these institutions that for other women involved, it was also consistent to be philanthropists, advocates of women's health care by women doctors, and antisuffragists.

In Melbourne, it was the issue of women's suffrage which rendered visible what was at times a significant tension between the philanthropic and feminist meanings of women's hospitals, and of the management of women's health by women. If anything, the Queen Victoria Hospital became less openly feminist after its initial fundraising ventures and its first few years of operation.[38] So, for example, in 1900 an official of the hospital unofficially circulated for signatures a petition against women's suffrage: employees, inpatients and outpatients were asked to sign. The United Council for Women's Suffrage was justifiably shocked and wrote: "we are reluctant to believe that such a thing could have happened in the Queen Victoria Hospital, the idea of establishing which originated with advocates of the enfranchisement of women, & which is at present largely supported by workers in the Women's Suffrage movement."[39] In 1912 the Women's Political Association in Victoria presented a petition for the enfranchisement of British women to the House of Commons, and asked the committee of the Queen Victoria Hospital to sign in their individual capacities. So distanced had it become from feminist politics that the committee declined. And it is sadly ironic that the committee which refused to support this petition for British women, had just finished organizing the erection of polling booths within the hospital for the use of staff and patients in the recent election.[40]

### Maternalism

Many of the potential contradictions between women's philanthropy and a more explicit feminism were collapsed into the discourse of maternalism in the interwar years. While maternalism reached a peak then, there is certainly a continuity in "women's health" meaning "reproductive health" over the period in question. In 1865, for example, a woman in the British feminist *Alexandra Magazine* wrote that the question of women doctors would soon be settled "if the full expression of the female mind could be heard on . . . *infant mortality.* . . . It is *the question,* not of the day, but of all time—the woman question—how are we to save our babies from the death that menaces them?"[41] However, the politics attributed to this issue shifted considerably. While in the late nineteenth century issues around women's reproductive health could be used to launch a feminist criticism and to refine a feminist theory of men's abuses, it proved difficult to sustain this into the twentieth century, when whole social movements, to say nothing of the state, were mobilizing around issues to do with women's bodies, but for different reasons. While criticism of male medical/sexual culture was always a stronger strand within feminism in England than in Australia, in both countries feminism and the work of women doctors were largely co-opted by this eugenic-driven maternalism.

Recently there has been considerable feminist rethinking of early twentieth-century maternalism as an enabling discourse for women. It has been suggested that maternalism was in part driven by women who reinterpreted the new interest in and importance of motherhood to press for state intervention in women's interests, for women's welfare and for measures which actually increased women's independence.[42] It is important to recognize, as much of this work does, the complexities of the boundaries between feminism and maternalism, although one of the problems is the renaming as "maternalist" campaigns and politics we used to think of as "feminist."[43] It is also important to qualify the relentless oppressiveness which many historians writing in the early and mid-1980s attributed to maternalism.[44] Yet, as far as these hospitals are concerned, it remains the case that they shifted fairly consistently towards a eugenic concern with the health of the nation/race.

By the turn of the century, Dr. Mary Scharlieb had become the most prominent surgeon at the New Hospital and had largely assumed Elizabeth Garrett Anderson's duties and leading role. Scharlieb's medical practice, her writing and her educational work were certainly driven by a sense of social progress, and even one which must be seen as woman-centered. While she never aligned herself with the early twentieth-century women's movement, she did identify herself as a eugenicist. Yet the difference was often unclear, as Scharlieb's statements about the social role of women doctors suggests: "I realised that one of a woman doctor's privileges and duties is to assist in preserving the health of the nation, and therefore in the prevention of disease, in the suppression of alcoholism and vice, and more especially in the prevention of infantile mortality and diseases in young children."[45] Even doctors, such as Louisa Martindale, who were intensely critical of male sexuality and its consequences for women's health in the feminism of the pre-war years, redirected this energy for social change into eugenics. In her 1922 book, *The Woman Doctor and Her Future,* Martindale quoted Schopenhauer admiringly: "'[Woman] is the creature to whom the Race is more than the Individual, the being to whom the Future is greater than the Present, and perhaps it is because of this inherent, deep-rooted, ineradicable quality of visionary foresight that no work attracts some women more than that of a life service in the cause of Eugenics or Research."[46]

Established in 1922, the Rachel Forster Hospital was created just when maternalism was gaining real momentum in Australia, and just when the professionalism of women's roles as health-care workers was being consolidated. In Australia, maternalism was an ideology bounded by racial issues, as all (and only) white women were targeted by pro-natalist policies such as motherhood and child endowments.[47] Women doctors in Sydney established their hospital at a time when maternal and infant welfare was attracting unprecedented at-

tention from the state, and when the swift increase in institutionalized childbirth was just beginning. It is no coincidence, of course, that the period in
which the state developed a real anxiety over population issues was also the
period which saw increased state control over hospitals, and childbirth shifting
into those hospitals. Women's hospitals, women doctors and the concept of
women's health were all strongly influenced by these developments.

What is striking about the public reception of the Rachel Forster Hospital is the extent to which its exclusively female medical staff was not seen to be
particularly problematical. While this certainly drew comment, indeed it was
sometimes called "The Women Doctors' Hospital," this fact barely required
explanation.[48] Unlike in Melbourne a generation earlier, no public debate
ensued over just why women needed women doctors. In many ways, the
motherhood ideology of which Russell has written had come to envelop so
many aspects of women's activities, and so potently to define being female,
that in the interwar period women doctors could be viewed as even more
natural "mothers of the race" than at the turn of the century.[49] Because
motherhood itself had become so "scientific" in the 1920s and 1930s, women
doctors were even more effective scientific mothers.

In their public discussion of women's health care by and for women, doctors involved in the Rachel Forster Hospital spoke rarely, and certainly more
coyly than earlier generations, of "cases where women should be attended by
women doctors." Some even spoke of a "prejudice against women doctors, the
difficulty of obtaining positions on the honorary staff being especially pro-
nounced."[50] But these were isolated public comments, not dwelt upon in
newspapers and never linked to a more fundamental feminist position. The
most striking difference between the Sydney hospital in the 1920s and earlier
institutions in Australia and England, is the almost complete erasure of criticism of male doctors, medical students included. Every now and then it was
said that "women would hesitate to attend an ordinary public hospital," as
Rachel Forster did at the first annual meeting, but unlike earlier ventures, no
reasons were offered as to why this might be so.[51] While the professionalization of medicine and the entrenchment of women health practitioners within
a medical hierarchy with a newly consolidated social status must account in
part for this refusal to view men and male doctors critically, this is also more
broadly characteristic of women's politics in the interwar period. It is a most
significant shift. Any feminism inherent in the practice of women's health care
being delivered by women was certainly compromised. While the committee

of the hospital always met at the premises of the Feminist Club in Sydney, what had feminism come to mean? An article in 1928 entitled "A Feminist and Proud of It" quoted the Minister for Health, Dr. Richard Arthur, in full support of the Rachel Forster Hospital: "I may say I am almost a Feminist, as I am in sympathy with so many women's movements."[52] "Feminism," for many, had come to mean simply the work of women.

For all the dominance of the discourse of maternalism in the interwar period, it seems at first glance that it did not entirely force a view of women's health as maternal/reproductive health. Women doctors at the Rachel Forster Hospital did not approach women's health in the reductionist way one might expect. Gynecological illnesses were by no means the focus of medical practice. Indeed, it was seen to be different from other women's hospitals in Sydney at the time, precisely because women's general illnesses were treated.[53] Unlike the New Hospital and the Queen Victoria Hospital at their foundations, women doctors at the Rachel Forster Hospital were certainly not specializing in gynecology. Indeed, throughout the 1920s and 1930s there was no such specialist attached to the hospital, although two women worked almost exclusively in the venereal disease clinic. According to the annual report for 1926, only around 20 percent of the inpatients at the Rachel Forster Hospital were admitted with any sort of genito-urinary or gynecological illness. At the Queen Victoria Hospital at the same time it was around 29 percent, a significant reduction from 60 percent gynecological patients in its opening years.[54] In some ways, then, these hospitals can be seen to question the conflation of women's health and reproductive health which maternalism supposedly intensified.

Yet other issues cut across this interpretation. Most obviously, all of these hospitals were increasingly functioning as places for institutional childbirth.[55] The Rachel Forster Hospital also connected its medical services with children far more than the other hospitals had in the late nineteenth century and at the turn of the century. Indeed, its location was chosen precisely because it was in a neighborhood crowded with children, and the hospital constantly publicized the fact that mothers could have their own health and that of their children treated at the same time. But perhaps more pertinently, what characterized maternalism, and what made it such a problematical discourse for women, was precisely the fact that it did not focus narrowly on childbirth. Interwar maternalism defined women as mothers in an all-encompassing way, enveloping all aspects of women's lives, not simply childbirth itself. And so, while

215

doctors at the Rachel Forster Hospital were not specifically concerned with a narrowly defined reproductive health, as the earlier doctors had been, in other ways womanhood and motherhood had come to be so conflated that it was virtually impossible for them to be prised apart: "motherhood" now figured in all aspects of the health of women, not simply in "diseases peculiar to women," to use a nineteenth-century phrase.

Like the hospitals themselves, the work of women doctors shifted in a general sense from a specific focus on women's gynecological health to a broader view of healthy motherhood. In the early twentieth century, medical women were vastly overrepresented in the plethora of new jobs in public health for women, in maternal and infant welfare, in education. To take just one example, Dr. Margaret Harper, one of the women involved in establishing the Rachel Forster Hospital, also opened in 1922 a home for the "education of mothers in infant feeding and mothercraft," funded by the Royal Society for the Welfare of Mothers and Babies. Her eminent career followed a classic path for women doctors of her generation, assuming amongst many other responsibilities, the first lectureship in Diseases of the New-born and Mothercraft at the University of Sydney.[56] In a positive sense, this can be seen as the legacy of nineteenth-century ideas about a feminine medical practice articulated by Blackwell and others. The Rachel Forster Hospital committee certainly stressed its commitment to the notion of preventive medicine.[57] However, divested of any particular concern about relations between women and men, and located within a discourse which privileged a concern about relations between current and future generations, the social mission, not to mention the material work, of earlier women doctors had been co-opted.

Through all the complexity of what a women-only hospital meant in the interwar years, one thing is certain: there was no pressure on any of these institutions to lose their women-only status. Rather, in one form or another there was a new imperative for them. At the Queen Victoria Hospital there was a fresh emphasis on the hospital as a female institution, as the slogan "by women, for women" was officially adopted in 1924 and displayed proudly on badges and on letterheads.[58] There was certainly a discourse of sexual difference at work, within which to situate these hospitals, but it was one fraught with difficulties. Interestingly, it was not until the 1960s and 1970s that the women-only status of all of these hospitals came under threat. Partly under the weight of "equality" rhetoric, moves were made to accept male nurses, followed by male patients and male doctors. While the simultaneous establishment of women's health centers is often seen as an initiative of second-wave feminism, it is clear that the delivery of women's health care by women has a remarkably continuous history. But historical study of such women's institutions creates an acute awareness of the way in which they were, and are, always firmly grounded in prevailing discourses, be they of the late nineteenth or the late twentieth century. Historical study of these hospitals also presents the issue, still problematical, of the difference between institutions for women and feminist institutions.

## NOTES

1. Quoted in Gwendolen H. Swinburne, *The Queen Victoria Hospital, A History: The First Fifty Years* (Melbourne: The Queen Victoria Hospital, 1951), 17 18.

2. Virginia Drachman, *Hospital with a Heart: Women Doctors and the Paradox of Separatism at the New England Hospital, 1862-1969.* (Ithaca and London: Cornell Univ. Press, 1984).

3. Russell argues that the very possibility of women entering the medical profession in Victoria was defined by a pervasive ideology of motherhood and of race survival, and that it was "possible to support women doctors with the same motherhood ideology as was directed against most women." Penny Russell, "'Mothers of the Race': A Study of the First Thirty Women Medical Graduates from the University of Melbourne" (B.A. Hons. thesis, Monash University, 1982), 5.

4. St. Mary's Dispensary, *Annual Report* (1867): 10.

5. Minutes of the Management Committee, Oct. 18, 1872, Oct. 19, 1875, Mar. 9, 1877, Elizabeth Garrett Anderson Hospital Records, Greater London Record Office.

6. Russell, "'Mothers of the Race,'" 19-24.

7. Monika Wells, "'Gentlemen, the Ladies have come to stay:' The Entry of Women into the Medical Profession in Victoria and the Founding of the Queen Victoria Hospital for Women" (master's thesis, University of Melbourne, 1987), 1.

8. See, for example, "Medical Women," *Australian Medical Journal* 10 (July 1865): 233; "Dr Mary Walker and Dr Elizabeth Blackwell and Miss Garrett," *Victoria Magazine* 8 (Jan. 1867): 232-40.

9. Although the turn-of-the-century Sydney Medical Mission, an inner-city dispensary and home medical service was primarily a cooperative effort of women in philanthropy and medicine. See M. Hutton Neve, *"This Mad Folly": The History of Australia's Pioneer Women Doctors* (Sydney: Library of Australia, 1980), 103-7.

10. Minutes of the Management Committee, June 3, 1872, Elizabeth Garrett Anderson Hospital Records.

11. Minutes of the Management Committee, Feb. 1, 1888, Feb. 22, 1888, Elizabeth Garrett Anderson Hospital Records.

12. Minutes of the Management Committee, Dec. 19, 1900, Queen Victoria Hospital Archives, Monash Medical Centre, Melbourne.

13. "Queen Victoria Hospital," *Age,* July 6, 1899.

14. "The New Hospital for Women," *The Sanitary Record* (July 1874): 56.

15. Catriona Blake, *The Charge of the Parasols: Women's Entry to the Medical Profession* (London: The Women's Press, 1990). Susan Kingsley Kent, *Sex and Suffrage in Britain, 1860-1914* (Princeton: Princeton Univ. Press, 1987).

16. See Regina Morantz-Sanchez, *Sympathy and Science: Women Physicians in American Medicine* (Oxford: Oxford Univ. Press, 1985), 185 ff.

17. New Hospital for Women, *Annual Report* (1879): 3.

18. "Human Vivisection: Interview with Dr. Elizabeth Blackwell," *Daily Chronicle,* May 22, 1894 (original emphasis).

19. "The New Hospital for Women," *Echo,* July 5, 1888.

20. Ida, "A Popular Proposal: A Diamond Jubilee Memorial," *Age,* Feb. 19, 1897.

21. *Leader,* Nov. 4, 1905, in album of newsclippings 1881-1917, Elizabeth Garrett Anderson Hospital Records.

22. "Queen Victoria Hospital: The Opening Ceremony," *Age,* July 6, 1899.

23. *Argus,* Mar. 20, 1901; "An Appeal," *Work and Leisure* 5 (1881): 849-90.

24. Russell, "Mothers of the Race," 37-38.

25. See Rosemary Fitzgerald, "The 'Double Cure': Female Medical Missions in Colonial India," paper presented to the Health and Empire seminar, Institute of Commonwealth Studies, University of London, Oct. 29, 1993.

26. *The Christian World,* Apr. 14, 1892, in album of newscuttings, 1881-1917, Elizabeth Garrett Anderson Hospital Records.

27. Letter in the *Standard,* Oct. 29, 1888, reprinted in New Hospital, *Annual Report* (1889):13.

28. *The Philanthropist,* Mar. 1897, in album of newscuttings, 1881-1917, Elizabeth Garrett Anderson Hospital Records.

29. *Argus,* Mar. 20, 1901.

30. St. Mary's Dispensary, *Annual Report* (1867): 6. Minutes of the Management Committee, 18 Oct. 1872, Elizabeth Garrett Anderson Hospital Records. Minutes of the Management Committee, June 7, 1897, June 16, 1897, Queen Victoria Hospital Archives.

31. J. McCormick to Hon. Sec., Queen Victoria Hospital, Oct. 17, 1899, Queen Victoria Hospital Archives.

32. Minutes of the Management Committee, Mar. 1, 1899, Aug. 2, 1899, Queen Victoria Hospital Archives.

33. New Hospital for Women, *Annual Report* (1875): 7.

34. Quoted in Swinburne, *The First Fifty Years,* 17-18.

35. Farley Kelly, "Vida Goldstein: Political Woman," in *Double Time: Women in Victoria—150 Years,* eds. Marilyn Lake and Farley Kelly (Harmondsworth: Penguin, 1985), 172.

36. See Janice N. Brownfoot, entry for Annette Bear Crawford, *Australian Dictionary of Biography,* vol. 7 (Melbourne: Melbourne Univ. Press, 1983), 230-31.

37. See Wells, "The Entry of Women," 117-19.

38. Russell, "'Mothers of the Race,'" 26. Wells, "The Entry of Women," 124.

39. Hon. Sec., United Council for Women's Suffrage to Queen Victoria Hospital Committee, 14 Aug. 1900, Queen Victoria Hospital Archives.

40. Minutes of the Committee of Management, June 30, 1912, Aug. 22, 1912, Queen Victoria Hospital Archives.

41. "The First English School of Medicine for Women," *Alexandra Magazine* (June 1865): 324 [original emphasis].

42. See Hilary Land, "Introduction," *Gender and History* 4 (1992): 284. Seth Koven and Sonya Michel, "Introduction: 'Mother Worlds,'" in Seth Koven and Sonya Michel, eds., *Mothers of a New World: Maternalist Politics and the Origins of Welfare States* (New York: Routledge, 1993), 2-3.

43. See, for example, Sonya Michel and Robyn Rosen, "The Paradox of Maternalism: Elizabeth Lowell Putnam and the American Welfare State," *Gender and History* 4 (1992): 364-65.

44. For example, in the Australian context, Russell, "'Mothers of the Race,'" Jill Julius Matthews, *Good and Mad Women: The Historical Construction of Femininity in Twentieth-Century Australia* (Sydney: George Allen & Unwin, 1984), and Kereen Reiger, *Disenchantment of the Home: Modernizing the Australian Family* (Oxford: Oxford Univ. Press, 1985).

45. Mary Scharlieb, *Reminiscences* (London: Williams and Norgate, 1925), 208.

46. Louisa Martindale, *The Woman Doctor and Her Future* (London: Mills and Boon, 1922), 133. For further discussion of English women doctors' involvement with feminism and eugenics, see Alison Bashford, "Edwardian Feminists and the Venereal Disease Debate in England," in B. Caine, ed., *The Woman's Question* (Sydney: Univ. of Sydney Press, 1994).

47. See Marilyn Lake, "Mission Impossible: How Men Gave Birth to the Australian Nation—Nationalism, Gender and Other Seminal Acts," *Gender and History* 4 (1992): 305-22.

48. "The Women Doctors' Hospital," *Daily Guardian,* 24 Aug. 1925.

49. Russell, "'Mothers of the Race,'" 5.

50. Minutes of the Committee of Management, June 13, 1923, Rachel Forster Hospital Records, Mitchell Library, Sydney.

51. Report of the First Annual Meeting, Minutes of the Committee of Management, June 13, 1923, Rachel Forster Hospital Records.

52. Unnamed newscutting, Mar. 23, 1928, album of newscuttings, Rachel Forster Hospital Records.

53. There was no doubt that this hospital was performing very special work, hitherto not provided for, in that it treated cases of women other than maternity & gynaecological, to which the other women's hospitals mainly confined themselves." Minutes of the Committee of Management, June 13, 1923, Rachel Forster Hospital Records.

54. Queen Victoria Hospital In-Patients Book, 1899-1924, Queen Victoria Hospital Archives.

55. Rachel Forster Hospital, *Annual Report* (1928): 3-4.

56. "The Welfare of Mothers and Infants," *Medical Journal of Australia* (Mar. 1922): 278. Victoria Cowden, entry for Margaret Harper, *Australian Dictionary of Biography*, vol. 9 (Melbourne: Melbourne Univ. Press, 1983), 204-5. Harper was one of many Sydney doctors who had gained early experience at the Queen Victoria Hospital, Melbourne.

57. See for example, Rachel Forster Hospital, *Annual Report* (1927): 8.

58. Wells, "The Entry of Women," 102.

# HALFWAY UP THE HILL

*Doctresses in Late
Nineteenth-Century American Fiction*

LILIAN R. FURST

*Between 1881 and 1891* the figure of the "doctress," as she was then
called, makes a prominent appearance in American fiction. During that
decade five novels offer divergent portraits of this newcomer on the social
scene. In chronological order they are *Dr. Breen's Practice* by William Dean
Howells (1881), *Doctor Zay* by Elizabeth Stuart Phelps (1882), Sarah Orne
Jewett's *A Country Doctor* (1884), *The Bostonians* by Henry James (1886), and
Annie Nathan Meyer's *Helen Brent, M.D.* (1891). In four of the five novels the
life, work, and status of the doctress is the main theme. Only in *The Bostonians* is the persona of the female physician, Dr. Mary Prance, not the central
heroine. However, as the only fully independent professional woman she is an
important character in a novel about the feminist movement.[1]

This spate of five novels in ten years suggests that the doctress had not
only attained public visibility,[2] but had also captured the imagination. Certainly access to medical education for women had been a highly controversial
issue in the United States after the middle of the century when they had
begun to try to gain admission to regular medical schools. Women had always
been informal healers within the kinship circle of family and neighbors. Many
early housekeeping manuals, such as Mrs. E. Smith's *The Compleat Houswife*
(1742) and the British Mrs. Beeton's *Book of Household Management* (1861)
combined medical with food recipes. Self-help books, notably Dr. William
Buchan's *Domestic Medicine; or a Treatise on the Prevention and Cure of Diseases
by Regimen and Simple Medicines* (1772), John G. Gunn's *Domestic Medicine*
(1830) and *The Maternal Physician* (1818) by "An American Matron," were all

clearly addressed to female readers. Women also became active in the later nineteenth century in various sectarian health reform movements such as the then fashionable water cures and notably in the Physiological Societies, which taught the "laws of life" and especially hygiene to female audiences as an extension of domestic proficiency. But this casual exercise of paramedical skills was superseded in the course of the nineteenth century by the gradual rise and increasingly powerful organization of medicine as a profession, and a decidedly *male* profession. Instruction by apprenticeship, such as Harriot and Sarah Hunter underwent in the early 1830s, gave way to training in medical schools, whose growth accelerated rapidly in the latter half of the century from 52 in 1850 to 75 in 1870, 100 in 1880, 133 in 1890, and 160 by 1900. The schools varied enormously in quality, so that serious efforts to improve medical education were initiated in 1870 by Harvard's President Eliot. The previous two-year program, consisting largely of theoretical, didactic lectures devoid of regular sequence, was expanded in 1871 into a three-year course in which anatomy, physiology, chemistry, and pathological anatomy, that is, the laboratory sciences, came to play an ever more important part. At about the same time hospitals moved from the periphery to the center of medical education and practice, changing from refuges for the homeless poor and insane into the physician's primary workshop. It was also in the 1870s and 1880s that medical men converged in agreement on the need for licensing and proper regulation of the profession. This stiffening and enforcement of the requirements is typified by the 1877 law in Illinois that empowered a state board of examiners to accept diplomas only from reputable schools.

The reform and institutionalization of medical education militated against women. As the historian Gerda Lerner has succinctly put it, "Women were the casualties of medical professionalization."[3] Whether such an oppression/victimization model is simplistic has been a matter of argument among historians, some of whom see women's attempts to enter into regular medicine as part of the larger nineteenth-century struggle for female self-determination. It was clearly a rebuff to such aims that women's repeated efforts to gain admission to medical schools met with scoffing rejection under a profusion of pretexts. Elizabeth Blackwell did achieve entrance to the medical school located in Geneva, New York in 1845 because students and faculty thought the application a joke and voted for it in jest; in 1849 she graduated at the top of her class. Another exceptional case is that of Marie Elizabeth Zakrzewska, who had been a brilliant midwife in Berlin and who graduated from the medical school in Cleveland in 1856. But by and large specious objections and excuses prevailed to exclude women from medical schools and hence from the profession. The very idea of a female doctor was considered to violate the norms of feminine behavior; women were regarded as unfit, physically and temperamentally, for the "blood and agony" of medical practice, which would compromise their innate delicacy; indeed, they were deemed constitutionally unfit for education after puberty, when all their energy should be directed to the development of the "pelvic power"[4] that would make them good mothers. That was the central argument of Dr. Edward H. Clarke in his 1873 treatise with the misleading title, *Sex in Education: A Fair Chance for Girls,* in which he asserted that intellectual activity during menstruation would surely lead to "neuralgia, uterine disease, hysteria, and other derangements of the nervous system."[5]

With the doors insolently slammed in their faces, the women began to organize their own medical colleges: the New England Female Medical College in 1848, the Women's Medical College of Pennsylvania in Philadelphia in 1850, the New York Women's Medical College (homeopathic) in 1863, the Homeopathic Medical College for Women in Cleveland in 1868, and, in the same year, the Women's Medical College of the New York Infirmary for Women and Children, the Woman's Hospital Medical College, in Chicago in 1870, and the New York Free Medical College for Women in 1871. None of these endeavors could have succeeded without the support and cooperation of some male physicians who were willing to act as instructors until the women themselves had acquired sufficient expertise and experience to teach their successors. Hands-on casework was also essential to medical training. As women were denied internships and residences, they founded first dispensaries and then hospitals for women and children, of which the earliest were the New York Infirmary for Women and Children, opened in 1857, and the New England Hospital for Women and Children in 1862. From these institutions the early pioneer women doctors were graduated, including three black women: Rebecca Lee in 1861, Rebecca Cole in 1867, and Sara McKinney Stewart in 1870. Some of the more affluent and ambitious went on to further training in those European universities that admitted women. Mary Putnam Jacobi, for instance, became the second woman to attain the M.D. in Paris in 1875. The University of Zurich, open to women since 1864, was another popular destination.[6] Back home, well prepared to practice, intending to serve women and children, the doctresses faced more difficulties in obtaining membership in the state medical associations. Such membership was not strictly a prereq uisite for practice; nevertheless, it had important practical implications as a symbol of legitimate acceptance as well as for referrals, admission to hospital staffs, in other words, for full integration into the profession. Curiously eva- sive terms such as "inexpedient" and "inopportune" were advanced for a while as grounds for rejection; the qualifications necessary for admission were de- clared to apply to males only. But in 1877 the state societies of Kansas, Michi- gan, and Rhode Island did take women; others followed, with Massachusetts in 1884 among the last.

This necessarily brief overview of women's struggle to enter the medical profession in this country[7] is the context for the novels under discussion. It is no coincidence that doctresses feature in American fiction of the 1880s be- cause by then they had begun to surface as a social phenomenon. They were by then, to adopt the metaphor in the title of this volume, half way up the hill. Nor is it coincidental that all the five novels are set in the Northeast— one in New York, and the other four in New England—for these were the prime centers of medical education for women, and had a far higher concen- tration of female physicians than anywhere else: in 1880 132 women were practicing in Boston alone, 14.9 percent of the city's medical force; by 1890 the figures had risen to 210 and 18.0 percent respectively (in the rest of the country the corresponding percentages are 2.8 for 1880, and 4.4 for 1890).[8] Clusters of women doctors were found elsewhere too: out west, where the pi- oneering spirit made the social climate less straitlaced, and in Washington, where some 90 women doctors formed part of a large and lively community of female professionals between 1870 and 1900, drawn to the capital by the postwar expansion of the federal government.[9]

The novels are interesting for the lively insight they give not only into the careers of the doctresses but also into the prevailing social attitudes toward them. A number of common preoccupations recur, although there are also considerable variations between them so that it is a spectrum of possibilities that emerges rather than a consensus. The novels portray doctresses at dif- ferent stages in their careers: Nan Prince in *A Country Doctor* is just going through her apprenticeship and early training; Grace Breen is on the verge of starting to practice, while the other three are already well established. Atalanta Zay singlehandedly runs a large rural practice in Maine; Mary Prance engages in both clinical and research medicine in Boston, and *Helen Brent, M.D.*

opens with the heroine's appointment to the presidency of a women's hospital and medical college after she has built a prodigious reputation.

A major source of diversity lies in the gendered perspective. Two of the works, *Dr. Breen's Practice* and *The Bostonians,* are authored by men, while the other three are by women. Here a clear dichotomy is apparent: the women are far more positive in their perception of the doctress, portraying independent, self-confident, successful practitioners. Elizabeth Phelps's Dr. Zay performs minor surgery with "a firm and fearless touch,"[10] goes out on night calls alone in her horse and buggy, is "sent for all over the county" (86), and earns $5,000 a year, though she could make much more if she did not treat the poor virtually for free. Helen Brent, described as "well known" and "popular,"[11] performs "difficult gynecological operations, the success of which had interested the entire medical profession—operations that required nerve, coolness, daring, skill, a steady hand, and a delicate one; and when they were over, she had never been known either to faint or to go into hysterics, as Dr. Manning had prophesied would be the conduct of the woman physician" (15). The young Nan Prince, too, in *A Country Doctor* shows a "a sort of self-dependence and . . . self-reliance"[12] together with an instinctive insight into people, and the "resource, bravery, and ability to think for one's self that make a physician worth anything" (184). In a revealing scene, during an outing with friends while she is still in medical school, she attends to a farmer who has dislocated his shoulder in a fall by taking off her boot and manipulating the joint back into position with a deft movement of her foot and arm (295).[13] By contrast, William Dean Howells's Dr. Grace Breen is an "inexperienced girl,"[14] timid, hesitant, in constant need of reassurance and approval from her mother, who undermines her as consistently as does the narrator (e.g., that "girl"). Self-deprecatory, lacking pride in achievement, in fact lacking in achievement, the pathetic Dr. Breen is the opposite to the commanding Dr. Zay and Helen Brent, who possess both dignity and panache. Midway between these extremes is James's Dr. Mary Prance, "a plain, spare young woman, with short hair and an eyeglass,"[15] an austere, dry, laconic observer of the feminist scene who pursues her studies far into the night, sharpening her instruments (probably for dissection) in a little physiological laboratory that she has set up in her back room (31). She is vehement in not wanting "the gentlemen doctors to get ahead of her" (37) nor in having anyone tell her "what a lady can do!" (38). At first the young Southern lawyer, Basil Ransom, sees her rather negatively, as a sexless creature who looks "like a boy, and not even like a good boy" (32), and is put off by "her flat, limited manner" (33). Gradually, however, he comes to appreciate that "this lady was tough and technical" (33), that she conducts business "with the greatest rapidity and accuracy" (331), that she is as successful as ambitious, has lucidity of mind to the point of "diabolical shrewdness" (319), and even a streak of humor.

Dr. Prance is always focalized through the eyes of Basil Ransom: "The little medical lady struck him as a perfect example of the 'Yankee female' . . . produced by the New England school system, the Puritan code, the ungenial climate, the absence of chivalry" (31). This and similar comments raise some vital issues of focalization: who is it that is seeing the doctress? what is the source of the information within the frame of the fiction? and what is the effect of the particular angle of vision? In *The Bostonians* the narrative disposition remains relatively simple, with a male figure acting as a surrogate for a male author, presenting an external image of the doctress (that is to say, we always see Dr. Prance through Basil's vision). At the opposite pole, the female author of *Helen Brent, M.D.* presents a kind of super-doctress, beautiful, strong, smiling, calm, always in control. In *Dr. Breen's Practice,* on the other hand, a male author takes a dualistic approach, both entering into Grace's thoughts and recording how others envisage her. A similar stance is adopted in *A Country Doctor,* where Nan Prince is first filtered through the perceptions of her guardian and mentor, Dr. Leslie; later, as she matures into adolescence and early womanhood, her own reflections on her medical aspirations are added. The most complex crossgendering occurs in *Doctor Zay,* where the doctress in this novel by a woman is consistently focalized, as in *The Bostonians,* through the observations of a man, Waldo Yorke, who has become her patient as a result of a serious accident that befalls him while his is in Maine on business. So here a disabled, and, what is more, a decidedly lackadaisical male is viewing a strong, indeed imperious female. This reversal of the customary nineteenth-century role order accounts for much of the work's piquancy.

The situation in *Doctor Zay* builds to a climax as Waldo slowly comes to the alarming realization that his competent, gentle attendant is not a nurse, as he naturally supposes when he recovers consciousness. The technique of suspense is cleverly deployed; Waldo's hostess, herself a patient and admirer of Dr. Zay, deliberately conceals the physician's gender. This graphic scene is so typical of the surprised discomfort evoked by the doctresses that it is worth quoting in full:

Only one person was in the room, a woman. He asked her for water. She brought it. She had a soft step. When he had satisfied his thirst, which he was allowed to do without protest, the woman gave him medicine. He recognized the familiar tumbler and teaspoon of his homeopathically educated infancy. He obeyed passively. The woman fed him with the medicine; she did not spill it, nor choke him; when she returned the teaspoon to the glass, he dimly saw the shape of her hand. He said,—

"You are my nurse?"

"I take care of you tonight, sir."

"I thank you," said Yorke, with a faint touch of his Beacon-Street courtliness; and so fell away again.

He moved once more at dawn. He was alarmingly feverish. . . . His agony had increased. He still moaned for water, and his mind reverted obstinately to its chief anxiety. He said,—

"Where *is* that doctor? I am too sick a man to be neglected. I must see the doctor."

"The doctor has been here," said the woman who was serving as nurse, "nearly all night."

"Ah! I have been unconscious, I know."

"Yes. But you have been cared for. I hope that you will be able to compose yourself. I trust you will feel no undue anxiety about your medical attendance. Everything shall be done, Mr. Yorke."

"I like your voice," said the patient, with delicious frankness. "I haven't heard one like it since I left home. I wish I were at home! It is natural that I should feel some anxiety about this country physician. I want to know the worst. I shall feel better after I have seen him."

"Perhaps you may," replied the nurse, after a slight hesitation. "I will go and see about it. Sleep if you can. I shall be back directly."

This quieted him, and he slept once more. When he waked, it was broadening, brightening, beautiful day. The nurse was standing behind him at the head of the bed. She said:—

"The doctor is here, Mr. Yorke, and will speak with you in a moment. The bandage on your head is to be changed first."

"Oh, very well. That is right. I am glad you have come, sir." The patient sighed contentedly. He submitted to the painful operation without further comment or complaint. He felt how much he was hurt, and how utterly he was at the mercy of this unseen, unknown being, who stood in the mysterious dawn there, fighting for his fainting life.

He handled one gently enough; firmly, too,—not a tremor; it did seem a practiced touch.

The color slowly struck and traversed the young man's ghastly face.

"Is *this* the doctor?"

"Be calm, sir,—yes."

"Is *that* the doctor's hand I feel upon my head at this moment?"

"Be quiet, Mr. Yorke—it is."

"But this is a woman's hand!"

"I cannot help it, sir. I would if I could, just this minute, rather than to disappoint you so."

The startled color ebbed from the patient's face, dashing it white, leaving it gray. He looked very ill. He repeated faintly,—

*"A woman's hand!"*

"It is a good-sized hand, sir."

"I—Excuse me, madam."

"It is a strong hand, Mr. Yorke. It does not tremble. Do you see?"

"I see."

"It is not a rough hand, I hope. It will not inflict more pain than it must."

"I know."

"It will inflict all that it ought. It is not afraid. It has handled serious injuries before. Yours is not the first."

*"What shall I do?"* cried the sick man, with piteous bluntness.

"I wish we could have avoided this shock and worry," replied the physician. She still stood, unseen and unsummoned, at the head of his bed. "I beg that you will not disturb yourself. There is another doctor in the village. I can put you in his hands at once, if you desire. Your uneasiness is very natural. I will fasten this bandage first, if you please."

She finished her work in silence, with deft and gentle fingers.

"Come round here," said the patient feebly. "I want to look at you." [*Dr. Zay*, 40-43]

This episode is a variant on the stock fairytale recognition scene, where the frog turns out to be a prince. Here things are more complicated: it is not merely that the prince (the doctor) turns out to be a frog (a woman), but that the entire system of social and moral values, on which the distinction between prince and frog rests, has to be thrown open to radical questioning. Yet even though Waldo's suspicious reluctance quickly yields to trust, he still feels the need to protect his mother in Boston from the knowledge that he is being cared for by a woman: "Write to my mother," he begs her, "Tell her not to worry. Don't say you are not a man" (48). Evidently he does not grasp the offensiveness of his request.

The motif of surprise at a woman practicing medicine recurs in one guise or another in all these novels, often linked to the underlying question of the propriety of such a career for a lady. The parameters of proper behavior for a lady were firmly drawn in the nineteenth century, and they excluded the active pursuit of a profession for pay outside the domestic sphere of the home. All the doctresses are transgressing a fundamental creed of the time; all are contrasted with what James calls "sweet *home-women*" (*The Bostonians*, 27; italics are author's). The foil to Dr. Zay is Mrs. Butterwell, with whom she lodges, and who represents the venerated ideal of the devoted housewife. Similarly, Helen Brent stands out against the socialites at New York tea parties, acknowledging that "her hopes, her aims, her theory of life were so irrevocably different from those of the women about her" (93). Yet these average, upper-class women are unmasked as hypocritical, shallow, and unscrupulous social climbers. Less pernicious but equally empty-headed is the circle of conventional women, friends of Nan's aunt, in *A Country Doctor*. They are deeply shaken by her nonchalant announcement that she is studying medicine. "What do you mean?" demands the aunt coldly before dismissing the idea as a "Nonsense, my dear" (249). Nan is reminded that it is "proper for young women to show an interest in domestic affairs" and that "a strong-minded woman is out of place" (279); she is further rebuked that for "a refined girl who has an honored and respected name to think of becoming a woman doctor" (281) is totally unnatural. While Nan is sufficiently resolute to brush these reproaches aside, Grace Breen is undone by the women's "distrust of a physician of their own sex" (*Dr. Breen's Practice*, 22). The young Mr. Libby's astonished question to Grace's sole patient, "You don't mean *that's* your doctor!" (17; italics are author's) is less hurtful to her than the rejection by other women. This is understandable in light of the pioneering women physicians' avowed aim, so eloquently articulated by the British Sophia Jex-Blake in her speech of 1869, "Medicine as a Profession for Women," that women should be trained "to attend medically to those of their own sex who need them," to give "sisterly help and counsel."[16]

The quality that redeems the doctresses from utter disgrace and that goes some way toward neutralizing their ambiguous social position is the acknowledgment that every one of them is a lady. Again, this is an absolutely crucial nineteenth-century concept that is categorically underscored in each novel. Even Dr. Prance in *The Bostonians,* despite her want of conventional femininity, is unequivocally seen to be a lady. Grace Breen has "a ladylike manner" (96), moderating her "business-like alertness" with "ladylike sweetness" (10). The adventurous Nan of *A Country Doctor* is, it is emphasized, by no means "mannish" (160); as "a young lady," she should, according to one of her elderly neighbors, "be made to look like the little lady she is" (129). That Dr. Zay "was unmistakably a lady" (17) is a real consolation for Waldo as he comes to terms with the revelation that his physician is female. It is reassuring to him that she has "the dress and carriage of a lady" (44). Her dress is given close attention: on calls she is unobtrusively modest in "blue, or black, or blue-black, or blue and black" (18) in winter, and cream or white in summer. But on social occasions, her colors are brilliant: a "parlor dress" of violet muslin with lace and satin ribbons at wrists and neck (155), or a ruby dress with a plush jacket and white lace. Likewise, Helen Brent, who wears a plain, stiff, black alpaca dress and large, wide, flat shoes in her professional guise, can, when she chooses, blossom into "a queenly lady" in a gown with a graceful train, a profusion of soft lace, and pretty kid slippers (175-76). She and Dr. Zay are idealized figures projected by a woman's imagination, able to combine "the decisive step" of "women of business" with "grace of movement and curves of femininity" (*Doctor Zay,* 97).

Just as being a lady makes social amends, so being useful acts as a moral justification. The urge to usefulness is potent in all the doctresses except the brisk Dr. Prance who, in her own words, doesn't "cultivate the sentimental" (33). Grace Breen, on the other hand, is obsessed by a Puritan sense of duty and a "severe morality" (39) that impels her to be "more useful to others" (12). Disappointed in love and rich enough not to have to work, she has chosen medicine "in the spirit in which other women enter convents, or go to heathen lands" (12). Perhaps she is the least successful of the doctresses precisely because her vocation is vaguely to be of service to womankind rather than specifically to study medicine, which she has found in part "almost insuperably repugnant" (12). Such hesitations are unknown to Nan, who has the support of a powerful role model in Dr. Leslie as well as of a family tradition in her father, a surgeon who died young. Still, Nan too is motivated as much by her drive to be useful as by her innate attraction to medicine: "she was filled with energy and a great desire for usefulness" (159), excited by the "renown some women physicians had won, and the avenues of usefulness which lay open to her on every side" (193). Her final riposte to her aunt's objections is simply that to study medicine "is the best way I can see of making myself useful in the world" (283). Dr. Zay is like Nan in having had a doctor father, whom she loved to watch in his laboratory. Her inspiration to go into medicine derives from both a personal experience and a public need: she had seen how decisively her mother had been comforted by women doctors in Boston and in Paris, and while spending summers at Sherman near her hometown of Bangor she realizes "how terrible is the need of a woman by women in country towns" (175). Although she concedes that women doctors "pay a price for our privilege" (123), she is sustained by her awareness that "the women all depend on me" (138). Helen Brent also knows the price paid by doctresses, but even more she knows that "I have a mission, a duty to perform" (40). Hers is the most encompassing calling: her "chief aim is make all women find themselves" (104) for she is "determined to leave the world better" (31) than she found it.

What then happens to these doctresses in the course of the novels' action? Except for Dr. Prance, who is a minor, static character, all of them face the dilemma of marriage. In this way the plots tie in with one of the paramount objections to women doctors, namely the clash of professionalism and marriage.[17] To the nineteenth-century mentality there was no happy solution to this conflict: for a woman to remain a spinster was thought to be unsatisfying, but if she married and had a family, she would be unable to attend to her patients properly. Actually a fifth to a third of female physicians at that time did marry, often fellow doctors; some continued their practices, others chose not to do so. The entire range of possibilities is illustrated in these novels. Nan Prince turns down the rising young lawyer, George Gerry. Because she finds him attractive, she has her moments of hesitant indecision, particularly during a sleepless night when "her old ambitions were torn away from her one by one, and in their place came the hardly-desired satisfaction of love and marriage, and home-making and housekeeping, the dear, womanly, sheltered fashions of life" (307). But in the clear light of day she understands that to marry would be to lose "the true direction of my life" (326), and that her part is "to make many homes happy instead of one" (327). Marriage, she realizes, would limit her potential for usefulness. As a contributor to *Alpha,* a journal edited by the physician Caroline Winslow, wrote in 1886: "A woman who has before her the broad avenues of usefulness, who has ambition and energy to develop her powers, will not be satisfied to tie herself down in the soul-cramping marriage. . . . [woman's] highest duty to herself and humanity demands her full development as a *Woman,* not as a *Wife* or *Mother.*"[18]

Helen Brent makes the same choice, though not without some bitterness. She has been shabbily treated by her lawyer fiancé, Harold Skidmore, who breaks their engagement when she takes her medical degree and goes off to Germany. The prototype of the new liberated woman, she argues vehemently that women should no more be expected to give up their profession when they marry than men. Yet her life, full, rich, and busy as it is, is not complete. At the end of the novel, after Harold's wife has left him, he writes to Helen that "some day there will come knocking at your gates a broken Harold, as a suppliant" (196). The somewhat mawkish sentimentality implicit in this adumbration of a happy ending was no doubt pleasing to readers of that period, but it seems to contravene the astringent, stalwart independence basic to Helen's character and to her professional success.

Grace Breen's marriage is another matter, for her commitment to medicine never appears to be strong. Beset by self-doubts both about her competence and her suitability to the profession, she takes marriage as a way out, possibly also as a compensation for the early disappointment that led her into medicine. She turns down the proposal of the mature Dr. Mulbridge, who suggests that they be "physicians in partnership" (322) as well as husband and wife. Her refusal becomes less puzzling when the terms in which he addresses her are taken into consideration. She has, in his words, shown herself to be "faithful, docile, patient, intelligent beyond anything I have seen" (228); but, he assures her, "you could never succeed alone" (223). He is right about her intelligence, for she tells him bluntly that he is "a tyrant" who wants "a slave not a wife" (254). Meanwhile she has sought the advice of young Mr. Libby about Dr. Mulbridge's proposal, which gives her opportunity to declare to him: "don't you see that I love *you?*" (248; italics are author's). So Grace Breen-Libby moves to the factory town where her husband manages his father's mills and where she treats his workers' sick children. The male narrator makes the final comment that "the conditions under which she now exercises her skill certainly amount to begging the whole question of woman's fitness for the career she had chosen" (271).

There is no such begging of questions with Dr. Zay, who ends up marrying her patient, Waldo Yorke, on her own perfectionist terms, in the conviction that the marriage can be "*divinely* happy" (248; italics are author's). She sorely tests Waldo, treating his love "like a fit of measles" (248), and sending him back to his law office in Boston to apply himself more diligently to his work. He returns after six months, the "new type of man" appropriate to the "new kind of woman," "a woman who diverged from her hereditary type" (244). She will, of course, maintain her practice, at once "a strong-minded doctor" and "a sweet woman" (254).

The endings of *Doctor Zay* and of *Helen Brent, M.D.* patently veer into the realm of romance, in a manner reminiscent of Jane Eyre's marriage to Mr. Rochester. All the novels have these romance elements, which nineteenth-century readers expected, indeed demanded. But on the whole the social context of the fictive doctresses climbing a long hill is predominantly realistic. The women conform to socio-historical demographic patterns by coming from financially comfortable middle-class settings, frequently from families progressive in outlook and with a medical tradition. Two of the five, Nan Prince and Atalanta Zay, are represented as orphans, freer from the directive constraints of blood relatives and with greater liberty to pursue their goal. Of Dr. Mary Prance's and Helen Brent's family circumstances nothing is known. However, the timorous Grace Breen, who has early lost her father, is very much under the control of a domineering and disapproving mother. All the doctresses portrayed in these novels receive an education in keeping with the options available at that period. Nan gets formal instruction in Boston after her apprenticeship with Dr. Leslie, and then goes to Zurich. Though offered an appointment at a city hospital, she prefers to go home to be a general practitioner, specializing in pediatrics, aspiring eventually to become her mentor's successor. Grace Breen, Helen Brent, and Atalanta Zay have all trained in New York; Dr. Zay has spent a further year in Zurich and Paris, while Helen Brent is the only woman whom Professor Schwetterberger has consented to instruct in Germany. In her speech on her accession to the presidency of the women's medical college she vows to provide women with "the very best training," upholding "the very highest scientific standards" (20). Significantly, three out of the five are devotees of homeopathy,[19] the gentler form of medicine, which uses minuscule doses of medication and was more favored by women physicians than the heroics of allopathy. They are also typical in envisaging themselves as ministering primarily to women and children; the bolder among them, Nan Prince and Dr. Zay, are not embarrassed by male patients either, whom they acquire either as a result of accidents requiring immediate attention or who are the elderly spouses of their female patients. But even Dr. Zay is forced to confess that she has never before treated a *young* man.

While the family background and medical training attributed to these doctresses is consonant with the possibilities open to women at that time, the information on their actual professional work is fairly scant. A surprising feature of all five novels is the far greater attention paid to the women's social dilemmas than to their medical activities. Nan in *A Country Doctor* accompanies Dr. Leslie on his rounds to patients, and on two occasions is able to give prompt and effective first aid. Dr. Prance in *The Bostonians* is seen attending to Miss Birdseye, taking her pulse and observing her with a cannily vigilant gaze as she approaches death. Despite her rejection of sentiment, "this competent little woman" shows a capacity for tact and compassion, addressing the old lady still "dryly" but also "gently" (328). On the other hand, when Grace Breen is faced with a critical medical situation, she reverts to the role of nurse, deferring to the superior judgment of Dr. Mulbridge, who is brought in to take charge of the case. Her lack of assertiveness, admittedly the behavior expected of nineteenth-century women, contravenes the boldness characteristic of the pioneer female physicians. Helen Brent, by contrast, is said to perform the most daring surgeries and becomes a leader in her field, yet not once throughout the novel is she shown dealing with a patient. Readers have merely the narrator's hyperbolic reports of Helen's amazing feats—hardly convincing evidence. Only Dr. Zay interacts with a patient, Waldo Yorke, dressing his wound, dispensing medication, and supervising his convalescence with exemplary skill. But even here the emphasis is on the growth of the romantic relationship that develops out of their professional rapport. This greater concentration on the doctresses' social lives is in keeping with the conventions of the novel of manners, the genre to which all these works belong. In the fictional representations the tendency either to deflate or to inflate is very evident. Grace Breen is presented in a negative, reductive manner, while Helen Brent, Atalanta Zay, and Nan Prince are to varying degrees idealized. The historical inevitably yields at one point or another to the fictive.

These five American novels have a counterpart in five British fictions that appeared at roughly the same period: Charles Reade's *A Woman Hater* (1877), G. G. Alexander's *Dr. Victoria: A Picture from the Period* (1881), the anonymously published *Dr. Edith Romney* (1883), *Mona Maclean: Medical Student* by "Graham Travers," the pseudonym of Margaret Georgiana Todd, who was Sophia Jex-Blake's biographer, and Arthur Conan Doyle's short story, "The Doctors of Hoyland" from his collection, *Round the Red Lamp* (1894). As in the United States, the sudden popularity of women physicians as fictive heroines is a concomitant of the battles raging in Great Britain most acutely from the later 1860s through the 1870s.[20] The thematic parallels between the doctress fictions on the two sides of the Atlantic are quite striking as the same issues are aired: surprise at the very idea of a woman practicing medicine, and even more at her competence, composure, and erudition; doubts as to the propriety of such a course; the contrast with "sweet *home-women;*" justification through usefulness in the form of service to fellow women; the recognition of the women's essentially ladylike behavior as a conduit to social acceptability; and the culminating problem of marriage. The British fictions are also like the American ones in showing the doctresses at various stages in their careers, and in adopting a range of gendered perspectives. Although the British figures, too, are basically true to social history norms, the lengthy narratives have a rather more marked proclivity to the melodramatic than the American examples in their highly involved, at times frankly creaking plots and substantial romance elements. The signal exception is Conan Doyle's sparkling, ironic tale, whose outline is similar to that of *Dr. Zay:* the male patient, in this instance the town's doctor, in an accident sustains a compound fracture of a leg, which is expertly handled by the young woman; her follow-up visits lead to a proposal of marriage and partnership. But the end has a distinctive sting in the tail, for this doctress prefers to accept the opportunity she has just been offered to do research at the Physiological Laboratory in Paris.

"There are many women with a capacity for marriage," she tells her suitor, "but few with a taste for biology. I will remain true to my own line."[21]

After the early 1890s doctresses ceased to feature as a curiosity in literature. It would be nice to be able to conclude that this denoted their assimilation into the social landscape with the acceptance of medical practice as a normal role for women. This is not, however, what happened. Ironically, the percentage of women students in American medical schools dropped precipitously from a high of 18.22 percent in 1893-94 to a low of 4.6 percent in 1944.[22] This sharp decline was a direct consequence of the closure of the women's medical colleges or their absorption into coeducational schools between 1884 and 1903.[23] Only the Women's Medical College of Pennsylvania remained an exclusively female institution. The appearance of doctresses in American fictions between 1881 and 1891 is the literary inscription of a brief early window of opportunity for women physicians.

NOTES

1. By contrast, the medical student, Ruth Bolton, in *The Gilded Age* (1873; Rpt. N.Y.: Trident Press, 1964) by Mark Twain with Charles Dudley Warner, is no more than a subsidiary figure. From a Quaker family in Philadelphia, Ruth rebels against the useless and dependent life that was the norm for women. She is a foil to the novel's heroine, Laura Hawkins, a socialite femme fatale in Washington. Ruth takes up medicine, against her mother's wishes, as "the only method of escape" from "the clutches of the old monotony" (179) of her dour, stiff home. Although medical study is draining for her, she shows "the utmost coolness," "skillful hands," and "a gentle firmness" (247) in tending a patient's wound. However, after nearly dying of a fever contracted in the hospital, Ruth ends up by admitting her love for Philip Sterling. Her future is left open, but presumably it is marriage. *The Gilded Age* also makes mention of a successful female practitioner, Mrs. Dr. Longstreet, who "has a great income" (344). The novel is not included in my study because its primary focus is satire of social mores.

2. Nevertheless, William G. Rothstein's 362-page book, *American Physicians in the Nineteenth Century* (Baltimore and London: The Johns Hopkins Univ. Press, 1972) mentions the existence of women physicians only once, in a footnote (300) recording that in 1900 17 percent of students in homeopathic medical schools were female, as against 5 percent in regular medical schools.

3. "The Lady and the Mill Girl: Changes in the Status of Women in the Age of Jackson," *Midcontinent American Studies of Journal* 10 (spring 1969): 6.

4. James Compton Burnett, M.D. in 1895; rpt. in *Victorian Women,* eds. Erna Olafson Hellerstein, Leslie Parker Hume, and Karen M. Offen (Stanford: Stanford Univ. Press, 1981), 94.

5. Rpt. in *Women, the Family, and Freedom,* eds. Susan Groag Bell and Karen M. Offen (Stanford: Stanford Univ. Press, 1983), I:429. Clarke was a complicated figure whose position was paradoxical: he did support women physicians even while advocating that girls could not stand the strain of higher education after puberty.

6. See Paulette Meyer, "They Met in Zurich," this volume.

7. For a fine, detailed account see Regina M. Morantz-Sanchez, *Science and Sympathy* (New York: Oxford Univ. Press, 1985).

8. Mary Roth Walsh, *"Doctors Wanted: No Women Need Apply": Sexual Barriers in the Medical Profession, 1835-1975* (New Haven and London: Yale Univ. Press, 1977), 186.

9. See Gloria Moldow, *Women Doctors in Gilded Age Washington: Race, Gender and Professionalization* (Urbana and Chicago: Univ. of Illinois Press), 1987.

10. *Doctor Zay* (Boston: Houghton Mifflin, 1882), 47.

11. *Helen Brent, M.D.* (New York: Cassell, 1894), 14.

12. *A Country Doctor* (Boston: Houghton Mifflin, 1984), 137.

13. The young physician in Louisa May Alcott's *Jo's Boys* (1886) strongly echoes Nan, even in name. Like her, Alcott's character administers prompt and appropriate aid in an accident and, like her also, she remains "a busy, cheerful, independent spinster," dedicating "her life to her suffering sisters and their children" ( *Jo's Boys* [New York: NAL, 1987], 277). Alcott's novel, directed at juvenile audiences, tends to simplify issues, and has therefore not been included.

14. *Dr. Breen's Practice* (Boston: Osgood, 1881), 76.

15. *The Bostonians* (New York: NAL, 1980), 23.

16. Sophia Jex-Blake, *Medical Women* (Edinburgh: Oliphant, Anderson, & Ferrier, and London: Hamilton Adams & Co., 1886; rpt. New York: Source Books, 1970), 44.

17. The marriage/profession problem is played out in *The Bostonians* in the central figure, Verena Tarrant, in the struggle between Basil Ransom and Olive Chancellor for her allegiance.

18. *Alpha* 8 (Dec. 1886) 13; italics are author's.

19. Homeopathy, brought to the United States from Germany in 1825, rapidly developed into a prosperous and progressive medical sect with an affluent, largely urban, upper- and middle-class clientele. Around the middle of the century several Institutes of Homeopathy were founded: the American Institute in 1841, the Medical College of Philadelphia in 1847, and similar institutions in Cleveland in 1850 and in Chicago and New York in 1860. By 1900 10,000 homeopaths were in practice, primarily in the northern states. Homeopathy reached its zenith in 1880 just as the

LATE NINETEENTH-CENTURY AMERICAN FICTION

doctresses were coming into prominence. Although the American Medical Association at first ostracized homeopaths as "irregulars" because of their exclusive dogma, the wealth and influence of the homeopathic clientele assured the group's success and longevity. But as late as 1878 the Fairfield County, Connecticut, Medical Society expelled a physician for consulting with his homeopathic wife. Through their support of homeopathy women were active in the first attack on the heroics (and brutalities) of conventional therapies. Cf. Rothstein, 152-74, 230-46, 299-300.

20. See Catriona Blake, *The Charge of the Parasols: Women's Entry to the Medical Profession* (London: The Women's Press, 1990), 207-10 for a chronological overview.

21. *Round the Red Lamp* (New York and London: Appleton, 1921), 294.

22. Walsh, 193 and 245.

23. Ibid., 180.

# [ 12 ]

# "LEAVING THE PRIVATE HOUSE"
### Women Doctors in Virginia Woolf's Life and Art

ELSA NETTELS

*The woman physician* was an important figure in Virginia Woolf's life and art, although only one novel, *The Years* (1937), portrays her. Two of Woolf's own doctors were women: Elinor Rendel, the niece of Lytton Strachey; and Octavia Wilberforce, distantly related to the Stephen family and the last doctor to be consulted by Virginia and Leonard Woolf.[1] During the 1930s, the novelist frequently saw her niece Ann, Adrian Stephen's daughter, who read natural sciences and physiology at Newnham College, Cambridge; Ann volunteered but was turned down for medical service in the Spanish Civil War, and in 1940 worked as a doctor in the Dublin Hospital.[2] Ann Stephen's medical career may have moved Virginia Woolf to choose the woman physician as her exemplary figure, to represent women of all professions in their century-long struggle to achieve recognition and financial independence, in Woolf's own words, to cross "the bridge which connects the private house with the world of public life."[3]

The quoted words and the exemplary doctor appear in Woolf's long essay, *Three Guineas,* published in 1938, nine years after the more famous book, *A Room of One's Own.* Originating from her lecture, "Professions for Women," given in London to the National Society for Women's Service in 1931, *Three Guineas* is Woolf's most relentless attack on the institutions of British patriarchy that suppress women and sacrifice their interests to the interests of men. On finishing *Three Guineas,* Woolf wrote in her diary (Oct. 12, 1937), "It has pressed and spurted out of me . . . like a physical volcano."[4] The essay, cast as a letter to a male correspondent who wishes to know how women can help to prevent war, develops through anecdote, quotation and rhetorical questions a tightly constructed argument: women can help to prevent war only by becoming independent thinkers, free to speculate and voice their own opinions. They can become independent thinkers and speakers only by becoming financially independent. They must be able to earn money; they must cease to be economically dependent on their fathers and brothers. In short, they must leave "the private house"—the domestic sphere where women have traditionally been confined. In the private house, women are financially dependent on men; money spent on education in the schools and universities is spent on the male children; women are prepared for only one career and that is marriage. Outside the private house is the public world, where women have gained entrance but where men still dominate in all spheres of activity—in Parliament, the universities, the press, the financial world, the church, and the professions of law and medicine.

In *Three Guineas,* Woolf refers to several women who in the nineteenth century defied convention to enter the public sphere as reformers and writers: Florence Nightingale; Josephine Butler, who led the fight against the Contagious Diseases Act; and Mary Kingsley, a popular lecturer and author of widely read books, published in the 1890s, on her travels in West Africa. But Woolf chose as her representative figure a pioneer woman doctor, Sophia Jex-Blake (1840-1912), who struggled against the forces of patriarchy all her life. In *Three Guineas,* Woolf devotes several pages, based on Margaret Todd's biography (1918), to Jex-Blake's lifelong campaign to open the medical profession to women, a campaign in which success on one front merely shifted the battle to another.

Her struggle, narrated in Todd's biography, began in childhood. Sophia's father, a proctor of Doctors' Commons, and in Virginia Woolf's words, "an admirable specimen of the Victorian educated man, kindly, cultivated and well-to-do" (TG, 64), from the beginning acted to curb his daughter's independent spirit. He sent his son to public school and the university but considered sufficient for his daughter's education "pious and half-educated schoolmistresses" who were "trained to try to make their pupils gentle, agreeable, submissive, docile."[5] When Sophia escaped their influence to study at Queen's College in London, her father strenuously opposed the idea of her taking money for tutoring in mathematics.

In Boston, where she assisted Dr. Lucy Sewell at the New England Hospital for Women, Jex-Blake's application to the Harvard Medical School was rejected twice by its faculty, in 1867 and 1868. At the University of Edinburgh, where she and four other women in 1869 finally gained admission to study medicine in classes apart from the male students, the women were thwarted and attacked by hostile students and faculty, by the press, and in the courts of law. Woolf cites one occasion, described by Charles Reade in *A Woman-Hater* (1877), when a mob of several hundred rowdy male students rioted to try to prevent the women from entering the Surgeon's Hall to take their examination in anatomy. In her book *Medical Women* (1886), Jex-Blake wrote that at Edinburgh the five women fought "a true battle of liberty against tyranny"—a battle in which they had to defend themselves "with the constant vigilance of the soldier in time of war."[6]

Virginia Woolf does not describe Jex-Blake's personality, but in reading Todd's biography she would have recognized a precocious child in some ways like herself—inventive, imaginative, strong willed but eager for parental approval. Todd characterized Jex-Blake as "a born chronicler"; "almost in babyhood she struggled laboriously to get on to paper her doings and dreams."[7] She kept a diary from the age of nine; in her adult years, she was an indefatigable letter writer.

Not surprisingly, the letters from which Woolf quotes in *Three Guineas* are those in which Jex-Blake, aged nineteen, defends and her father opposes her taking wages of five shillings an hour for tutoring at Queen's College. Her father insists that she wants for nothing and will never be in want; that to take money she does not need would condemn her as greedy and would damage her reputation. Jex-Blake's letter in response, which Todd quotes in full, is notable for its calm, firm tone and masterly deployment of argument. The letter is a compelling defense of the basic right affirmed in *Three Guineas,* the right of women as well as men to earn their own living. Jex-Blake cites the opinion of the college authorities that she is the person best qualified for the tutorship. She observes that her brother accepts pay for his work and asks, "why should the difference of my sex alter the laws of right and honour?" She claims her right to "the honest . . . and perfectly justifiable pride of *earning.*" She rejects as absurd her father's offer to give her money if she will refuse to take it from the college, and she scorns the opinions of those who would criticize her for accepting "well-earned wages."[8]

Jex-Blake does not accuse her father of seeking to keep her dependent on him until she marries with his approval, but the root of his objection is clear to Virginia Woolf. "He wished to keep his daughter in his own power. . . . The case of Mr. Jex-Blake shows that the daughter must not on any account be allowed to make money because if she makes money she will be independent of her father and free to marry any man she chooses. Therefore the daughter's desire to earn her living rouses two different forms of jealousy. Each is strong separately; together they are very strong" (TG, 132-33).

No less pertinent was the effect upon Sophia of her father's appeal to what Woolf called "the womanhood emotion," roused by his insinuation that for his daughter to work for money would be unladylike and unwomanly (TG, 133). As Woolf herself had been forced to kill the "Angel in the House" in order to become a writer,[9] so Sophia Jex-Blake struggled to "kill the lady" by citing women of families "better and older than mine" who approved her plan to earn money (TG, 133). She did not then wholly succeed in her struggle to emancipate herself from claims, the falsity of which she perceived. In her diary she noted bitterly that in promising to tutor for one term without pay, out of deference to her father's wishes, she had yielded to no purpose: "Like a fool I have consented to give up the fees for this term only—though I am miserably poor. I am sorry. It was foolish. It only defers the struggle."[10]

Jex-Blake's power to define the cause and fight the battle made her an exemplary figure in a twofold sense: she was unique, preeminent, heralded at her death as the leader of a crusade who "more than anyone else . . . compelled the gates of the medical profession to be opened to women."[11] To Virginia Woolf she was also a representative figure deserving of study because "Her case is so typical an instance of the great Victorian fight between the victims of the patriarchal system and the patriarchs, of the daughters against the fathers" (TG, 64).

Two questions suggest themselves: Why did Woolf choose a physician rather than, say, a writer or a suffragist, as her typical figure? Why did she choose to study the professional woman in her position as daughter? Throughout *Three Guineas,* she refers to women as "the daughters of educated men," signalling her concern not only with women of her own class but also with women in their filial roles, as daughters, not as wives. We recall that the best known novels about women physicians, those by Americans, all pose the conflict not as a struggle against parental opposition but as a choice between a medical career and marriage. Nan Prince in Sarah Orne Jewett's *A Country Doctor* (1884) and Nan Harding in Louisa May Alcott's *Jo's Boys* (1886) refuse their ardent suitors and remain single. Grace Breen in William Dean Howells's *Dr. Breen's Practice* (1881) and the title character of Elizabeth Stuart Phelps's

*Dr. Zay* (1882) do marry at the end, after prolonged inner conflict. But all four novels embody the power of patriarchy in the suitor, not the father. Why did Woolf cast the fight in terms of "the daughters against the fathers?"

We begin to answer this question by remembering that Virginia Woolf was an Englishwoman and the daughter of Sir Leslie Stephen, as illustrious a Victorian father as any she cited in *Three Guineas*. In England, where traditions of centuries separated the spheres of the sexes as well as the social classes, the position of the father defined the position of the daughter and invested him with authority to a far greater extent than in the United States, where class divisions were viewed as barriers to be overcome, not natural hierarchies to be accepted. In the United States, too, the economic motive was often determinant. Several of the most distinguished of the pioneer women physicians in America, including Josephine Baker, Elizabeth Blackwell, Alice Hamilton, and Harriot Hunt, saw it as their duty to train for a profession when the illness or death of the father left a wife and small children dependent on the elder daughter's power to earn money.[12]

Virginia Woolf's own experience as a daughter prompted her to compare the rule of the father within the private house and the rule of men over women in public life. In *Three Guineas,* when she describes women such as Mary Kingsley, denied the formal education given to her brothers, Woolf could be describing herself, educated at home while her two brothers were maintained at Cambridge. It is true that Woolf scorned the visible signs and symbols of university power and authority—the robes and hoods, the degrees and processions. She refused an honorary doctor of letters from Manchester University, vowing in her diary (March 25, 1933), "Nothing would induce me to connive at all that humbug" (DVW, 4:148). Six years later she refused a doctorate from the University of Liverpool (DVW, 5:206). But the knowledge of her exclusion never lost its bitterness. As she explained to the composer Ethel Smyth, she made herself "fictitious and legendary" in *A Room of One's Own* only because critics would have dismissed her argument as personal grievance had she said outright, "Look here am I uneducated, because my brothers used all the family funds which is the fact."[13]

As Virginia Woolf's letters and diaries make clear, her intellectual and emotional bond with her father was extraordinarily strong. Her letters in the months after his death, February 22, 1904, express intense longing for his presence. The magnitude of her intellectual debt to her father makes his influence impossible to repudiate. At the same time, his psychological demands upon her, especially after her mother's death in 1895, made the debt a burden that moved her to write twenty-four years after he died that had he lived, "his life would have entirely ended mine. What would have happened? No writing, no books;—inconceivable" (DVW, 3:208). Naturally the women who most interested her were those in whose lives she read narratives of resistance to and escape from paternal authority. Either the importunate suitor does not figure at all, as seems to have been true of Jex-Blake,[14] or the suitor liberates the daughter from the father's power, as Robert Browning in *Flush* (1933) saves Elizabeth Barrett as well as her pet cocker spaniel from the power of "tyrants and dog-stealers."[15]

There are several reasons why Woolf chose medicine to illustrate the fight of the daughters against the fathers. Medicine ideally is an art of healing and nurturing that requires compassion, intuition, and sensitivity—qualities traditionally identified with women. At the same time, female medical students faced a unique kind of resistance because their study of anatomy and surgery was considered particularly unsuitable for women. As Jex-Blake's books and letters prove, medicine was probably the severest test of a woman's courage and resolve.

Virginia Woolf's idea of the woman physician and the severity of her struggle was shaped by her own view of the British medical establishment, above all by her experiences as the female patient of male doctors. From the age of thirteen, when she suffered the first of recurrent mental and physical breakdowns, periods of madness, and months of convalescence, she knew at firsthand the power of doctors to reinforce women's socially sanctioned roles as wives and mothers, to discourage professional ambitions and compel women's submission to masculine authority in the interests of their health. Subjected to the regimen of the nursing home in Twickenham where she was three times confined and for weeks forbidden to read or write or see visitors, Virginia Woolf saw her doctors as adversaries, "tyrannical" and "short-sighted" as she described Sir George Savage (1842-1921), for many years the family physician of the Stephens and the Woolfs.[16] As Thomas C. Caramagno has pointed out, the efforts of Leonard Woolf, doctors, and nurses, often hired for months at a time, probably saved Virginia Woolf from permanent confinement in an asylum.[17] Nevertheless, by the time she wrote *Three Guineas,* she had for years identified medicine as the profession which embodied the coercive power of patriarchy at its most absolute and far-reaching. To fight "the battle of Harley Street" (TG, 64) as Jex-Blake did, was to fight on the ground where men seemed most invulnerable, their victims most helpless.

Virginia Woolf's recognition of the power of doctors did not rest on any admiration of their knowledge. Indeed, what made the power of the medical establishment so disturbing was that doctors, in her view, knew so little yet behaved like omniscient despots. That doctors were ignorant was a recurrent charge in her letters and fiction. After her father's death, she vowed to Violet Dickinson, "I never shall believe, or have believed, in anything any doctor says—I learnt their utter helplessness when Father was ill. They can guess at what's the matter, but they cant put it right."[18] Thirty years later, when a male specialist prescribed treatment which both she and Elinor Rendel questioned, Woolf complained to Ethel Smyth, "the truth is doctors know absolutely nothing, but as theyre paid to advise, have to oblige."[19] In her first novel, *The Voyage Out* (1915), she portrayed two male doctors who not only fail to save the life of Rachel Vinrace but enjoy perfect unawareness of their incompetence. The first doctor, Rodriguez, dirty, shifty, and malicious, is farcical in his assurance that the dying girl "is not seriously ill." The second, ironically named Lesage, who relies on his "curt speech" and "sulky masterful manner" to overawe others, perceives the gravity of Rachel's illness but apparently knows nothing more.[20]

In Sir William Bradshaw in *Mrs. Dalloway* (1925), her most detailed fictional portrait of the male doctor, Virginia Woolf dramatizes the power of the British medical establishment at its most sinister and benighted. Bradshaw, the son of a shopkeeper, has risen to become the preeminent nerve specialist of Harley Street and the most powerful servant of the ruling class, invested by his professional authority with the power to define insanity and shut away the deviant. "Sir William not only prospered himself but made England prosper, secluded her lunatics, forbade childbirth, penalised despair, made it impossible for the unfit to propagate their views . . . "[21] Signifying his power are the kinds of symbols of patriarchy for which Woolf expressed such scorn: a knighthood, a photograph in his consulting room of Lady Bradshaw "in Court dress" (MD, 97); outside, a motor car, "low, powerful, grey with plain initials interlocked on the panel" (MD, 94). With forty-five minutes allotted to each patient, his life is regulated by "the clocks of Harley Street," which "counselled submission, upheld authority" (MD, 102).

Bradshaw is portrayed with one prospective patient, a shell-shocked victim of the First World War, Septimus Warren Smith, whose manic-depressive symptoms are those Virginia Woolf herself suffered: headaches, insomnia, aversion to food, illusory voices, hallucinations, paranoia, suicidal impulses, intense excitement and euphoria alternating with despair and debilitating fatigue. Bradshaw's treatment of Septimus quickly belies his reputation for "sympathy; tact; understanding of the human soul" (MD, 95). He cuts off Septimus's attempt to communicate his anguish and sense of guilt; mouths platitudes ("Nobody lives for himself alone" [MD, 98]), and mentally refers to Septimus as "that fellow" whose shabbiness offends him. Woolf describes his speciality as "this exacting science which has to do with what, after all, we know nothing about—the nervous system, the human brain" (MD, 99). But Bradshaw, who never doubts himself, prides himself on the accuracy of his diagnosis, which he makes with lightning speed, seconds after Septimus and his wife Rezia enter his room. When Rezia protests at his decree that her husband shall be separated from her and confined in a rest home which Bradshaw will visit once a week, the doctor brooks no opposition, refusing even to consider any other course: "There was no alternative. It was a question of law" (MD, 96-97).

It is the intrusion of the bumbling general practitioner, Dr. Holmes, that drives Septimus to suicide several hours later. But in Bradshaw Woolf incarnates the will of the Goddess Conversion, who disguises her lust for power as self-sacrifice or service to humanity but "feasts on the wills of the weakly, loving to impress, to impose, adoring her own features stamped on the face of the populace" (MD, 100). Foreshadowing the identification in *Three Guineas* of the tyrannies of patriarchy and of fascism, Woolf here identifies the doctor's craving "for dominion, for power" with the power of imperialist governments over the subject peoples of Asia and Africa (MD, 100). The irony that imperialist rivalry and conquest precipitated the war which shattered the mind of Septimus Smith and drove him to Harley Street and Bradshaw never occurs to his doctors.

Bradshaw is set apart from all the other characters in the novel, the only one who repels all those who encounter him. To Clarissa Dalloway, he seems "obscurely evil," "without sex or lust . . . but capable of some indescribable outrage—forcing your soul" (MD, 184). Bradshaw is the only character labeled and fixed by the narrator in pages of exposition. He is the only character of importance who is given no inner life, no interior monologue. The absence of consciousness through which his absolute self-assurance could be breached at once dehumanizes him and gives him a fraudulent aura of godlike omniscience.

This portrait of the male doctor, showing abuse of power at its most uncontrolled and frightening, makes most urgent the question Woolf poses in *Three Guineas:* How is the professional woman to succeed in the man's world without doing what successful men have done? How can women keep themselves from becoming greedy, domineering and despotic, unscrupulous in the competition for power and prizes? The "battle of Harley Street" fought by Jex-Blake in the nineteenth century—so typical it could be "the battle of Cambridge University at the present moment" (TG, 66)—proved to Woolf that professions have "a certain undeniable effect" upon those entrenched in them. "They make the people who practice them possessive, jealous of any infringement of their rights, and highly combative if anyone dares dispute them. Are we not right then in thinking that if we enter the same professions we shall acquire the same qualities?" (TG, 66). In short, "how can we enter the professions and yet remain civilized human beings?" (TG, 75). Woolf's answer was to urge women to retain the position and virtues of outsiders, to prefer "obscurity and censure" to "fame and praise" (TG, 80), to refuse corrupting employment by institutions that would demand allegiance to their own interests, to reject all "badges, orders, or degrees" (TG, 80). By these refusals women could bring to their professions the tolerance and patience and integrity fostered by exclusion.

Woolf's answer to her question in *Three Guineas* helps to explain her portrayal of the one woman physician in her fiction, Peggy Pargiter, who appears in the final section, "Present Day," of *The Years.* Peggy, in her late thirties, belongs to the third generation of the upper middle-class London family whose history in the novel spans some fifty years, from the 1880s, when the patriarch Abel Pargiter ruled his household of four daughters and three sons, while maintaining a mistress nearby, until the 1930s, when his children and grandchildren, including Peggy, gather for a party and family reunion. While Woolf was writing *The Years* she was attended by Dr. Elinor Rendel, with whom, on one occasion at least, she talked "about the period and professional women, after the usual rites with the stethoscope" (Feb. 4, 1931, DVW, 4:9). But nothing of their conversation, no facts abut the training or practice of a woman physician appear in *The Years.* At the party which concludes the novel, Peggy encounters her father, her brother, cousins, aunts, and uncles; she is never seen with patients in an office or a hospital.

In this and in other ways, she differs from women physicians portrayed by the American novelists. Peggy has apparently succeeded in her profession; a former teacher, "her master," calls her "my most brilliant pupil,"[22] but she has little joy in anything. Unlike the women of earlier fiction, such as Phelps's Dr. Zay, James's Dr. Prance in *The Bostonians* (1886), and Alcott's Nan Harding, who exude energy, determination and confidence in the value of their work, Peggy seems depressed and weary in spirit, as if the struggle for place had exhausted her. To herself and others at the party she seems withdrawn and morose—"a lonely, bitter and disillusioned human being" as one critic of the novel describes her; "the liberated woman who has extricated herself from the joy of human relationships," according to another.[23]

Although Peggy feels isolated and detached at the party, "plated, coated over with some cold skin" (Y, 350), she is not completely liberated from feelings bred by the proper upbringing of an educated man's daughter, who in adolescence was chided for using slang and excluded from the after-dinner talk of politics (Y, 202, 203). At the party, it is her father's presence that evokes her keen pleasure in knowing herself praised by "her master"; "The nerve down her spine seemed to tingle as the praise reached her father" (Y, 362). When she lashes out at her brother North for the conventional life she imagines he will lead—"You'll marry. You'll have children. What'll you do then? . . . Write little books to make money . . . instead of living . . . living differently" (Y, 390-391), she betrays her own sense of failure and guilt for *not* conforming, for failing to achieve society's ideal of womanhood: she does not wish to marry; "she would have no children" (Y, 396).

Peggy's self-doubts and her skepticism about the medical profession set her apart from the all-knowing male doctors like Holmes and Bradshaw. Peggy does not downgrade her own abilities as does Howells's Dr. Grace Breen, but she refuses to be an oracle and she repeatedly disclaims the kind of authority others would impute to her: "she was daily impressed by the ignorance of doctors" (Y, 329). She tells her uncle, who is also her patient, that "doctors are great humbugs," although she admits, "We've learnt a few little tricks" (Y, 357). When her aunt Eleanor asks her what dreams mean, she responds, "How often have I told you? Doctors know very little about the body; absolutely nothing about the mind" (Y, 384-85).

Although—or perhaps because—she rejects the doctor's mantle of omniscience, she has far greater insight than Woolf's fictional male doctors into the mental states and emotions of other people. She accuses herself of coldness;

she compares "the laboratory; the professions" to the medieval monastery where one seeks to escape the pain of feeling ("not to live, not to feel," Y, 355), but the very desire for refuge attests to the acuteness of her feelings and her awareness of the feelings she evokes in others.

More than any other character in the novel, Peggy exemplifies Woolf's desire to capture the essence of human character and to recognize the unique complexities that defy labels. As Woolf created her characters, so Peggy mentally composes a picture of her aunt Eleanor, seeking the right words, "trying to add another touch to the portrait," then rubbing out the words because "she's not like that—not like that at all" (Y, 334). Like Clarissa Dalloway, she reflects on the sacred mystery of separate identities, "two sparks of life enclosed in two separate bodies" (Y, 334). As she watches her aunt Delia, she asks herself the central question of Woolf's essay "Mr. Bennett and Mrs. Brown": "But what makes up a person?" and she concludes that material facts—"wavy hair," "a dress with gold spots," the presence of three children—cannot express the woman (Y, 353).

One cannot imagine such thoughts passing through the minds of Holmes and Bradshaw. Equally alien to Woolf's fictional male doctors is Peggy's habit of self-analysis, her determination to identity the true source and nature of her feelings. Thinking of her cousin Sara, she recognizes a thrill of bitterness and asks, "Why was she bitter?" Did she envy her cousin or disapprove of her friendships "with men who did not love women"? (Y, 327). The sight of her father's worn shoes gives her "a direct spontaneous feeling" which she analyzes: "Part sex; part pity. . . . Can one call it 'love'?" (Y, 351).[24] Like Septimus, she is haunted by the horror of the world's brutality and suffering; she wonders how anyone can be happy "in a world bursting with misery" (Y, 388); then she wonders if she is indulging in a self-gratifying pose: "Was she not seeing herself in the becoming attitude of one who points to his bleeding heart?" (Y, 388). When she gazes at the sky filled with stars she rejects the conventional words that immediately invade her mind: "inscrutable, eternal, indifferent": "But I don't feel it. . . . So why pretend to?" (Y, 360).

Peggy's self-knowledge and honesty acquire added significance in light of Woolf's analysis in *Three Guineas* of the failure of educated men to recognize the source of their resistance to their daughters' aspirations. She begins by applying to all professions statements in *The Ministry of Women* made by Professor Laurence Grensted of Oxford, who traced the refusal of Anglican churchmen to admit women to the priesthood to "infantile fixation," a powerful subconscious motive or "non-rational sex taboo" that perpetuated the domination of men over women (TG, 125-26). In particular, Woolf emphasized Grensted's assertion that the motive was so powerful because it was subconscious. To her, the strength of the opposition of Elizabeth Barrett's father to his daughter's marriage proved its origin "in some dark place below the level of conscious thought" (TG, 130). Likewise, the resistance of Sophia Jex-Blake's father to her earning money originated "in the levels below conscious thought" (TG, 131).

In a reversal of roles, Virginia Woolf, the patient of male doctors, used medical terminology to expose the patriarchal will to power as a disease which, "though unnamed, was rampant" in the nineteenth century (TG, 135). The "case" of Sophia Jex-Blake's father, "very easily diagnosed," was typical; in almost every biography of an educated man's daughter one found "the familiar symptoms" (TG, 132, 135) of paternal opposition to her marriage or her career. Eventually many of the fathers in private gave way, Woolf noted, but when they banded together in professions they became more deeply "infected" by "the fatal disease," which became "still more virulent outside the house than within" (TG, 138).

Virginia Woolf freed Peggy from the arrogance, complacency, and moral blindness that afflicted the male doctors of her fiction. But why did she not show her woman physician engaged in her medical practice, succeeding where the men failed, helping to heal the minds and bodies of her patients, saving them by the insight, imagination and skill so conspicuously lacking in the male doctors?

One answer is suggested by Woolf's descriptions in her diary of the doubt and anguish she suffered during the composition of *The Years*. In 1932, she began writing what she called an "Essay-Novel," in which chapters in the fictional history of the Pargiters would alternate with expository sections on feminism, politics, education, and other issues raised by the events of the narrative. After writing some one hundred thousand words in half a year (DVW, 4:132), she removed the essay parts from the narrative, finding it impossible to "control this terrible fluctuation" between fact and fiction (DVW, 4:350). Fear that the novel was "hopelessly bad" tormented her during the months that she revised the book and brought her close to a mental breakdown. Peggy, the focal character in the last part of *The Years*, seems to be the conduit of Woolf's sense of exhaustion, which moved her to write after correcting the proofs: "I wonder if anyone has ever suffered so much from a book as I have from The Years. . . . It's like a long childbirth" (DVS, 5:31).[25]

In any case, both *The Years* and *Three Guineas,* which develops essay material deleted from the novel, show Virginia Woolf impressed by the persistence, not the diminishing, of gender inequality, far more moved to demonstrate the power still exercised by men in the professions than to celebrate the success of women in overcoming that power. In *Mrs. Dalloway,* Doris Kilman tells her pupil Elizabeth Dalloway that "law, medicine, politics, all professions are open to women of your generation" (MD, 130), but Woolf had evidence to defend her claim in *Three Guineas* that masculine hostility to women in the professions or "priesthoods" remained a powerful force. In her diary she cited the experience of Dr. Janet Vaughan, the daughter of a childhood friend and the holder of a postgraduate appointment in clinical pathology at the Hammersmith Hospital, who was dismissed from her post on the grounds that "no woman can do research work" (DVW, 4:283). Woolf's friend Ray Strachey, the sister of Adrian Stephen's wife Karin, and the author of several books on women in the professions, noted that the Sex Disqualification Removal Act of 1919 did not insure that women would be found qualified to enter any profession, insisting that "a wide gap" remained "between legislation and action."[26] In *Careers and Openings for Women* (1935), she cited medicine as "one of the well-established careers" for women, offering them better opportunities than law or accounting or engineering. But she noted that nearly all the London teaching hospitals still refused to admit women students and that government authorities were likely to dismiss women doctors if they married.[27]

Hilary Newitt, in her book *Women Must Choose* (1937), from which Virginia Woolf took notes while writing *Three Guineas,* observed that women faced more obstacles than men in entering and rising in the medical profession and that the legislation passed in 1919 had not led to a marked increase in the number of women physicians.[28] Census returns cited by Ray Strachey show that from 1921 to 1931 the number of women doctors increased by 557, to a total of 2310; the number of nurses increased by 24,528, to a total of 118,909.[29] E. Moberly Bell, in *Storming the Citadel* (1953), documents discrimination against women physicians persisting after the Second World War. Until 1950 women doctors in military service were denied commissions and membership in the Royal Army Reserve of Officers. Government authorities continued to support proposals to pay women less than men, to withhold promotion from women and to force women to retire earlier than men.[30] The evidence presented by all these writers refutes Nigel Nicolson's contention that the argument of *Three Guineas* was "to a large extent anachronistic" because the battle was won, because "the professions *were* opening to women; to give but one example of the trend, both Virginia's doctors in middle and later life were women."[31]

It would be interesting to know Virginia Woolf's impressions of her first woman physician, Elinor Rendel, but beyond noting her visits and diagnoses Woolf says nothing about her—her personality, her views of the medical profession, her experiences as a doctor. She remains a shadowy presence—a name more than a figure. But Octavia Wilberforce, Woolf's second woman physician, emerges clearly in Woolf's descriptions of her and in her own letters and autobiography.

Like Sophia Jex-Blake, Octavia Wilberforce was born into an upper middle-class family that disapproved of her professional ambitions. She, too, was a student in London, where she lived alone in boarding houses and was aided by friends. Like Jex-Blake, she remained single, believed that the woman physician should not marry, and was single-mindedly devoted to her profession. When Leonard and Virginia Woolf first met her, on January 8, 1937 (Octavia Wilberforce's birthday), she was practicing in Brighton, near the Woolf's house in Sussex, and living with the actress Elizabeth Robins, Henry James's friend and the first to play Ibsen's heroines on the London stage, in the 1890s. Elizabeth Robins was forty-seven when she met Octavia Wilberforce, then twenty-one. She supported the young woman in her struggle against her family and was like a mother to her. The Woolfs met Octavia when they went to Brighton to discuss a book by Elizabeth Robins that the Hogarth Press had agreed to publish. Virginia Woolf was then almost fifty-five, Octavia Wilberforce was forty-nine.

Had Virginia Woolf known of Octavia Wilberforce when she was writing *Three Guineas,* she might well have presented her case as a notable example of the fight "of the daughters against the fathers," a case of parental opposition more remorseless than that suffered by Sophia Jex-Blake. In her autobiography, Wilberforce describes "the atmosphere of nagging coercion"[32] surrounding her at home, recounts her parents' effort to force her into marrying a man she did not love, and details the cruel misogyny of her father, a magistrate and County Council member, who refused to pay for her medical training, cut her out of his will, and continued to deride her and women doctors in general after she had entered the London School of Medicine for Women. "He said I was a fool and would never get on" (OW, 60). During her Christmas vacation in 1915, she recalled, her family "subjected [her] to every kind of abuse" (OW, 79) because she refused the office of the youngest child, the care of her parents at home, and instead proposed to free herself from "Slavery to the Family" (OW, 56). At tea with the Woolfs she described her early years, which Virginia Woolf later summarized in her diary: "she had 9 in family; and they coerced her, though unwanted, through pressure of antiquated family feeling and propriety, to stay at home. Only through a great struggle did she break off and become a doctor" (DVW, 5:49).

The two women liked and esteemed each other; the first meeting led to visits back and forth between the two households, during which Leonard Woolf privately consulted with Octavia about his wife's health. Octavia admired Virginia Woolf's work and Virginia cared for her approval, noting in her diary after the first visit: "O said I must have great knowledge of other peoples lives to write AR of O [*A Room of One's Own*]. That pleased me" (DVW, 5:50). In May, 1940, Octavia Wilberforce attended the lecture, "The Leaning Tower," on the poets of the 1930s, that Virginia Woolf gave in Brighton to the Workers' Educational Association. She discussed Woolf's recently published biography of Roger Fry with her and urged Elizabeth Robins to read *Night and Day* (1919).[33] In the most literal sense Wilberforce was the nurturing physician. Concerned for the health of both Leonard and Virginia Woolf, whose "extreme thinness" worried her (OW, 161), she regularly took to them Jersey milk and cream and cheese from the dairy she maintained during the war.

Virginia Woolf resisted the idea of becoming Dr. Wilberforce's patient, although at Leonard's urging she agreed to an examination, which took place the day before her suicide. But she was attracted to Octavia and referred to her as "a new lover" and "a far away lover" in teasing letters to Vita Sackville West and Ethel Smyth.[34] She proposed to write a "living portrait" based on conversations with Octavia, feeling that in her "reticence and power combined" she was "very paintable, as the painters say."[35] (Octavia was somewhat taken aback by the proposal, uncertain whether or not to agree to it. "I'm not at all sure I would like it," she wrote to Elizabeth Robins, by then in the United States.[36]) Just four days before her suicide, Virginia Woolf returned to the subject in her diary: "Octavia's story. Could I englobe it somehow? English youth in 1900" (DVW, 5:359).

Woolf did not write the portrait but her first description of Octavia Wilberforce captures her character: "a very fresh coloured healthy minded doctor, in black, with loops of silver chain, good teeth, & a candid kind smile which I liked" (DVW, 5:49). This was a faithful sketch of a woman who could have sat for William James's picture in *The Varieties of Religious Experience* (1902) of "the religion of healthy mindedness," set in opposition to "the sick soul." Octavia Wilberforce's letters to Elizabeth Robins in America reveal a woman of resolute spirit, robust in mind and body, practical, compassionate, valiant in the face of the nightly threat of death during the German air raids. She was invigorated by the crisis, proud of "the stubborn undaunted spirit" of the British people, convinced that the war was salutary in rousing "this rather apathetic race" and banishing hypochondriacal fears. "War cures neurotics in most cases," she stated.[37]

Woolf's insight into the firm and forthright character of the doctor was understandably greater than Wilberforce's insight into the tortured psyche of the writer. Octavia's words, prompted by Leonard Woolf's account of Virginia's anguish and despair—"If only the world of writers could be disciplined into doing so much and then stop and relax"[38]—are not those of one who has stepped over the edge or looked too long in the face of the fire. Her instincts were sound when she recognized the morbidity of Virginia Woolf's obsessive preoccupation with her parents and tried to dispel it. But she failed to take seriously Woolf's fear that she had lost the power to write and thought she exaggerated for effect. "I'm quite unperturbed that you say you can't write," she assured Woolf in a letter dated January 26, 1941. "The longer you feel like that the better you'll write when you do get really going" (OW, 172). These words, so well-meant, seem rather like Dr. Holmes's assurance to Septimus that "there was nothing whatever the matter with him" (MD, 92).

But to judge Octavia Wilberforce by statements that in hindsight seem obtuse is to give a false impression of her and of Virginia Woolf's view of her. Woolf's letters convey admiration of her character, gratitude for her acts of friendship, and fascination with her struggle within the private house for freedom and independence. It was Leonard, not Virginia Woolf, for whom Octavia Wilberforce was primarily important in her capacity as a physician. What Virginia Woolf wished to represent in her "living portrait" of Octavia Wilberforce was not the medical doctor but the young woman and the life that had formed her: "English youth in 1900."

Had Virginia Woolf known Octavia Wilberforce when she wrote *The Years* would she have made the doctor the model for Peggy Pargiter? It is unlikely. The doctor in Brighton, inspirited by faith in the worth of her fight to save lives, tireless in "healing the sick by day, and controlling the fires by night,"[39] might well have joined the company of Alcott's and Jewett's stalwart physician heroines. She did not belong with the characters of *The Years*, thwarted or crippled by the codes of the Victorian family. And when Peggy enters the novel in the 1930s, achievements such as hers are overshadowed by the growing power of fascism and the imminence of war. To Peggy, who more than any other character in *The Years* expresses Woolf's point of view, private happiness and pride in personal accomplishment are impossible when "on every placard at every street corner was Death; or worse—tyranny; brutality; torture" (Y, 388).

In Octavia Wilberforce Virginia Woolf knew a woman who drew strength from opposition and adversity, a physician who left the private house and succeeded in the public world, apparently without loss of integrity or compromise of principle. She would seem to have accomplished what Woolf defined as the most difficult task facing the woman in a male-dominated profession: to establish herself without succumbing to the jealousy and rivalry Woolf believed endemic to the professions. But Virginia Woolf knew that the success of individual women, even those as dauntless as Sophia Jex-Blake and Octavia Wilberforce, did not destroy or even fundamentally change the patriarchal system she attacked in *Three Guineas*. Nor did Woolf intimate that her women physicians caused her to take a more favorable view of the medical profession: her early memories of nursing homes and rest cures and consultations in Harley Street were too powerful to be displaced. She commemorated women physicians because in their struggle to leave the private house she saw the opposition of the fathers at its most relentless, the daughters' fortitude most severely tried.

NOTES

1. The second wife of Octavia Wilberforce's great-grandfather, William Wilberforce (1759-1833), was the sister of Virginia Woolf's great-grandfather, James Stephen (1758-1832).

2. This information about Ann Stephen's medical career was given to the author by Hermione Lee, in a letter, June 1, 1993.

3. *Three Guineas* (New York: Harcourt, Brace, and World, 1938), 18. Hereafter abbreviated TG, with page references given in parentheses.

4. *The Diary of Virginia Woolf,* Vol. 5, *1936-1941,* edited by Anne Olivier Bell, assisted by Andrew McNeillie (London: The Hogarth Press, 1984), 112. In her diary, Virginia Woolf proposed several titles for her essay: "On Being Despised," "The Next War," "What Are We to Do," and "Answers to Correspondents." *The Diary of Virginia Woolf,* vol. 4, *1931-1935,* edited by Anne Olivier Bell, assisted by Andrew McNeillie (London: The Hogarth Press, 1982), 6 n.8, 300, 346, 348, and vol. 5, 3. Hereafter abbreviated DVW, references to these volumes of the diary and to Vol. 3, *1931-1935,* edited by Anne Olivier Bell, assisted by Andrew McNeillie (London: The Hogarth Press, 1982) will be given in parentheses.

5. Margaret Todd, *The Life of Sophia Jex-Blake* (London: Macmillan, 1918), 29, 49. Woolf's notes on Todd's biography appear on three pages in Vol. 7 and on one page in Vol. 26 of Holograph Reading Notes in the Berg Collection of the New York Public Library. For other accounts of Jex-Blake's career, see Beatrice Levin, *Women and Medicine* (Metuchen, N.J.: Scarecrow Press, 1980); Ray Strachey, *Struggle: The Stirring Story of Women's Advance in England* (New York: Duffield, 1930); Mary Roth Walsh, *"Doctors Wanted: No Women Need Apply": Sexual Barriers in the Medical Profession, 1835-1975* (New Haven, Conn.: Yale Univ. Press, 1977); Anne Witz, *Professions and Patriarchy* (London: Routledge, 1992).

6. Sophia Jex-Blake, *Medical Women: A Thesis and a History* (Edinburgh, 1886), 60, 59. In Charles Reade's *A Woman-Hater* ([New York: P. E. Collier, n.d.], 201-24), a fictional character, Rhoda Gale, identified as one of the students with Jex-Blake at Edinburgh, narrates the struggle in detail.

7. Todd, vii.

8. Todd, 67-72. Parts of the correspondence are quoted in TG, 64-65.

9. "Professions for Women," in *Women and Writing,* edited and with an introduction by Michele Barrett (New York: Harcourt Brace Jovanovich, 1979), 58-60.

10. Todd, 72. Quoted by Woolf in TG, 65.

11. Quoted by Todd, 541, from the obituary in the *Pall Mall Gazette.*

12. See S. Josephine Baker, from *Fighting for Life* in *Written by Herself: Autobiographies of American Women: An Anthology,* edited by Jill Ker Conway (New York: Vintage Books, 1992), 146; Elizabeth Blackwell, *Pioneer Work in Opening the Medical Profession to Women* (London: Longmans, Green, 1895), 28; Alice Hamilton, *Exploring the Dangerous Trades* (Boston: Little, Brown, 1943), 38; Harriot Hunt, *Glances and Glimpses* (Boston: John P. Jewett, 1856), 55.

13. Letter of June 8, 1933, *Letters of Virginia Woolf, vol. 5, 1932-1935,* edited by Nigel Nicolson and Joanne Trautmann (New York: Harcourt Brace Jovanovich, 1979), 195.

14. During her student years in London, Jex-Blake wrote in a letter, "I believe I love women too much ever to love a man," Todd, 65. In *Medical Women* she advises women against combining medical practice and marriage, but to "deliberately take their choice *either* to marry or to devote themselves to a learned profession" (212).

15. *Flush: A Biography* (New York: Harcourt, Brace and World, 1933), 73.

16. Letter to Violet Dickinson, Oct. 30, 1904, *Letters of Virginia Woolf, Vol. 1, 1888-1912,* editor, Nigel Nicolson; assistant editor, Joanne Trautman (New York: Harcourt Brace Jovanovich, 1975), 147. Virginia Woolf was at Jean Thomas's mental nursing home at Twickenham for six weeks in the summer of 1910; for several weeks in the winter of 1912; and for several weeks in the summer of 1913. Quentin Bell, *Virginia Woolf: A Biography,* 2 vols. (New York: Harcourt Brace Jovanovich, 1972), 1:164-165, 182; 2:12-13.

17. Thomas C. Caramagno, *The Flight of the Mind: Virginia Woolf's Art and Manic-Depressive Illness* (Berkeley: Univ. of California Press, 1992), 16, 23. The orthodox conservative views of Savage are detailed on pp. 9-21.

18. Letter to Violet Dickinson, Oct. 30, 1904, *Letters,* 1:148.

19. Letter to Ethel Smyth, May 31, 1934, *Letters,* 5:307.

20. *The Voyage Out* (London: The Hogarth Press, 1933), 412, 417.

21. *Mrs. Dalloway* (New York: Harcourt Brace Jovanovich, 1925), 99. Hereafter abbreviated MD, with page references given in parentheses.

22. *The Years* (New York: Harcourt, Brace, 1937), 362. Hereafter abbreviated Y, with page numbers given in parentheses.

23. Mitchell A. Leaska, "Virginia Woolf, the Pargeter: A Reading of *The Years,*" *Bulletin of the New York Public Library* 80 (winter 1977): 195; Sharon L. Proudfit, "Virginia Woolf: Reluctant Feminist in 'The Years,'" *Criticism* 17 (winter, 1975), 70.

24. Mitchell Leaska ("Virginia Woolf, the Pargeter," 195) quotes an earlier, more explicit version of this passage from the Holograph dated Aug. 5, 1934: "Her father had come in. Now that was odd she added; making another entry in her [mental] notebook; . . . love of father and daughter. Spontaneous. Rather suspect, all the same. Of mixed origin. Do I love my father sexually? she looked at Morris. No: there was a great deal of pity in it. Why does one always notice one's father's shoes? she asked." (author's ellipsis)

25. The composition of *The Years* is most fully discussed by Grace Radin, *Virginia Woolf's* The Years: *The Evolution of a Novel* (Knoxville: Univ. of Tennessee Press, 1981).

26. Ray Strachey, *Our Freedom and Its Results* (London: The Hogarth Press, 1936), 133.

27. Ray Strachey, *Careers and Openings for Women: A Survey of Women's Employment and a Guide for Those Seeking Work* (London: Faber and Faber, 1935), 164, 230.

28. Hilary Newitt, *Women Must Choose: The Position of Women in Europe To-day,* with a preface by Storm Jameson (London: Victor Gollancz, 1937), 227, 260.

29. Strachey, *Careers and Openings for Women,* 45.

30. E. Moberly Bell, *Storming the Citadel: The Rise of the Woman Doctor* (London: Constable, 1953), 181, 187.

31. Nigel Nicolson, Introduction, *The Letters of Virginia Woolf,* 5:xv.

32. *Octavia Wilberforce: The Autobiography of a Pioneer Woman Doctor,* edited by Pat Jalland (London: Cassell, 1989), 26. Hereafter abbreviated OW, with page references given in parentheses.

33. Letters to Elizabeth Robins, Dec. 23, 1940; Feb. 16, 1941, Fales Collection, Elmer Holmes Bobst Library, New York University. Quotation of unpublished letters by Octavia Wilberforce in the Fales Collection is by permission of Mabel Smith and New York University.

34. Letters of Jan. 19, 1941, to V. Sackville West; letter of Feb. 1, 1941, to Ethel Smyth, *The Letters of Virginia Woolf, vol. 6, 1936-1941* (New York: Harcourt Brace Jovanovich, 1980), 462, 465.

35. Letter of Mar. 4, 1941, to Octavia Wilberforce, *Letters,* 6:477.

36. Letter of Mar. 6, 1941, to Elizabeth Robins, Fales Collection.

37. Letters to Elizabeth Robins, Sept. 13, 1940; Dec. 6, 1940, Fales Collection.

38. Letter of Feb. 16, 1941, to Elizabeth Robins, Fales Collection.

39. Letter of Mar. 13, 1941, to Elizabeth Robins, *Letters,* 6:479.

# CONTRIBUTORS

*Alison Bashford,* lecturer in women's studies at the University of Sydney, Australia, has published in the fields of nineteenth-century medical history and the history of feminism, and is currently completing her first book, *Gender, Embodiment, and Victorian Medicine.*

*Lilian R. Furst* is Marcel Bataillon Professor of Comparative Literature at the University of North Carolina, Chapel Hill. Most of her publications are in nineteenth- and twentieth-century European literature, but she now works in the field of literature and medicine. She co-edited with Peter W. Graham *Disorderly Eaters: Texts in Self-Empowerment* (1992), and she has published articles on country physicians in *Nineteenth-Century French Studies* and on the medical background to *Middlemarch* in *Nineteenth-Century Literature.* Her book *The Etiquette of Power between Doctors and Patients: 1830 to the Present* will be published by the University Press of Virginia.

*William Kerwin,* assistant professor of English at Florida International University, has recently defended a dissertation at the University of North Carolina entitled "Framing Healers: Social Medicine and English Renaissance Drama," which focuses on social issues that helped to shape medical practice, and the meanings playwrights attach to these issues. He has also acted as instructor in social medicine at the University of North Carolina's Medical School.

*Gunilla T. Kester* is an independent scholar, writer, poet, and translator. A recipient of both the Fulbright Scholarship and the Scandinavian-American Fellowship, she completed her Ph.D. at the University of North Carolina in Chapel Hill in 1991 with a dissertation on contemporary African-American literature, a subject on which she has since written a number of articles. Her book, *Writing the Subject:* Bildung *and the African American Experience* was published by Peter Lang in 1995.

*Paulette Meyer* is a doctoral degree candidate in history at the University of Minnesota, where she helped to develop and teach a new sequence of courses in comparative world history. While writing her dissertation on women physicians in nineteenth-century Germany, she has taught classes at Southwestern State University in Marshall, Minnesota, and at Humboldt State University in Arcata, California. Recently she created a new course for science students at Humboldt State University in the history of biology.

*Regina Morantz-Sanchez* is professor of history at the University of Michigan. She is editor of *In Her Own Words: Oral Histories of Women Physicians* (1982) and author of *Sympathy and Science: Women Physicians in American Medicine* (1985). Her most recent articles are "Entering Male Professional Terrain: Dr. Mary Dixon Jones and the Emergence of Gynecological Surgery in the Nineteenth-Century United States" in *Gender and History,* and "Making It in a Man's World: The Late Nineteenth-Century Career of Mary Amanda Dixon Jones" in *The Bulletin of the History of Medicine* (both 1995). She is writing a book entitled "Conduct Unbecoming of a Woman: Gender, Professionalization, and the Emergence of Gynecological Surgery in the Late Nineteenth-Century United States."

*Nancy P. Nenno* is currently a visiting assistant professor at Wellesley College. She received her Ph.D. from the University of California at Berkeley. She specializes in twentieth-century German literature and film, gender studies, and cultural studies. A portion of the research for this essay was conducted while she was a 1993-94 Fulbright fellow in Berlin.

*Elsa Nettels,* J.B. and Mildred Hickman Professor of Humanities at the College of William and Mary, is the author of *James and Conrad,* which won a SAMLA Studies Award, *Language, Race, and Social Class in Howells's America,* and *Language and Gender in American Fiction.*

*Holt N. Parker* is associate professor of classics at the University of Cincinnati. He has been awarded the Women's Classical Caucus Prize for Scholarship, an NEH Fellowship and the Rome Prize from the American Academy in Rome. He is currently editing the manuscript of Metrodora, the earliest surviving work by a woman doctor.

*Michael Solomon* is associate professor of Spanish and comparative literature at Emory University, Atlanta, Ga. His book, *The Literature of Misogyny in Late Medieval Spain* (forthcoming from Cambridge University Press), treats the

260

relation between medical practices and antifeminist writing. He has published various articles on medicine and literature and has edited and translated an edition of the fifteenth-century Catalan medical treatise on sexual hygiene, *The Mirror of Coitus* (*Speculum al foderi*).

*Debra L. Stoudt*, associate professor of German at the University of Toledo, has published articles on the letters and sermons of the medieval German mystics and on the medical and alchemical manuscripts of sixteenth-century Heidelberg. Currently she is working on a monograph on the *Twelve-Volume Book of Medicine* of Ludwig V.

*Esther Zago* is an associate professor at the University of Colorado at Boulder, where she teaches mostly medieval literature in the Honors Program. After receiving a classical education in her native Italy, she took a Ph.D. in comparative literature at the University of Oregon. She has published monographs and essays on the medieval origins of fairy tales, the revival of romanesque architecture in America, Christine de Pizan, Boccaccio, and French prose romances, and also on Italo Calvino and Elsa Morante. Currently she is working on a book on the transmission and reception of French medieval animal fables.

# INDEX